The Contested Boundaries
of American Public Health

Critical Issues in Health and Medicine

Edited by Rima D. Apple, University of Wisconsin–Madison, and
Janet Golden, Rutgers University, Camden

Growing criticism of the U.S. health care system is coming from consumers, politicians, the media, activists, and health care professionals. Critical Issues in Health and Medicine is a collection of books that explores these contemporary dilemmas from a variety of perspectives, among them political, legal, historical, sociological, and comparative, and with attention to crucial dimensions such as race, gender, ethnicity, sexuality, and culture.

Emily K. Abel, *Suffering in the Land of Sunshine: A Los Angeles Illness Narrative*

Emily K. Abel, *Tuberculosis and the Politics of Exclusion: A History of Public Health and Migration to Los Angeles*

Susan M. Chambré, *Fighting for Our Lives: New York's AIDS Community and the Politics of Disease*

James Colgrove, Gerald Markowitz, and David Rosner, eds., *The Contested Boundaries of American Public Health*

Cynthia A. Connolly, *Saving Sickly Children: The Tuberculosis Preventorium in American Life, 1909–1970*

Edward J. Eckenfels, *Doctors Serving People: Restoring Humanism to Medicine through Student Community Service*

Julie Fairman, *Making Room in the Clinic: Nurse Practitioners and the Evolution of Modern Health Care*

Gerald N. Grob and Howard H. Goldman, *The Dilemma of Federal Mental Health Policy: Radical Reform or Incremental Change?*

Bonnie Lefkowitz, *Community Health Centers: A Movement and the People Who Made It Happen*

David Mechanic, *The Truth about Health Care: Why Reform Is Not Working in America*

Karen Seccombe and Kim A. Hoffman, *Just Don't Get Sick: Access to Health Care in the Aftermath of Welfare Reform*

Rosemary A. Stevens, Charles E. Rosenberg, and Lawton R. Burns, eds., *History and Health Policy in the United States: Putting the Past Back In*

The Contested Boundaries
of American Public Health

Edited by

James Colgrove, Gerald Markowitz, and David Rosner

Rutgers University Press

New Brunswick, New Jersey, and London

MT

Library of Congress Cataloging-in-Publication Data

The contested boundaries of American public health / edited by James Colgrove,
Gerald Markowitz, and David Rosner.
    p. ;   cm. — (Critical issues in health and medicine)
  Includes bibliographical references and index.
  ISBN 978–0-8135–4311–6 (hardcover : alk. paper)
  ISBN 978–0-8135–4312–3 (pbk. : alk. paper)
  1. Medical policy—United States. 2. Public health—United States. I. Colgrove,
James Keith. II. Markowitz, Gerald E. III. Rosner, David, 1947– IV. Series.
[DNLM: 1. Public Health—United States. 2. Attitude to Health—United States.
3. Dissent and Disputes—United States. 4. Federal Government—United States.
WA100C7612008
RA395.A3C732 2008
362.10973—dc22   2007033568

A British Cataloging-in-Publication record for this book is available from the British Library.

Manufactured in the United States of America

6/18/08

Contents

Acknowledgments   vii

Introduction: The Contested Boundaries of
Public and Population Health   1
James Colgrove, Gerald Markowitz, and David Rosner

Part I   Public Health in a Free-Market Society   13

Chapter 1   Public Health and Economics: Externalities,
Rivalries, Excludability, and Politics   15
Sherry Glied

Chapter 2   The Limits of Relying on Employers in an Intersectoral
Public Health Partnership   32
Dennis P. Scanlon and Marianne M. Hillemeier

Chapter 3   Speaking for the Public: The Ambivalent Quest of
Twentieth-Century Public Health   57
Nancy Tomes

Part II   Contested Boundaries   83

Chapter 4   Environmental Health as a Core Public Health Component   85
Phil Brown

Chapter 5   Paternalism and Its Discontents: Motorcycle Helmet Laws,
Libertarian Values, and Public Health   110
Marian Moser Jones and Ronald Bayer

Chapter 6   Prevention Strategies and Public Health: Individual and
Structural Prevention in Homelessness   127
William McAllister, Mary Clare Lennon, and Işıl Çelimli

Chapter 7   Dealing with Humpty Dumpty: Research, Practice,
and the Ethics of Public Health Surveillance   160
Amy L. Fairchild

Chapter 8   Health Production: A Common Framework to Unify Public
Health and Medicine   176
Alvin R. Tarlov

Part III   Public Health in the Post-9/11 World   201

Chapter 9   The Challenge of 9/11 to the Ideologies of
               Population and Public Health   203
               David Rosner and Gerald Markowitz

Chapter 10   Public Health Preparedness: Evolution or Revolution?   226
               Nicole Lurie, Jeffrey Wasserman, and
               Christopher D. Nelson

Chapter 11   Blown Away: Health Care, Health Coverage, and
               Public Health after 9/11 and Katrina   239
               Beatrix Hoffman

               Conclusion. Public Health Takes on Gun Violence:
               A Dialogue on Contested Boundaries   257
               Mark Rosenberg and Jeremy Travis

               Contributors   281

               Index   285

Acknowledgments

This book grew out of a series of meetings and seminars organized through the Robert Wood Johnson Foundation Investigator Awards in Health Policy Research Program. In 2003 Gerald Markowitz and David Rosner gave a presentation about their work on the history of public health in America to the annual meeting of the RWJF investigators in Aspen, Colorado. The audience became deeply involved in a lively discussion of a fundamental question: What was it, after all, that we defined as "public health"? Before the presentation was completed, Lynn Rogut and David Mechanic suggested that we consider organizing a group of RWJF scholars to participate in a series of seminars to address this issue. At the next scholars retreat a number of investigators had a breakfast meeting to begin to define the parameters of this project. This initial group included Steve Kunitz, David Mechanic, Rosemary Stevens, Keith Wailoo, Beatrix Hoffman, Amy Fairchild, Ron Bayer, Scott Burris, Amani Nuru-Jeter, Alvin R. Tarlov, Bruce Link, Mary Clare Lennon, Nancy Tomes, Dennis Scanlon, Jim Knickman, Eric Klinenberg, Zita Lazzarini, and John Lynch. We would like to thank the Robert Wood Johnson Foundation, especially David Mechanic and Lynn Rogut, for their support.

The following spring and summer, a series of public seminars featuring presentations by authors of the chapters in this book was held at Columbia University's Mailman School of Public Health. We would like to thank Allan Rosenfield, the dean of the school; Andrew Davidson, the executive vice dean; and Richard Parker, chair of the Department of Sociomedical Sciences, for their support of this project.

We are grateful to Doreen Valentine, our editor at Rutgers University Press, for her support of the volume and her many thoughtful comments on the manuscript, and to Rima Apple and Janet Golden, editors of the Critical Issues in Health and Medicine series. We thank Bobbe Needham for her expert copy editing.

We would like to thank others who have been helpful and supportive of this effort: Nitanya Nedd, Alison Bateman-House, Sarah Vogel, Barron Lerner, Gerald Oppenheimer, Nancy Stepan, Betsy Blackmar, Samuel Roberts, Eric Foner, Pamela Smith, Marcia Wright, Sarah Phillips, Alan Brinkley, Alice Kessler-Harris, Basil Wilson, Michael Blitz, Betsy Gitter, Carol Groneman, Eli Faber, Fritz Umbach, Andrea Balis, Josh Freeman, Mary Gibson, and Ruth Heifetz.

Chapter 5 was originally published in the *American Journal of Public Health* and is reprinted with permission from the American Public Health Association. Chapter 7 originally appeared in the *Journal of Law, Medicine, and Ethics* and is reprinted with permission from the journal. Chapter 9 is excerpted from David Rosner and Gerald Markowitz, *Are We Ready? Public Health since 9/11*, © 2006, The Regents of the University of California, published by the University of California Press, and is reprinted with permission. Chapter 10 was copyrighted and published by Project HOPE/*Health Affairs* as Nicole Lurie, Jeffrey Wasserman, Christopher Nelson, "Public Health Preparedness: Evolution or Revolution?" *Health Affairs* 25(4): 935–945, 2006. The published article is archived and available online at www.healthaffairs.org.

Figure 2.1 originally appeared in *Health and Work Productivity: Making the Business Case for Quality Health Care*, edited by Ronald C. Kessler and Paul E. Stang, The John D. and Catherine T. MacArthur Foundation Series on Mental Health and Development (Chicago: University of Chicago Press, 2006), and is reprinted with permission.

Of course, we want to thank our families: Robert Sember, Molly Rosner, Kathlyn Conway, Zachary Rosner, Andrea Vasquez, Bill Markowitz, Tobias Markowitz, Elena, Steve, Mason, and Ceci Kennedy, Isa Vasquez, and Anoton Vasquez.

The Contested Boundaries
of American Public Health

Introduction

The Contested Boundaries of
Public and Population Health

On the surface there appears to be widespread agreement on the overall mission of public health, as reflected in such comments . . . as "public health does things that benefit everybody," or "public health prevents illness and educates the population." But when it comes to translating broad statements into effective action, little consensus can be found. Neither among the providers nor the beneficiaries of public health programs is there a shared sense of what the citizenry should expect in the way of services, and both the mix and the intensity of services vary widely from place to place.

—Institute of Medicine, 1988

For more than a century, the activities subsumed under the rubric "public health" have reduced illness, suffering, and death and improved society's quality of life. Yet in spite of—or perhaps because of—its importance, the field of public health remains poorly understood, its accomplishments often unrecognized and undervalued. Public health is typically distinguished from health care by its focus on the prevention of illness rather than on the cure and its intervention at the level of populations rather than of individual patients. Its institutional forms include a sometimes bewildering array of public and private entities in the governmental, academic, charitable, and (occasionally) business sectors. Its activities are carried out by a heterogeneous workforce whose members' backgrounds include medicine, nursing, epidemiology, statistics, law, education, engineering, and natural and social sciences (Szreter 2003; Fox 2001; Rosner 1995; Hamlin 1998; Rosenkrantz 1972).

The diffuse and often amorphous nature of the work of public health professionals impedes wide understanding and support. And because the influences on illness and well-being are so numerous and varied, the potential reach of public health activities can seem endless, lacking any clear boundary. At different moments in history, all of the following have been seen as legitimate forms of public health action: housing reform; street cleaning and sanitation; mass education about nutrition, obesity, sexual intercourse, and drug use; hospital and clinic care; curbs on handgun availability; and prevention of and response to bioterrorism. Negotiations over what constitute the legitimate boundaries of public health have involved a wide range of constituencies: government officials and their staffs at municipal, state, and federal levels; representatives of philanthropic and social welfare agencies; civil servants; hospital and clinic administrators and staffs; and activists and consumer groups. Venues for these discussions have included legislative hearings in political capitals, community forums, scholarly and academic debates, and articles and commentaries in the mass media.

Dialogue has been extensive but consensus elusive. There is no agreement, for example, about how far public health efforts should go in attempting to modify aspects of lifestyle such as diet and exercise, and whether the field's mandate extends to intervening in broad social and economic conditions, such as regulating environmental and occupational toxins or advocating for more equitable distribution of wealth in society. In recent years, some academics and policy makers, adopting the rubric "population health," have sought to push the limits of public health activity by focusing more extensively on such determinants of health as income, employment, housing, and education.

This book explores a seemingly straightforward question that is central to debates about how best to prevent illness and enhance the well-being of society: What are the boundaries of public health today and how have they changed over time? Underlying this inquiry is a set of related questions that are both empirical and philosophical: What are the field's core functions? What conditions, behaviors, and environmental influences should it seek to affect? What strategies and practices should it use in carrying out its mission? Which disciplinary perspectives are most critical to this work? Who is responsible for these activities? What do policy makers and public health intellectuals think the boundaries can be and should be? How have historians described these shifting boundaries over time?

The answers to these questions have profound consequences. Twenty years ago, the Institute of Medicine report quoted at the beginning of this introduction warned of a system in "disarray," in part because of the lack of consensus about what the appropriate functions of public health were and where its responsibilities lay (Institute of Medicine 1988). A follow-up report in 2003, though noting some improvement, once again described failures of coordination, consistency, and vision (Institute of Medicine 2003). Some have argued that the lack of consensus about what public health should be and do prevents the United States from achieving its health goals. But this collection of essays demonstrates that the boundaries of public health are constantly being renegotiated. A consensus, if formed, would necessarily be fragile and temporary.

The challenge of mapping the boundaries of public health begins with the field's very definition. In its 1988 report, the Institute of Medicine defined public health as "what we, as a society, do collectively to assure conditions in which people can be healthy." Such a capacious understanding echoes the spirit of the World Health Organization's 1948 constitution, which defined health as "a state of complete physical, mental and social well-being and not merely the absence of disease or infirmity." As the field has embraced the concept of population health, with its claims that a fundamental reordering of social hierarchies may be essential to bringing about lasting improvements in health, debates about scope and reach have grown more contentious, both within and outside the profession. In 1998, the title of a widely discussed article in the *Lancet* by three Boston University professors posed the question: "Should the mission of epidemiology include the eradication of poverty?"—which the authors answered with a firm no (Rothman, Adami, and Trichopoulos 1998). Libertarian and anti-statist commentators have also criticized broad notions of protecting the public's health. The conservative legal scholar Richard Epstein of the University of Chicago sharply rebuked what he saw as paternalistic efforts directed toward illnesses related to "personal" behavior such as smoking, illicit drug use, poor diet, or reckless driving. "There are no non-communicable epidemics," Epstein declared—a view that could scarcely be more at odds with the thinking of some of the most influential figures in contemporary public health who are committed to addressing what they consider epidemics of obesity, hypertension, diabetes, and other chronic, noncontagious conditions (Epstein 2003, S154). In the statistics about the leading sources of preventable illness in this country today, these professionals see an imperative to act, even if it means taking the field boldly into areas in which it has not traditionally been active (Frieden 2004).

Views about the proper sphere of public health, while they are often a proxy for a broader set of political beliefs about the roles of the state, civil society, and individuals in assuring the common welfare, do not always track neatly onto liberal and conservative ideologies. Civil libertarians on the political Left have objected to many public health proposals that threatened to intrude on individual autonomy, such as the potentially coercive responses to the spread of HIV and moves by employers to restrict the hiring of cigarette smokers. And many on the political Right have embraced public health as a partner in the fight against bioterrorism, seeing its disease surveillance functions as an essential tool in thwarting the efforts of extremists.

If the broad question of how far public health should extend its ambit has produced controversy, so has the issue of what strategies it should use in carrying out its mission. The field's core activities, such as collecting and analyzing statistics to track patterns of disease, producing and disseminating health education messages, and performing sanitary engineering related to clean water and sewage, are generally well accepted. But even these apparently straightforward practices can provoke controversy. Should surveillance include the collection of individual patients' names and potentially stigmatizing information? Should health education include efforts to address problems that some people do not consider diseases in the formal sense, such as violence and obesity? Does the field's sanitation mission include the regulation of industrial toxins and hazardous substances such as lead paint, when such oversight may impinge on free enterprise?

Some of the most successful strategies in public health have been the most contentious. Taxation, for example, has proved to be a highly effective way of reducing consumption of unhealthy products such as cigarettes. But some have argued that "sin taxes" are ethically unacceptable because they are regressive, disproportionately burdening the poor, while others have claimed that the use of taxation to achieve public health goals is an unacceptable form of coercion under any circumstance, a subterfuge designed to impose de facto prohibition without naming it as such (Sullum 1998). "The power to tax," Supreme Court justice John Marshall famously wrote, "involves the power to destroy" (*McCulloch v. Maryland* 1819). Similar questions surround the use of litigation to advance health policy. Lawsuits against tobacco companies were one of the most powerful tools for bringing about changes in tobacco marketing, and cases against manufacturers of lead paint, after years of stalemate, appear to be gaining success in forcing companies to bear the costs of abating their product. As a result, some public health advocates have urged similar legal actions against the fast-food industry for its role in fostering obesity—a strategy that, even though it is only in its incipient stages, has already provoked furious controversy and legislation in several states to indemnify fast-food companies from "McLawsuits" (Mello, Studdardt, and Brennan 2006).

The Historical Roots of an Uncertain Mission

Throughout the nineteenth and early twentieth centuries, public health activities were essential to the growth and stability of cities and states. Epidemic diseases such as cholera, smallpox, and typhoid threatened the health of young and old alike and disrupted the economic well-being of the growing industrial and commercial centers throughout the country. Quarantine, isolation, surveillance, smallpox vaccination, and the provision of pure water, sewerage systems, and street cleaning made public health departments central to municipal and state reform efforts.

Ironically, however, the very success of these interventions, combined with the perception of the growing effectiveness of clinical medicine, led to a slow decline in the perceived importance of public health departments (Rosenkrantz 1972; Rosner 1995; Tomes 1998). By the 1920s, the diseases that had spurred the development of modern public health organizations were on the wane, while chronic, noninfectious illnesses—against which there was no clear course of public health action—were growing in importance. Around the same time, public health split institutionally from the practice of clinical medicine. The medical profession claimed authority over the domain of most individual patients, while public health retained narrow responsibility for a few perennially unpopular categories of care that the medical profession didn't want to provide: services for the indigent, treatment of sexually transmitted diseases, and control of once-epidemic but increasingly vestigial contagions such as tuberculosis and smallpox. The cleavage between the environmentally focused prevention of illness and its biomedical treatment and cure sowed the seeds of much of public health's modern-day discontent. The field was left with a poorly defined mandate that lacked a base of popular support. Leaders of the field, unwilling to risk further erosion of their limited political backing, failed to advocate more forcefully for their interests and thus contributed to the accretion of power by the medical profession (Farley 2004).

During the middle decades of the twentieth century, new medical technologies such as antibiotics for the treatment of bacterial infections overshadowed traditional public health practices such as sanitation, sewerage, and clean water provision. The development of curative therapies exacerbated the shift in spending priorities from public to personal health services. The mirage of a society freed from infections by the ministrations of individual physicians—rather than by public health activities—dominated the popular imagination. The diminishing stature of the field and the growing power of hospitals and specialized physicians as the bulwark against disease led to a conundrum for those concerned with the maintenance of the public health infrastructure. Requests by state and city health officials for more funding and resources to address fissures in the public health system were often seen as self-interested appeals. As components of public health's original mandate were moved into departments of sanitation, environmental protection, housing, and hospitals, what public health professionals considered their core functions became more isolated and specialized. The public and the political leadership no longer understood or sympathized with public health officials' goals or activities (Farley 2004). Nevertheless, total government spending for public health increased as part of the growth of the public sector more generally.

In the view of some critics, public health officials were to a considerable extent responsible for their own predicament. They had defined their mandate narrowly and shrunk from political engagement with powerful interests such as corporations and businesses that created unhealthful environments. They had failed to confront medical specialists interested in defining preventive interventions as clinical and hence reimbursable. Paul Cornely perhaps most memorably made this critique in a 1971 address to the American Public Health Association. Newly elected as the group's first African American president, Cornely leveled a blistering attack at what he saw as the complacency of his profession. It had been "a mere bystander" to profound changes in the health care system that had taken place in the 1960s; its members wasted their time on "piddling resolutions and their wording." Public health, he charged, "remained outside the power structure" (Cornely 1971). Cornely's address was a clarion call for more aggressive action against a host of health problems integral to modern industrial society.

The power of corporate interests, however, and a more general cultural ethos favorable to capitalism and consumption limited the profession's ability to shift its focus to lifestyle conditions. Although successive surgeons general used their office's bully pulpit to warn of the dangers of smoking beginning in the 1950s, for example, the overall strategy of much of the public health community remained one of accommodation to the powerful tobacco industry well into the 1970s (Fairchild and Colgrove 2004). Illustrating the decentralized and democratic nature of public health action in the United States, some of the most critical victories in the fight against tobacco-related sickness and death were won by actors outside official public health agencies: community activists who pressed for laws banning public smoking and, later, state attorneys general, whose lawsuits in the 1990s would win restrictions on tobacco advertising and promotion, as well as reimbursement to states for the costs of caring for sick smokers.

Complicating the mission of public health was the rise in the 1970s of a powerful discourse of "personal responsibility" for health and disease. Prominent academics and policy makers argued that blame for an unhealthy society rested on the personal habits of individuals and questioned the extent to which the government should intervene to fight problems such as smoking, substance use, and sexually transmitted disease (Knowles 1977). This trend dovetailed with the rise of the limited-government ideologies that characterized the era of Ronald Reagan in the United States and Margaret Thatcher in Britain. Amid attacks on the "nanny state," it was difficult to argue that public health officials should seek to prevent illnesses that were—so the story went—the result of people's own poor choices. Similar, the antiregulatory climate ensured that efforts to curb environmental and occupational toxins gained little traction.

At the same time, the stature of public health professionals, like that of most other institutions and authorities, underwent a sharp erosion in a social climate where expert judgments were increasingly met with cynicism and mistrust (Mazur 1977). Spurred by the rise in social protests and driven by issues of race, gender, and sexuality, activists charged that the institutions responsible for dealing with patterns of morbidity in society were instruments of an oppressive structure fundamentally inimical to public health. The reputation of public health suffered severe blows from the revelation in 1972 of the notorious Tuskegee syphilis experiment conducted by the U.S. Public Health Service since the late 1920s and the collapse in 1976 of the Centers for Disease Control's ill-fated plan to protect the nation from swine flu.

The recognition of AIDS in 1981 upended the prevailing view that infectious disease no longer represented a significant problem. The new threat gave public health the chance to demonstrate the enduring relevance of its traditional tools for fighting contagion, such as surveillance and case finding. But the social landscape had fundamentally shifted. With the rise of empowered community groups and social mobilization by affected populations, public health professionals could no longer use paternalistic or authoritarian approaches without provoking resistance. Efforts to close gay bathhouses, for example, brought public health officials into conflict with the well-organized and politically astute gay community, which saw in the move an ominous threat to hard-won individual liberties (Bayer 1989).

From "Public" to "Population" Health

In the 1980s and 1990s many public health theorists and researchers developed the concept of population health as an alternative analytic tool to expand the increasingly marginalized and restricted purviews of traditional public health.

The roots of population health extend as far back as the social medicine movement in the 1930s led by Richard Titmuss, Jerry Morris, Mervyn Susser, and others in the United Kingdom, and to Marc Lalonde in Canada in the 1970s. For these thinkers, population health, compared to traditional public health, placed a greater emphasis on addressing the nonmedical determinants of health; gave a higher priority to reducing inequalities in health outcomes; and had a more prominent focus on resource allocation and redistributive policies to remedy these disparities (Kindig and Stoddart 2003). The approach was strongly influenced by empirical research on population cohorts such as the ongoing Whitehall studies of British civil servants and by books such as *Why Are Some People Healthy and Others Not? The Determinants of Health of Populations* (Evans, Barer, and Marmor 1994). These studies suggested that inequality itself, and not simply material deprivation, exerted a powerful influence on health.

For many liberal scholars, the idea of expanding the boundaries of public health activities to include social and environmental issues seemed both progressive and scientifically accurate. But population health as a field was neither monolithic nor uniformly liberal. At the same time that some proponents were underscoring the importance of the social determinants of health, others were claiming that individual behavior and genetic and other personal "risk factors" were more important than public health activities in determining health status. Conservative policy makers used these findings as arguments against welfare state policy, devaluing the role of government. Other researchers, in turn, challenged the neoconservative orthodoxy that personal risk factors accounted for morbidity and mortality.

The liberal version of population health was both a repackaging of venerable public health ideals and an attempt to substantively reorient the field toward more explicit political activism. Its most vocal supporters readily conceded that it was not a new concept but a reembrace of ideas that had long informed many progressive views of public health. John Frank of the Canadian Institute for Advanced Research, one of the leading think tanks promoting the concept, noted that the approach "is not so much a shift as it is a validation of and return to our historical roots" embodied by such nineteenth-century visionaries as Rudolph Virchow, Edwin Chadwick, and John Griscom, who saw connections between the most basic aspects of people's material existence—their diet, houses, and jobs—and their health status (Frank 1995, 164). In this respect the concept resembled the movement to link health and human rights, which was also emerging during the 1990s, in part from the civil libertarian challenge to the threat of coercive measures to stem the spread of AIDS. These ideas, too, had a long and distinguished pedigree (Oppenheimer, Bayer, and Colgrove 2002).

In spite of the extensive attention from theorists and researchers over the past fifteen years, the impact of the population health approach remains ambiguous. As Kindig and Stoddart argued in 2003, much public health activity, at least as it is practiced in the United States, does not have the broad mandate envisioned in population health, "since major determinants such as medical care, education, and income remain outside of public health authority and responsibility, and current resources do not even allow adequate attention to traditional and emerging public health functions" (382). Policy makers differ in their views about how the concept is to be operationalized—"Population health," said Milbank Fund president Daniel Fox, "is what people say it is"—while many in the public health rank and file, preoccupied with simply trying to sustain their existing programs in an often hostile political climate, have only a vague understanding of what the new terminology entails and what it might mean for their daily work (Fox, Kramer, and Standish 2003, 21).

Though liberal practitioners of public health, and now of population health, have claimed a more sociologically informed and enlightened view of how health outcomes are determined, their political and institutional weakness has prevented them from transforming their vision into reality. The reach of public health—at least that of the field's progressive wing—has usually exceeded its grasp. Understanding why this has been so—why a professional group supposedly possessed of a sophisticated body of technical knowledge about patterns of illness in society continues to have limited ability to alter those patterns— requires confronting the unresolved question of where the boundaries of public health lie.

Whether it goes by its traditional name, public health, or the more contemporary label, population health, the field faces critical challenges in the new century. Its institutional and political position is more in flux—and more precarious—than at any point in its history. In the fearful and uncertain environment of post–September 11 America, as basic public health functions such as surveillance, contact tracing, and quarantine came to be viewed as essential to national defense, some public health administrators and advocates hoped they could recapture the authority they believed public health had in a bygone era. Some observers called for a revamping of the nation's health insurance system so that more of the population was covered as a means of improving the surveillance of disease; some called for an expansion of the scope of traditional public health activities so that the barriers between prevention and care would be reduced; some called for the integration of social services into the health care and public health systems. Yet others cautioned that simply increasing financial resources would do little to address long-term problems. And many worried that the new prominence of public health as a component of the national defense threatened to divert attention from routine interventions of proven value that prevented a far greater toll in morbidity and mortality. Indeed, where some health officials saw the potential for strengthening, others saw an ominous "militarization" of public health. The pull toward serving as an adjunct of national defense—toward a top-down approach, an aggressive use of police powers, and a focus on forestalling catastrophic events rather than on routine health maintenance—made many in the field uncomfortable. Jeffrey Koplan, former head of the Centers for Disease Control and Prevention, pointed out in an interview on June 20, 2004, that the trajectory of public health for the prior two generations had been to forge ties based upon mutual trust between officials and communities. Activities such as surveillance, disease reporting, and tracking could take on an ominous aspect for community groups who were newly concerned with civil liberties and intrusions on privacy. Employees of the U.S. Public Health Service, said Koplan, "are wearing uniforms more frequently and increasingly thinking of themselves as part of the uniformed services. This might seem like a superficial issue but causes morale issues and affects recruitment of new individuals and retention of people who have other options. It has an effect on the quality of the workforce" (Markowitz and Rosner 2004). Differing orientations toward the role of public health in national defense have created new fissures in an already splintered professional group.

Exploring the Boundaries

The genesis of this volume lies in the shared interests of investigators funded by the Robert Wood Johnson Foundation. A diverse groups of scholars involved with research on health policy realized that their projects shared an underlying commonality: They all raised questions about the conceptual and professional boundaries of public and population health. The disciplinary perspectives represented here include history, economics, political science, medicine, and sociology. All the authors approach the set of related questions descriptively and analytically with a common task: to understand what are—and should be—the field's chief goals and activities.

   The aim of this volume, it should be stressed, is not to provide a definitive map of the boundaries of public and population health. Such an attempt, as these authors make clear, would be fruitless given the fundamental nature of the disagreements that prevail. Rather, these scholars seek to make explicit a set of assumptions that are often unstated or concealed; to describe and analyze the varying perspectives of the many constituencies involved in setting public health priorities; and to underscore the extent to which definitions of public and population health are intertwined with political realities.

Since the terrorist attacks of September 11, 2001, public health has been pulled in new directions that hold both promise and peril. As the limitations of surveillance and laboratories became apparent, politicians, administrators, and the general public gained a new appreciation of the vital role that public health agencies could play in emergencies. The uncertainty of the moment of political crisis, combined with the potential for new infusions of funding to support bioterrorism prevention, have presented the public health community with an opportunity to revitalize and rethink the health agenda for the nation. Where these efforts will lead and what shape public health will take in the coming decades remain to be seen.

References

Bayer, Ronald. 1989. *Private Acts, Social Consequences: AIDS and the Politics of Public Health*. New York: Free Press.

Cornely, Paul B. 1971. The Hidden Enemies of Health and the American Public Health Association. *American Journal of Public Health* 61:7–18.

Epstein, Richard A. 2003. "Let the Shoemaker Stick to His Last": A Defense of the Old Public Health. *Perspectives in Biology and Medicine* 46:S138–S159.

Evans, Robert G., Morris L. Barer, and Theodore R. Marmor, eds. 1994. *Why Are Some People Healthy and Others Not? The Determinants of Health of Populations*. New York: Aldine de Gruyter.

Evans, Gregory R. James M. Crutcher, Brooke Shadel, et al. 2003. Terrorism from a Public Health Perspective. *American Journal of Medical Science* 323:291–298.

Fairchild, Amy, and James Colgrove. 2004. Out of the Ashes: The Life, Death, and Rebirth of the "Safer" Cigarette in the United States. *American Journal of Public Health* 94: 192–204.

Farley, John. 2004. *To Cast Out Disease: A History of the International Health Division of the Rockefeller Foundation (1913–1951)*. New York: Oxford University Press.

Fox, Daniel M. 2001. The Professions of Public Health. *American Journal of Public Health* 91:1362–1364.

———. 2003. Commentary: Populations and the Law: The Changing Scope of Health Policy. *Journal of Law, Medicine, and Ethics* 31:607–614.

Fox, Daniel M., Mary Kramer, and Marion Standish. 2003. From Public Health to Population Health: How Law Can Redefine the Playing Field. *Journal of Law, Medicine, and Ethics* 31:21–23.

Frank, John W. 1995. Why "Population Health"? *Canadian Journal of Public Health* 86: 162–164.

Frieden, Thomas R. 2004. Asleep at the Switch: Local Public Health and Chronic Disease. *American Journal of Public Health* 94:2059–2061.

Hamlin, Christopher. 1998. *Public Health and Social Justice in the Age of Chadwick: Britain, 1800–1854*. Cambridge: Cambridge University Press.

Institute of Medicine. 1988. *The Future of Public Health*. Washington, D.C.: National Academies Press.

———. 2003. *The Future of the Public's Health in the Twenty-first Century*. Washington, D.C.: National Academies Press.

Kindig, David, and Greg Stoddart. 2003. What Is Population Health? *American Journal of Public Health* 93:380–383.

Knowles, John H. 1977. The Responsibility of the Individual. *Daedalus,* winter, 57–80.

Mazur, Allan. 1977. Public Confidence in Science. *Social Studies of Science* 7:123–125.

McCulloch v. Maryland. 1819. 17 U.S. 316.

Mello, Michelle M., David M. Studdardt, and Troyen A. Brennan. 2006. Obesity—The New Frontier of Public Health Law. *New England Journal of Medicine* 354:2601–2610.

Oppenheimer, Gerald, Ronald Bayer, and James Colgrove. 2002. Health and Human Rights: Old Wine in New Bottles? *Journal of Law, Medicine, and Ethics* 30:522–532.

Rosenkrantz, Barbara. 1972. *Public Health and the State: Changing View in Massachusetts, 1842–1936.* Cambridge, Mass.: Harvard University Press.

Rosner, David, ed. 1995. *Hives of Sickness: Epidemics and Public Health in New York City.* New Brunswick: Rutgers University Press.

Rothman, Kenneth J., H. O. Adami, and Dimitri Trichopoulos. 1998. Should the Mission of Epidemiology Include the Eradication of Poverty? *Lancet* 352:810–813.

Satel, Sally. 2001. Public Health? Forget It. Cosmic Issues Beckon. *Wall Street Journal,* December 13.

Sullum, Jacob. 1998. *For Your Own Good: The Anti-Smoking Crusade and the Tyranny of Public Health.* New York: Free Press.

Szreter, Simon. 2003. The Population Health Approach in Historical Perspective. *American Journal of Public Health* 93:421–431.

Tomes, Nancy. 1998. *The Gospel of Germs: Men, Women, and the Microbe in American Life.* Cambridge, Mass.: Harvard University Press.

Part I

Public Health in a Free-Market Society

The chapters in this section consider what is arguably the central conundrum of public health in America: Though it is an enterprise with an essentially collectivist orientation premised on an activist state, it operates within a political and civic culture whose preeminent values are individualism, limited government, and private sector initiative. These authors analyze the ways this social context has shaped and constrained what public health can accomplish. Sherry Glied applies the analytic frameworks of neoclassical economics to construct a definition of the boundaries of public health. Glied rejects the narrow notion, advanced by some libertarian thinkers, that public health should concern itself only with those functions the private sector cannot or will not provide. Instead, she contends, an examination of the political economy of public health reveals that a broadened mandate is essential. Dennis Scanlon and Marianne Hillemeier also approach the issue from the perspective of economics, with a more specific question: What is the role of private employers in shaping public health? Employer-based health insurance has been a critical component of the nation's health care system for the past half century, but little attention has been given to what businesses can or should do to advance public health. Nancy Tomes examines the historical evolution of the profession within a market-oriented culture in which members of the public have been conceptualized as "consumers" of health care. In this context, a major challenge for public health practitioners has been to advance their claim as the group best qualified to speak on behalf of those consumers and their interests. This role, Tomes argues, "has required the profession to bite the hand that feeds it: to point out the defects of business as usual, while being dependent on that business for funding and authority."

Public Health and Economics

Externalities, Rivalries, Excludability, and Politics

The scope of activities under the jurisdiction of public health departments has broadened to include many that seem far removed from control of the list of communicable disease that the U.S. Public Health Service published in 1921 (U.S. Public Health Service 1921). The term "public health" itself has been conflated with the expression "population health" or even the idea of prevention more generally. Addressing population health or prevention, in turn, is as readily a responsibility of large private insurers or of individual physicians as of any public entity. Public health departments today face increased responsibility for a growing share of the endless threats to the population's health and, at the same time, a loss of a distinctive mission in a world populated by HMOs, insurers, and a host of other private organizations.

This predicament means that the budgets of city, state, and federal public health agencies are perpetually under attack, even while the agencies' duties expand. In the wake of 9/11, health departments around the country complained that new antiterrorism responsibilities—even where supported by new funding—were siphoning already inadequate funds away from real public health problems. Is there a distinction between public health and population health or prevention? What part of those pieces are the core functions of public health?

Perhaps surprisingly, one place to look for an answer to the question of the boundaries of public health is in neoclassical economics. Economics, as a discipline, has displayed no more than passing interest in the subject of public health. Yet, it is possible to construct a fairly clear definition of the core activities of public health through some simple extensions of the basic economic model of health.

The Production of Health

The basic economic model of health, which I will use as the basis for a theory of public health, is the theory of health production that was developed by Michael Grossman in 1972.[1] In Grossman's model, health is a flow of benefits generated by a nontradable capital good, health capital. Individuals determine how much health capital to produce (and how to produce it) by making subjectively rational tradeoffs between this health capital and goods not related to health. These tradeoffs depend on the prices of the inputs to health capital, on individual preferences, and on each individual's initial endowments of income, time, genes, and so on.

In this model, the flow of health generated by health capital is valuable both in terms of investment and in terms of consumption. As an investment, having better health yields fewer sick days and a longer work life. These benefits, in turn, generate higher income, which can be used to purchase other nonhealth goods and services. As a consumption good, better health is a benefit for its own sake. The consumption value of health means that health would have substantial economic value even if had no effect on productivity or economic output.

The Grossman model is unreservedly individualistic. Health, because it is not tradable, is less "public" than almost any other good or service. Within this formal model, the health of the population is simply the sum of the health produced by all the individuals within that population.

The value of the population's health as an investment good, in terms of the output that health produces, has been quantified. Burton Weisbrod's 1961 book *The Economics of Public Health*, for example, emphasizes the substantial value of health in terms of economic productivity.[2] The value of the population's health as a consumption good has also been measured. Recent estimates by Nordhaus (2005), for example, suggest that the consumption value of improvements in health since 1900 has grown about as rapidly as the growth in real income. The cost of producing health can also, in principle, be measured. It includes the cost of all actions taken to improve health—including the costs of medical care consumed, time spent in all activities associated with the production of health, whether intended to prevent disease or to treat it, and the lost utility associated with treatment and preventive actions (including, for example, the enjoyment lost from not smoking).

Population health, as it arises in this model, is in no sense "public health." Grossman's original model offers no obvious role for the public sector. Of course, as Arrow (1963) points out, there are many market failures around medical care and medical insurance. Efficiency may best be served by having government intervene in these markets to make them function better. But medical care is just one among many inputs into the production of health in the Grossman model, and health can certainly be produced without any medical care at all.[3] Intervention in the medical care market may improve the efficiency of the economy, but it doesn't naturally comprise "public health."

Adding a Public Element to the Production of Health

The Grossman model focuses on the production of individual health. Within the framework of this model, we can imagine a host of situations where there are interactions among the individuals within the population. Consider some simple ones. I get immunized against measles, hence the prevalence of measles—and your risk of measles infection—declines. I smoke cigarettes near you, and your risk of lung cancer increases. I dump sewage into the local river that feeds the municipal water supply, increasing the incidence of water-borne disease in the city population. I examine New York City mortality statistics and publish a paper showing that many children ages three to eight die from window falls, and you install window guards to protect your children. Taking this logic further, in an extension along lines suggested by Lester Thurow (1971), I make a contribution to build a medical facility for homeless people, and you are no longer saddened by the fact that people are going without care. In economic terms, we call these situations problems of "public goods" (more specifically, "nonrival goods" and "nonexcludable goods") and "externalities."

Economists often use the terms "public goods" and "externalities" interchangeably, but they are not quite the same. Externalities are all situations where my actions have a positive (positive externality) or negative (negative externality) effect on your well-being or your ability to produce other goods and services, and where you have not been compensated for these effects of my actions. The reduction in risk that you, a stranger, obtain from my choosing to be vaccinated against measles is an externality. Economic theory suggests that the market is likely to produce too much of goods that cause negative externalities and too few of goods that cause positive externalities.

Public goods (or bads) are goods (or bads) that are nonexcludable and nonrivalrous in consumption. Goods are nonexcludable if it is not feasible to exclude some people from consuming a good that others are consuming. If you stop someone from dumping sewage into our collective water supply, it will be impossible to exclude me from the benefits of your action. If a good is nonexcludable, there is an inherent "free rider" problem. Since even nonpayers can consume the good, no one wants to pay for it. Everyone has an incentive to have someone else incur the costs of the good while benefiting from the outcomes. In the case of nonexcludable bads, any action that I take to eliminate the bad will also redound to everyone else's benefit. For this reason, goods that are nonexcludable will tend to be underproduced. Likewise, bads that are nonexcludable will tend to be overproduced.

Goods are nonrival if one person's consumption of a good does not diminish the amount available to another. Providing the good to one additional consumer would provide that consumer with some gain but would cost nothing at all. If goods are nonrivalrous, it may be possible to exclude someone from using them, but it would be highly inefficient to do so. Once a researcher has conducted a study showing that window guards reduce mortality, others can obtain that information at very little additional cost. The economy will not produce the most efficient possible outcomes if externalities and public goods exist. These situations generate a need for the use of the coercive power of the state in some way. In many, even most, potential cases of externalities, the externality problem can be, and usually is, resolved efficiently if the government develops an enforceable system of property rights.[4] Thus, there is generally no externality problem associated with visitors smoking in your private home. You have an enforceable property right to constrain the behavior of visitors within your home. Should you wish to prohibit smoking within your home, the police power of the state stands ready to enforce your prohibition.

In cases of public goods—externalities where the good (or bad) is nonexcludable and nonrivalrous—it is generally not possible to achieve economically efficient outcomes simply by allocating and enforcing individual property rights. For example, it would be difficult to assign property rights in the air we breathe. Moreover, while we may all have a legal right to breathe clean air, no single one of us has much incentive to devote much time and effort to the enforcement of this right. If one of us did take action to keep the air clean, everyone else would benefit without incurring any costs at all. Similarly, we would all benefit if information on the causes of death were collected and made available, but no individual would rationally make the investment to collect these data themselves.

Lester Thurow's argument about charity follows along these same lines. We all benefit (psychically) if poor people receive adequate medical care. But, on the whole, we'd be just as happy if someone else spent their money doing it as if we did it ourselves (barring anticipation of rewards in some world to come). Thus, Thurow argues, redistribution is also a public good. Society inevitably does too little of it.

In the context of Grossman's model of the production of health, these externalities and public goods related to health offer a role for the public sector. In practice, governments divide up the responsibilities among departments and agencies. Governments develop systems of allocating individual property rights, including health-related property rights, and enforce these through their legal system. Purely redistributive activities fall most naturally into the purview of the U.S. Treasury Department.[5] The remaining "public goods" situations related to health comprise the traditional focus of health departments.

The actions of health departments in response to the existence of these public goods feed back into the framework of individual health production. Health departments may provide goods and services directly, often at minimal cost to the user. Health departments may use tax dollars to subsidize services provided by other providers, again effectively lowering prices. They may exert a direct coercive effect on individual behavior, through regulation of activities generally (smoking regulations, for example) or restricting the behavior of individuals (isolation of disease carriers). These coercive actions effectively raise the price (whether financial or nonfinancial) of the regulated activity substantially. More recently, health departments have joined with other areas of government to tax public bads. The taxes raise the prices of these bads.

Once the new set of prices induced by health department action has been introduced, the prices enter the individual production function for health, and individuals once again make individually rational decisions. If the public health activities are indeed optimal, individual decisions will now lead to what are both individually and socially efficient choices (though these may include choices to engage in unhealthy activities).

Public health activities interact with private decisions and may even increase the return to private investments in health. This potential increase in the payoffs to individual investments in health that follows public investments means that addressing the insufficiency of public goods can have multiplier effects on population health. Dow, Philipson, and Sala-i-Martin (1999) and Cutler and Miller (2005a) demonstrate such spillovers, improvements in health outcomes following public health interventions that exceed those directly generated by the interventions themselves.

The new set of prices induced by the health department may also affect different people differently (depending on how responsive they are to prices). Those who are very responsive to changes in financial costs—generally those of lower incomes—will tend to be more affected by these interventions. Thus, the actions of public health departments often have a redistributive component, whether intentionally or unintentionally.

Pure(r) Public Goods

The economic model suggests a definition of public health as that subset of governmental activities that addresses health-related public goods. This definition potentially encompasses a great deal, since many activities have some public good components, although the public good component is often trivial. To see this, consider a ridiculous example: If I have my teeth whitened, all other riders on the subway may receive slightly more utility from my smile. It is hard to believe that this external effect leads to an important efficiency loss from too little tooth whitening. Traditional health department activities tend to be those that address those public goods problems where the free market leads to greatest underproduction.

Nonrivalrous Goods

Much of the traditional work of public health consists of the collection, tabulation, and analysis of routine epidemiological data. The information that results from these disease surveillance activities is not naturally embodied in a drug or treatment or product. In consequence, it is entirely nonrivalrous in consumption, and, in practice, nonexcludable as well. Once the information has been collected and made available to one user, it can be made available to all other users at no additional cost. While it might be possible, with considerable effort, to exclude nonpayers from gaining access to these data, such a prohibition would be inefficient, because the incremental cost of access is zero. Moreover, exclusion is likely to prove difficult. Anyone who did purchase the information could make it available to others at no personal cost, because my health has no direct effect on the health of others. If a good is nonrival, society is better off if we do not limit access to it.

These properties of epidemiological information suggest that, in many cases, no private market would likely arise to collect and tabulate it for the population as a whole. An insurer might wish to monitor the health status of its enrollees and might survey their health conditions (although the evidence suggests that few insurers do). Even this engaged insurer, however, would be unlikely to have an interest in the general health status of the overall population, including those not now or ever likely to be covered by its policies.

Without any incentive to promote a private market, information of this sort will tend to be underproduced without public intervention. The production of this information by a health department can improve the technology available to each individual to produce health. Knowledge of disease risks allows people to make better choices with the endowments they have available to them. As Glied (2001) shows in the case of childhood injury epidemiological data, the gains from public health information can be very large.

The gains from public health production of epidemiological surveillance information are greatest in the cases where that information cannot be tied to some known private good. If surveillance information can be embodied in an excludable, nonrival good or service—for example, where the results of epidemiological surveys can be used to design and market products—the gains from public production of the information will be correspondingly small. The efficiency benefits of the *public* production of surveillance information are greatest in situations where the outcome of the investigation and the potential value of that outcome are not clearly linked to any private good.

Like the production of surveillance information, tracking infectious disease carriers and subsidizing or coercing them to cease infecting others constitutes a service that is nonrivalrous and nonexcludable. People who spread disease confer negative externalities on others. Unless treatment is available, disease carriers may not wish to know that they are infected. Once informed of their status, some infected people will behave altruistically and avoid infecting others. But others will have little incentive to reduce their own disease-spreading activities.

Identifying and isolating a disease carrier to protect one person benefits all others who might have been exposed at no additional cost. The widespread benefits of tracking disease carriers and subsidizing their treatment mean that no single susceptible individual has much incentive to do it. Instead, faced with the possibility that others are disease carriers, uninfected individuals have an incentive to change their own behavior to avoid contact with potential susceptibles. This risk-avoidance behavior is personally costly and may, in certain circumstances, increase the general prevalence of disease, by reducing the number of potential uninfected contacts (see Michael Kremer's analysis of HIV, 1996).

Public Goods Monopoly Infrastructure

Another traditional role for health departments has been the development and maintenance of large-scale public health physical infrastructures, particularly municipal water supply and sewage treatment systems. The careless disposal of sewage is a clear example of a public bad. Dumping generally occurs in public property or rivers and lakes that serve large populations. Thus, poor private sewage disposal generates a collective negative externality.

Health departments address this negative externality through the development and subsidization of sewage treatment systems. In this situation, the role of public health goes beyond the construction of the facility. The operation of the facility must continue to be subsidized over time so that people do not have an incentive to revert to less costly, externality-causing alternatives. Often, tax-based subsidization of such facilities is coupled with systems of penalties designed to coerce people to use only these disposal options.

Water filtration and clean water systems perform a public health function that parallels that of sewage treatment, although their economic characteristics are rather different. Use of untreated water is primarily a private bad; there is no externality to correct in this case. Moreover, the benefits of water treatment are excludable. Households can be (and generally are) charged for their local water utilization.

Water treatment systems, however, have a low (though not zero) degree of rivalry. A network of water pipes can provide service to additional subscribers at very low cost. Municipal water systems are natural monopolies. A single water supply and treatment facility can produce water much more efficiently than can multiple competing systems. The economic role of health departments in this case is to own or regulate a region's monopoly water treatment system. The early twentieth-century debates over whether municipalities ought to develop their own water treatment facilities or contract for the provision of water reflects the economic ambiguity of the public role in the provision of clean water. In their analysis of the genesis of municipal water filtration, Cutler and Miller (2005b) conclude that the observed public role in water treatment reflects, primarily, the advantage of local governments in financing such large-scale natural monopoly public investments.

Benefits Conferred on Both Current and Future Generations

Many health risks, including those associated with sewage and unclean water, can be avoided by taking precautions (avoiding crowded places, washing hands often, staying out of restaurants, cooking all eggs to hard-boiled). Taking such precautions is costly. The expense of taking such precautions means that an entrepreneur who develops a less costly avoidance strategy—think of antibacterial hand cleansers—can reap benefits. The existence of a market for avoidance strategies often obviates the need for public intervention.

In some cases, however, an intervention that reduces avoidance costs has "permanent" payoffs—costs must be incurred today, but returns are experienced both by the current and by all future generations. The payoffs from these public health investments are not "excludable" to these future generations. In effect, future generations free ride on current investments. The existence of benefits to future generations, who do not participate in either private or public decision making today, implies that there will be too little private investment in such activities today.

Many public health investments in the development of clean water and sanitary sewage disposal systems have this characteristic. For example, during the 1890s, the municipality of Chicago reversed the flow of the Chicago River so that the city's water supply would no longer be contaminated by sewage (Blake 1956). This action continues to benefit the residents of Chicago today, a century later.

The advancement of public health knowledge offers another example of such payoffs to future generations. Research that identifies disease risk and protective factors today will continue to be useful into the indefinite future. The development of the germ theory of infectious disease, for example, provided considerable benefit to the generation alive at its introduction but also continues to provide benefit today (Deaton 2005).

Another case of future benefit concerns the complete eradication of disease. As Tomas Philipson points out, the eradication of smallpox provides immensely more benefit than would control of the disease. Future generations are entirely spared the need to take precautions against developing smallpox (Philipson 1995, 2000). At the same time, the eradication of the disease means that there is no private good (not even a vaccination) that can be sold to these future generations.

Future benefits may also arise through the avoidance today of public bads. Control of indiscriminate use of antibiotics today, for example, primarily benefits future generations by stemming the rise of new antibiotic-resistant strains of disease. Future generations, however, cannot compensate today's antibiotic users for these potential benefits.

Broadening the Definition of Public Health: Impure Public Goods

Traditional public health activities—surveillance, research, sanitation, clean water—tend to have a very substantial "public goods" component. The unfettered private market would be unlikely to provide these goods, so in the absence of public involvement, they would tend to be underproduced. The welfare of all of society can be improved through adequate provision of these goods and services.

But many of the activities that comprise the broader swath of public health today have a much smaller pure public goods component. Some—such as the delivery of personal health care services related to noninfectious disease (preventive or otherwise)—don't have much of a public goods component at all. The only "public good" present in this component of the Medicaid program, for example, is redistribution.[6]

In cases of "impure" public goods—goods where there is a substantial element of "privateness" or excludability present—the consequences of public intervention are not clear-cut. Public health intervention may have unanticipated consequences that mitigate the health and efficiency effects of the intervention.

These unanticipated consequences are a natural outcome of the processes under-lying the health production function model. Changing a price in this model will generate a reoptimization of individual behavior that may undo the public action. Since prices affect different people differently, these public health actions will also have a redistributive function. Redistribution, rather than efficiency enhancement, is often the main economically beneficial effect of these activities.

When Is a Public Good Not Public?

Not all public goods (or bads) require government intervention to ensure adequate provision. In many situations, activities with a "public good" or "public bad" component are complementary to activities where excludability is not a problem.[7] Consider restaurant inspection.

There is a substantial demand for information about the (overall) quality of restaurants and, recent evidence suggests, about their health characteristics as well (Jin and Leslie 2003). In 1998, the Los Angeles Health Department began requiring restaurants to post the results of annual inspections in their windows. Jin and Leslie (2003) show that, after the results of the scores were made pub-lic, customers became significantly less likely to patronize restaurants with a grade of B or lower (a B restaurant has a hygiene score of 80–89 on a scale where an A grade is 90–99 and a failing grade is below 60).

Information about the health quality of restaurants is a nonrivalrous public good—once I invest in learning about the quality of a restaurant, the informa-tion can be provided at no additional cost to everyone else. Thus, no individual would spend much time inspecting restaurant kitchens. This pattern would appear to suggest that information on the health quality of restaurants must be provided publicly. But this is less clear once the impact of the decline in res-taurant health quality is incorporated in the full health production model.

Without restaurant inspections, food poisoning would rise and fewer people would eat out. A private company could profit by developing a credible restau-rant inspection system and selling it to restaurants. Restaurants that paid the price of inspection would be permitted to post their grades in the window and to advertise that their quality was high. The value of the restaurant inspection company would depend on the extent to which restaurant customers viewed the reports as credible.

In the world of product safety, many analogous private quality assurance systems exist. Underwriters Laboratory, Good Housekeeping, and Best's Insurance Reports are paid by product manufacturers to develop information that is valuable to consumers. In these cases, quality-monitoring activities, although they have public goods elements, are produced at high levels because they enable more of a complementary private product to be sold.

Public health provision of these pure quality-monitoring services and coercive actions to close down failures are likely to have relatively little impact on the overall health of the public. Public provision substitutes for—or crowds out—the private producer and so provides little new information. In fact, the quality of municipal restaurant inspection systems may be lower than would be that of the corresponding private system. Municipal restaurant inspection systems have a monopoly on quality monitoring, and restaurant owners cannot respond to a decline in the credibility of these systems by refusing to purchase them.[8]

The main function of public provision of this information and mandatory participation in these systems is redistributive. Some (low-income) consumers will not be willing to pay a premium for eating in a restaurant that participates in a private quality monitoring system. These consumers may eat in unmonitored restaurants and suffer unfortunate health consequences. After public provision of restaurant inspection information, the low-quality producers will no longer be available. Whether low-income consumers are better off or not depends on who pays the cost of the quality monitoring system and on what happens to the underlying price of the goods themselves. If, as is typically the case, the price of restaurant inspections and of maintaining the quality of restaurant hygiene at standard levels is borne by restaurants, the price of eating out will rise. Low-income consumers may now be priced out of the market, improving their health but, perhaps, diminishing their overall well-being. Alternatively, they may turn to lower-cost, less-regulated producers (street vendors, for example) and experience more, rather than fewer, health problems.

Many health department activities have the property that they are complementary to private activities. There exists a thriving private market in the dissemination of information. News media survive because consumers want information (a public good) and this information is complementary to advertising markets. Public health messages brought to the attention of the news media, and likely to be of interest to the public, will tend to be disseminated broadly (often too broadly) by the media (Philipson and Posner 1994). While the public health impact of the development and initial dissemination of this information is often dramatic (see, for example, the impact of the surgeon general's report on smoking), the empirical evidence suggests that later public dissemination efforts have somewhat less impact. Dissemination activities, again, tend to have a redistributive focus, rather than an efficiency focus.

Substitution between Public Goods and Individual Actions

Most standard economics textbooks (and virtually all health economics texts) use immunization as the classic example of a positive externality. Each of us benefits from the immunization decisions of others, and we would all like to free ride on others' immunization choices. The textbook theory suggests that in the presence of such externalities, market equilibrium may generate inadequate levels of immunization. The arguments around immunization also apply to preventive actions taken to prevent the spread of sexually transmitted diseases or HIV. Use of condoms by one (uninfected) person reduces the prevalence of disease and hence the risk faced by other potential (uninfected) sex partners.

The textbook model suggests that these positive externalities should be off-set by subsidies for socially responsible behavior. Immunizations—or condoms—should be offered at less than market price to increase utilization. In the context of the health production model, however, the consequences of such subsidies are not quite so straightforward.

Recent economics work points out that this textbook analysis misses a further feedback loop (Philipson 1995, 1996; Ahituv, Hotz, and Philipson 1996). In the health production model, the decision to be immunized depends on both the price of immunization (or condom use) and on the benefits of this behavior. The benefits of preventive behavior, in turn, depend on the underlying prevalence of disease. Reducing the price of prevention generates a lower prevalence of disease and this, in turn, reduces the benefits of prevention, off-setting the initial price reduction.

This feedback loop makes it very difficult for individual prevention of infectious disease to drive prevalence to zero. As disease prevalence falls, whether in the case of measles or HIV, a growing literature shows that the level of precautions taken falls as well. Depending on the responsiveness of behavior to the price of prevention and to the benefits of prevention, subsidies may or may not reduce risk of disease. In either case, however, subsidies redistribute the risk of disease. Subsidies will tend to shift the prevalence of illness away from those who were centrally concerned with the price of prevention (poor people) toward those who were centrally concerned with disease prevalence.

In the case of diseases with high prevalence, this feedback loop is likely to be very important. Private benefits from reducing risk will be very large and the social benefit from intervention correspondingly smaller. Conversely, in the case of diseases with low prevalence that are nearly eradicated, private benefits from preventive action will tend to be small and the social benefits of interven-tion very large, particularly if they lead to disease eradication.

Public Goods Generated by Social Insurance

As infectious disease prevalence has fallen, health departments' focus has increasingly turned toward the prevention of chronic disease. Chronic disease clearly affects the health of the population. A chronic disease—or a chronic disease risk factor—is only a public health problem, however, to the extent that it generates externalities.

The importance of externalities in motivating intervention in the case of chronic disease has generated numerous empirical economic studies assessing the external costs of tobacco use, alcohol use, physical inactivity, and most recently obesity. The seminal work in this genre (Manning et al. 1991) examined the external costs of tobacco and alcohol use.

In some of these cases—most notably, the substantial external costs of alcohol-related automobile accidents—the external costs identified are classic public bads. In the case of obesity and physical activity, and tobacco as well, the external costs are largely those associated with public and private insurance programs (such as Medicare and Medicaid) that cover the disability and medical costs of those who become ill in consequence of the risky behavior (and the offsetting benefits to private and public pension programs of premature mortality).

The external costs of illness associated with insurance programs can be, in principle—and often are, in practice—internalized through variable premiums. Life insurers have long charged higher premiums to smokers, as do non–group health insurers. A growing economics literature on obesity appears to indicate that the external costs of obesity are mainly borne by obese individuals themselves, through lower wages that may offset their higher medical costs (Cawley 2004; Bhattacharya and Bundorf 2005).

Social insurance programs do not typically charge variable premiums based on risk behaviors or lifestyles. In the health production model, the failure to charge variable premiums in social insurance programs reduces the costs of engaging in unhealthy behavior.[9] In this context, taxation of the unhealthy behavior merely corrects for the existing and inefficient subsidy to unhealthy behavior generated by social insurance. Perhaps taxing the unhealthy activity has lower administrative costs than would assessing premiums appropriately.

Taxing bads to correct social insurance externalities may confer welfare benefits, but this is likely just a second-best solution to the existence of the initial distortion. Moreover, the strategy of using public health taxes to undo the redistributive function of social insurance may act to erase the progressive benefits of social insurance itself (Remler 2004).

The Political Economy of Public Goods

Economic theory suggests a set of conditions that define when public health action is most beneficial—when these actions are most irreplaceable. Public health activities enhance efficiency most when they address issues where there is a serious "free rider" problem of nonexcludability or where a good is entirely nonrivalrous (both from the perspective of suppliers and purchasers). Not all free rider problems or problems of nonrivalry warrant public health interference, however. Public health action is not as necessary when the private market will generate the same activities. The private market may do so either because of complementarities between public health activities and private excludable goods markets or because public health actions substitute for the effects of the prevalence of disease itself. Public health does perform an economically useful function when it stems externalities generated by other social programs, but this is only a second- best activity necessitated by the distortions introduced through the social programs themselves. Public health is at its best when it is producing basic epidemiological or risk factor research, or putting into place measures that will benefit future generations.

This set of criteria, however appealing, places the actual enterprise of public health in a rather unfortunate position. Public health, economic theory says, is most useful and beneficial when nobody can observe cash savings because of the actions of public health; when public health activities don't even try to reduce taxes; when the potential benefits of public health actions are unclear; and when the potential beneficiaries of public health activities aren't even born yet!

The political participation that generates public health itself, however, is a public good. Mobilizing to protect public health requires costs that generate benefits—public goods—of service to the entire population. The economic definition of public health requires that it target areas that, by definition, have no apparent constituency to support them and where the outcomes of the activities themselves are not readily predictable and countable. Often, the more observable an activity is, the less essential its public health function.

Public health, as a common good, suffers not only on the demand side, where all other public goods produced by government must also face the problem of a lack of constituency. The production of public health is an activity that is inherently local, labor intensive, and fragmented. Unlike, for example, the concentrated suppliers of national defense services, the public health workforce is a diffused constituency that must overcome its own collective action problems to lobby government for increased funding. The core functions of public health have no lobby but the good government types and altruistic sanitarians.

In this context, the expansion of the boundaries of public health is, in economic terms, a survival strategy. By providing prevention services and addressing population health needs more broadly, it creates constituencies who benefit directly, immediately, and observably from the services, information, and subsidies provided by public health. The benefits of these activities are so readily apparent, however, mainly because they substitute for obvious private activities. The danger is that these sideshow activities will overtake the main stage. The expansion of the scope of public health—rather than creating budgetary space for core activities—may leave us with a public health system that provides services redundant to the private market, while neglecting those public health functions where public action is truly indispensable.

Acknowledgments

I thank Joshua Graff Zivin, Dahlia Remler, and Dennis Scanlon for many useful suggestions.

Notes

1. Note that medical care is a subset of health generally. Arrow's earlier paper (1963) addresses market failures in the medical care market, not the production of health generally.
2. A large subsequent literature measures the (investment) value of health lost due to specific illnesses, the "burden of disease."
3. Some might argue that the Grossman model's assumption of rationality is false or that people exhibit bounded rationality. Individual irrationality would mean that the outcomes of a private market in health production were not necessarily economically efficient. The resulting inefficiency would not, however, provide any obvious role for government. To make the case for public intervention here, one would need to show, at a minimum, that individuals who tend to make irrational choices about their own health production will be more rational in their decisions around the election of a government that will then make health production decisions on their behalf (see Pauly 1988 for a discussion of this point).
4. Ronald Coase (1960) shows that under certain (strong) assumptions, it doesn't matter to efficiency how the property rights are allocated so long as they are all determined.
5. Economic theory suggests that redistributive objectives are most efficiently accomplished through the redistribution of income. Redistributing income changes the endowments available for health production and improves equity while allowing each individual to make subjectively optimal choices about how much health to purchase. This theory assumes that people seek to redistribute overall well-being, not only health or health care.
6. As noted earlier, economists would argue that redistribution is better accomplished through the tax system than through the health department.
7. Tyler Cowen (2005) notes that lighthouses, the textbook example of a public good, were actually owned privately in much of England during the nineteenth century. Local ports paid for the operation of lighthouses in order to increase shipping traffic to the port.
8. The private sector might respond by providing a more rigorous monitoring system.

9. Some proponents of the health production model believe that this implicit subsidy accounts for the higher smoking rates observed in many European countries that have high cigarette tax rates and comprehensive social insurance programs.

References

Ahituv, Avner, V. Joseph Hotz, and Tomas Philipson. 1996. The Responsiveness of the Demand for Condoms to the Local Prevalence of AIDS. *Journal of Human Resources* 31:869–897.

Arrow, Kenneth. 1963. Uncertainty and the Welfare Economics of Medical Care. *American Economic Review* 53:941–973; reprinted in 2001, *Journal of Health Politics, Policy, and Law* 26, 5 (October):851–883.

Bhattacharya, Jay, and M. Kate Bundorf. 2005. *The Incidence of the Healthcare Costs of Obesity.* NBER Working Papers 11303. Washington, D. C.: National Bureau of Economic Research.

Blake, N. M. 1956. *Water for the Cities: A History of the Urban Water Supply Problem in the United States.* Syracuse, N.Y.: Syracuse University Press.

Cawley, John. 2004. The Impact of Obesity on Wages. *Journal of Human Resources* 39, 2 (Spring): 451–474.

Coase, R. H. 1988. The Problem of Social Cost. *Journal of Law and Economics* 3, 4:1–14.

Cowen, Tyler. 2005. Public Goods and Externalities. *Library of Economics and Liberty.* www.econlib.org/library/Enc/PublicGoodsandExternalities.html. *Retrieved September* 30, 2005.

Cutler, David, and Grant Miller. 2005a. The Role of Public Health Improvements in Health Advances: The Twentieth-Century United States. *Demography* 42, 1 (February): 1–22.

———. 2005b. *Water, Water, Everywhere: Municipal Finance and Water Supply in American Cities.* NBER Working Papers 11096. Washington, D. C.: National Bureau of Economic Research.

Deaton, Angus. 2005. *The Great Escape: A Review Essay on Fogel's "The Escape from Hunger and Premature Death, 1700–2100."* NBER Working Papers 11308. Washington, D.C.: National Bureau of Economic Research.

Dow, William H. Tomas J. Philipson, and Xavier Sala-i-Martin. 1999. Longevity Complementarities under Competing Risks. *American Economic Review* 89, 5 (December): 1358–1371.

Glied, Sherry. 2001. The Value of Reductions in Child Injury Mortality in the U.S. In *Medical Care Output and Productivity,* ed. David M. Cutler and Ernst R. Berndt, 511–538. Chicago: University of Chicago Press.

Grossman, Michael. 1972. On the Concept of Health Capital and the Demand for Health. *Journal of Political Economy* 80, 2 (March–April): 223–255.

Jin, Ginger Zhe, and Phillip Leslie. 2003. The Effect of Information on Product Quality: Evidence from Restaurant Hygiene Grade Cards. *Quarterly Journal of Economics* 118, 2 (May): 409–451.

Kremer, Michael. 1996. Integrating Behavioral Choice into Epidemiological Models of AIDS. *Quarterly Journal of Economics* 111, 2 (May): 549–573.

Manning, Willard G., Emmett B. Keeler, Joseph P. Newhouse, Elizabeth M. Sloss, and Jeffrey Wasserman. 1991. *The Costs of Poor Health Habits.* Cambridge, Mass.: Harvard University Press.

Nordhaus, William D. 2005. Irving Fisher and the Contribution of Improved Longevity to Living. *American Journal of Economics and Sociology* 64, 1 (January): 367–392.

Pauly, Mark V. 1988. Is Medical Care Different? Old Questions, New Answers. *Journal of Health Politics, Policy, and Law* 13, 2 (Summer): 227–237.

Philipson, Tomas. 1995. The Welfare Loss of Disease and the Theory of Taxation. *Journal of Health Economics* 14, 3 (August): 387–395.

———. 1996. Private Vaccination and Public Health: An Empirical Examination for U.S. Measles. *Journal of Human Resources* 31, 3 (Summer): 611–630.

———. 2000. *Economic Epidemiology and Infectious Diseases Handbook of Health Economics.* 1B:1761–1799.

Philipson, Tomas, and Richard A. Posner. 1994. Public Spending on AIDS Education: An Economic Analysis. *Journal of Law and Economics* 37, 1 (April): 17–38.

———. 1995. A Theoretical and Empirical Investigation of the Effects of Public Health Subsidies for STD Testing. *Quarterly Journal of Economics* 110, 2 (May): 445–474.

Remler, Dahlia. 2004. Poor Smokers, Poor Quitters, and Cigarette Tax Regressivity. *American Journal of Public Health* 94, 2 (February): 225–229.

Thurow, Lester C. 1971. The Income Distribution as a Pure Public Good. *Quarterly Journal of Economics* 85, 2 (May): 327–336.

Weisbrod, Burton. 1961. *The Economics of Public Health.* Philadelphia: University of Pennsylvania Press.

The Limits of Relying on Employers in an Intersectoral Public Health Partnership

With the multiplication of factories the improvement in the lot of the laboring man has become a vital question of the day. . . . The health of society in general is both directly and indirectly menaced by insanitary conditions in any industry.

—C.F.W. Doehring, 1903

America's businesses and employers have the opportunity to promote health and prevent disease and disability in their own workforces. Employers are also a critical source of health care payment for personal health care services. Furthermore, because businesses are closely involved with communities, they can collaborate in partnerships that monitor, identify, and address community health problems.

—Institute of Medicine, 2003

The two epigraphs, written a hundred years apart, illustrate the often schizophrenic view of employers in the history of public health. On the one hand, employers have been blamed for numerous public health problems, ranging from injuries resulting from unsafe and unsanitary working conditions in factories to poor air quality in cities—an undesirable byproduct of manufacturing and commerce. On the other hand, many analysts have recognized that personal and community health is directly tied to income, housing, and health insurance benefits, which are supported by jobs provided by employers and a strong tax base in communities. While it is perhaps not surprising that employers could be viewed as both villain and champion in the eyes of special interest groups and the media, this schizophrenic view has also characterized public health policy circles. For example, the Institute of Medicine's landmark 1988 report, *The Future of Public Health in America*, hardly mentioned employers, yet they received their own chapter and were identified as key public health partners in the IOM's 2003 follow-up report, *The Future of the Public's Health in the Twenty-first Century*.

So which is it—villain or unjustly vilified? Problem or partner? We explore in this chapter both where employers have fit with respect to public health historically, and where employers should fit in the future. We use the recommendations from the 2003 IOM report (see the sidebar for a summary of the report's recommendations) regarding an enhanced role and new responsibilities of employers as the launching point for our discussion, and we assess the feasibility and logic of placing more ownership for our nation's health squarely on the shoulders of the employer community.

Specifically, we examine the following questions in this chapter:

- Why was there an increased emphasis, between the 1988 and 2003 IOM reports, on the role of employers in protecting and promoting public and population health?
- What role have employers played historically in assuring public and population health? What do recent trends in employer health related activities tell us about the likelihood of employers becoming a key public health partner?
- Should employers assume an enhanced responsibility for our nation's health? What is the appropriate expectation—and boundary—between the responsibilities of private employers, individuals, and government, as represented by public health agencies?

Factors Influencing the Expanded Employer Role between the 1988 and 2003 IOM Reports

In *The Future of Public Health* the IOM in 1988 analyzed the state of "disarray" in U.S. public health activities in the 1980s and presented a plan of action that it hoped would lead to stronger public health capability. Although the report referred to a multidimensional public health system with roles for both public and private entities, it focused almost exclusively on governmental public health agencies. It mentioned private-sector groups, including employers, only in passing, such as a brief reference to the involvement of business coalitions in worksite health promotion programs in some states (198). The report's plan of action defined the mission of public health as "fulfilling society's interest in assuring conditions in which people can be healthy" (7), described the governmental role in fulfilling this mission, and delineated responsibilities unique to each level of government. Additional recommendations related to effective implementation of this plan included revisions to the existing statutory framework, structural and organizational modifications for agencies, strategies to build additional agency capacity, and improved education for public health professionals.

In its 2003 report, *The Future of the Public's Health in the Twenty-first Century*, the Institute of Medicine issued the following recommendations regarding employers' role for protecting the public's health in the new millennium:

> The corporate community and public health agencies should initiate and enhance joint efforts to strengthen health promotion and disease and injury prevention programs for employees and their communities. As an early step, the corporate and governmental public health community should:

a. Strengthen partnership and collaboration by:
  - Developing direct linkages between local public health agencies and business leaders to forge a common language and understanding of employee and community health problems and to participate in setting community health goals and strategies for achieving them, and
  - Developing innovative ways for the corporate and governmental public health communities to gather, interpret, and exchange mutually meaningful data and information, such as the translation of health information to support corporate health promotion and health purchasing activities.

b. Enhance communication by:
  - Developing effective employer and community communication and education programs focused on the benefits of and options for health promotion and disease and injury prevention, and
  - Using proven marketing and social marketing techniques to promote individual behavioral and community change.

c. Develop the evidence base for workplace and community interventions through greater public, private, and philanthropic investments in research to extend the science and improve the effectiveness of workplace and community interventions to promote health and prevent disease and injury.

d. Recognize business leadership in employee and community health by elevating the level of recognition given to corporate investment in employee and community health. (13–14).

The 1988 IOM report stimulated a variety of responses by policy makers, public health agencies, and educational institutions aimed at systematic improvement (IOM 2003). Concerns about public health capacity continued to intensify, however, and in February 2001 the IOM convened the Committee on Assuring the Health of the Public in the Twenty-first Century (Fox 2001). The committee's report, issued in 2003, prominently featured employers and business as essential actors in an intersectoral public health system. This expansion of the role ascribed to employers in impacting public health over the fifteen years that had elapsed since the IOM's earlier report was likely due to a confluence of factors that included deterioration in health benchmarks, salient deficiencies in public health infrastructure, widespread adoption of a multiple determinants framework for conceptualizing population health status, and increasing alignment of employers' interests with traditional public health goals.

Deterioration in U.S. Health Benchmarks

The impetus to broaden the focus of the public health system to explicitly include employers came in part from recognition that, despite governmental reform efforts, many indicators of population health continued to fall far short of their potential. Among countries surveyed by the Organization for Economic Cooperation and Development, for example, U.S. life expectancy declined from nineteenth place in the early 1970s to twenty-eighth by the turn of the century, and the U.S. infant mortality rate fell from fifteenth to thirty-first (United Nations Development Program 2003).

Several specific public health issues that motivated the IOM's 1988 call for reform remained prominent or had intensified by 2003. HIV/AIDS infection prevalence skyrocketed, for example, from approximately 35,000 persons in 1986 to as many as 1,185,000 by the end of 2003 (Centers for Disease Control and Prevention 2004). Lack of access to health care for the indigent continued to be a troubling reality, with 20.7 million Americans reporting in 2003 they had delayed medical care in the past year and another 15 million saying they did not receive needed medical care due to cost (Schiller, Adams, and Nelson 2005). While rates of smoking declined somewhat between the IOM reports, more than one in five Americans were smokers in 2003 (Jiles et al. 2005), and as a result smoking remained a prominent contributor to premature mortality as well as to chronic health problems (Mokdad et al. 2004). Furthermore, by 2003 wide-ranging disparities in health status and health care utilization and quality by race/ethnicity and socioeconomic status were increasingly recognized as persistent threats to achieving optimal population health within the existing public health environment (Agency for Healthcare Research and Quality 2003; U.S. Department of Health and Human Services 2000).

Chronic Deficiencies in the Public Health Infrastructure

The events of September 11, 2001, and the subsequent anthrax attacks focused public attention on the need for increased public health capacity to respond to threats of bioterrorism and other potential health disasters (Salinsky 2002). As Fee and Brown (2002) note, however, public health infrastructure issues, including organizational inefficiencies, jurisdictional irrationalities, and chronic underfunding, have been ongoing problems for many years. While additional funding for public health infrastructure was allocated in the wake of the terrorist attacks, concerns remained that much of this money went to preventive efforts for very low probability events, with little benefit in terms of overall public health capability (Cohen, Gould, and Sidel 2004).

The 1988 IOM report stimulated some notable initiatives to improve public health infrastructure over the 1990s, including the development of a core set of public health functions which laid the foundation for public health workforce development strategies included in *Healthy People 2010* (U.S. Department of Health and Human Services 2000), as well as for the development of the National Public Health Performance Standards Program (Centers for Disease Control and Prevention 1998). In addition, new program initiatives such as the university-based Centers for Preventive Research, the National Public Health Training Network, and the National Electronic Disease Surveillance Network have contributed to increased public health capacity. Despite these accomplishments, however, the 2003 IOM report concluded that many of the infrastructure-building recommendations in the original report remained unaddressed. The demonstrable lack of support and advocacy for government-based public health infrastructure improvements lent support to a broadened focus incorporating employers and additional private-sector resources.

Adoption of a Multiple Determinants Framework
for Conceptualizing Population Health

Another stimulus toward an inclusive vision for the U.S. public health system was the gradual evolution from a simplistic view of health as merely the absence of disease to an increasingly comprehensive conceptualization of health and the mechanisms underlying population health status. In 1990, Evans and Stoddart published their influential model that depicts health as shaped by determinants in the social, physical, and genetic environment, in addition to health care use.

In a similar vein, Dahlgren and Whitehead (1991) developed a conceptual framework of health influences with age, sex, and hereditary factors at its center and progressively more distal contextual factors in layers radiating outward. Their model was noteworthy in explicitly citing working conditions and unemployment as important influences on health status. In 2000, the Institute of Medicine itself issued a report on intervention strategies for health promotion, framing these approaches within a multilevel model of health influences that included social relationships, living conditions, neighborhoods and communities, institutions (including medical care), and social and economic policies.

These conceptual models share a broad-based, ecological view of the determinants of health. Because many of these determinants are beyond the control of public health agencies and health care professionals, they imply that achieving optimal population health will require additional coordinated strategies that actively engage private-sector influences such as employers and business.

Increasing Alignment of Employers' Interests with Traditional Public Health Goals

Many employers have long understood that the health of their employees has an important impact on their businesses' bottom lines. Healthy workers are more productive than others because they are absent less often and are more efficient and focused while at work (Burton et al. 2005; Collins et al. 2005; Lerner et al. 2003). They also require proportionately lower expenditures for medical care coverage, disability payments, and workers' compensation (Goetzel et al. 2004; Stewart et al. 2003). In recognition of these realities, companies are increasingly instituting workplace health promotion and disease prevention programs. Employers have also been at the forefront of developing and using performance and value measures in health care. While there is some evidence to suggest that such programs can produce savings in medical costs (Goetzel, Juday, and Ozminkowski 1999), much remains to be learned about the effectiveness of specific intervention strategies and the best structure for programs in various types of workplaces (Institute of Medicine 2003).

More broadly, the 2003 IOM report makes the case that it is in the best interests of major employers to invest in community health, as well as in health promotion among their own employees. Corporate investment in community health infrastructure, the report argues, will likely result in a larger pool of productive workers, many of whom will want to work for an employer perceived as socially responsible and known for civic leadership. Furthermore, involvement with social issues can positively affect business performance in terms not only of employee recruitment and retention but also of heightened employee morale, positive community support for the corporation and its needs, and improved supplier relationships (IOM 2003).

The task set for employers by the IOM committee is a tall one, and, as we will see, it is not clear that employers are interested in embracing this expanded role.

Understanding Employers' Involvement in Health Care

Historical and Conceptual Framework

Employers have historically played an important role in the health of Americans. Taken from Ron Kessler and Paul Stang's *Health and Work Productivity* (2006), figure 2.1 illustrates many health-related activities that most employers are involved in. These can be classified as those related to occupational health and safety and required by law (e.g., workers' compensation, compliance with Occupational Safety and Health Administration standards); those related to

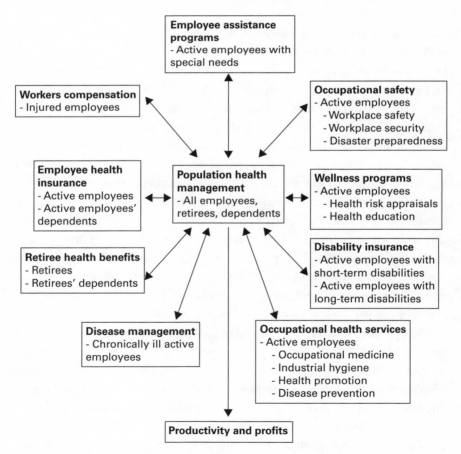

Figure 2.1 Employer Health Programs and a Population Health Management Approach

reducing absenteeism and enhancing the productive capability of workers (e.g., wellness and employee assistance programs); and those viewed as necessary to compete for workers in the labor market (e.g., the provision of health insurance benefits). For example, since the passage of the Occupational Safety and Health Act of 1970, employers have worked with the federal government to prevent job-related death, injury, and illness among their employees. Additionally, employers provide workers' compensation to employees who suffer a job-related injury or illness. However most of the programs identified in figure 2.1 are not connected as the figure suggests, but operate in silos—a point we return to later in the chapter.

Thus, while employers participate in many health-related activities, they are involved in some because of legal requirements and in others in the belief their involvement will benefit their business—either directly, via productivity, or indirectly, as a draw for workers in the labor market. The reason for employer involvement in health-related programs is important to delineate at the outset because the IOM's recommendations largely focus on employers *voluntarily* partnering with the public health system, which would primarily involve changes in health-related activities not required by law, and thus, we argue, changes that must ultimately fit the economic objectives of employers.

Economic Framework

In order to assess the likelihood and value of employers joining an intersectoral public health partnership, it is useful to have a framework for understanding why employers are involved in health care issues to begin with, particularly when such involvement seems outside the core business for most employers. Grounded in economics, our framework begins with the underlying motivation of any for-profit firm: the desire to maximize profits. With minor changes, this framework also fits not-for-profit firms or organizations in which profit maximization is not a strict objective.

In their simplest form, profits are a function of a firm's total revenues and total costs, where costs are a function of the various inputs and the prices of the inputs that are used to produce the core goods/services sold by the firm. While the specific inputs and mix of inputs that go into producing a firm's core goods/services vary (e.g., steel, tires, and paint for an auto manufacturer, food and advertising for a restaurant), one pivotal input is labor, with some firms (e.g., service firms) relying disproportionately more on labor than do other firms.

Thus, for many firms, profit is highly dependent on the amount of labor hired and the price (i.e., wage) paid for that labor. In addition, productivity itself is highly dependent on the skill of the labor hired, and the capability of hired

workers can vary significantly based on experience, education, motivation, training, and other factors. Thus, many firms perceive differences in the expected productivity levels of job applicants and seek to hire applicants who will contribute
most productively to the firms' objectives. Likewise, job applicants look for the
best compensation package (wages and benefits). The key questions here are how
and why the health-related activities of employers impact both the ability of
firms to hire labor and the productivity of the labor once it is hired. An understanding of these relationships requires knowing why responsibility for health
care and health-related benefits became associated with employers in the first
place.

Employer-sponsored health insurance benefits for employees and their
beneficiaries, as well as for retirees, accounted for 7.6 percent of total labor
compensation in 2006 (Bureau of Labor Statistics 2006). That many employers
provide health insurance benefits, which thus are tied to employment, is an
artifact of federal policy in World War II, which froze workers' wages to ensure
an adequate supply of labor for the government's war effort (Fronstin 2001;
Moran 2005; Rosner and Markowitz 2003; Starr 1982). What the government
did not anticipate was that employers, in an attempt to compete for scarce
workers, would offer benefits such as health insurance in addition to wages. By
2005, 60 percent of employees received some form of health insurance benefit
or offer of health insurance from their employer (Kaiser Family Foundation and
Health Research and Education Trust 2005).

Aside from historical reasons, the standard economic view of employer-
sponsored health benefits hypothesizes that employers will offer health insurance because employees demand it in lieu of higher wages. From this perspective
employers make a decision on total compensation and are viewed as being indif-
ferent about how total compensation is divided between wages and benefits,
arriving at a decision that reflects the average preference of the labor force. Thus,
all else remaining constant, as benefit costs increase, this model predicts that
wages will stay stagnant or rise more slowly to ensure that the sum of both components equals the targeted compensation amount (Pauly 1999). Because of het-
erogeneity among workers' preferences, this model also helps to explain why
firms differ in whether they offer and subsidize employee health insurance.

As illustrated in figure 2.1, however, employers are also involved in providing health-related programs and benefits for workers once they are employed. For
example, disease management, wellness, and employee assistance programs are
becoming common for many midsize to large employers (Short, Mays, and Mittler
2003). The theory of the profit-maximizing firm also explains why employers provide these programs. Specifically, evidence illustrates that U.S. employers have a

direct financial interest in ensuring that their workers are healthy and productive. In a recent study by the Commonwealth Fund, labor time lost due to health reasons represented lost economic output totaling an estimated $260 billion per year (Davis et al. 2005). Thus, by developing or contracting and paying for programs aimed at keeping workers healthy, productive, and on the job, firms believe they enhance productive efficiency and thus maximize profits.

Firms' decisions regarding whether to offer various health-related benefits and the level at which to subsidize these benefits also take into account how the federal government treats these expenditures and the rules associated with providing health benefits. Specifically, the IRS treats employer and employee health insurance contributions as tax exempt in the computation of corporate income tax and employees' personal income, thus effectively making the cost of one dollar in health insurance benefits less than one dollar to both the firm and the employee. In addition, sections of the Federal Omnibus Employee Retirement Income Security Act (ERISA) of 1974 allow certain employers to self-insure their health benefits programs, and to choose benefit packages that are exempt from state mandates—additional advantages to the firm. Such considerations are important for understanding employer involvement in health-related activities and reduce the cost and uncertainty associated with providing health-related benefits, thus making the decision to do so more attractive to firms.

In summary, voluntary employer involvement in health-related programs can be viewed as a business decision: For recruitment, retention, and productivity reasons, the benefit of involvement outweighs the cost.

Recent Trends in Employers' Health-Related Activities

Providing Health Insurance in Inflationary Times

In 2003, private-sector health insurance accounted for 36 percent of national health expenditures in the United States (Smith et al. 2005), covering 159 million Americans under age sixty-five and supplementing Medicare coverage for 15 million elderly people (Fronstin 2004). In a recent survey of U.S. employees, 60 percent stated that health insurance was the most important employer benefit (Employer Benefits Research Institute 2004).

But with health benefits consuming a larger part of employee compensation in an era of rising health care costs, the employer-based health insurance system has come under assault. For example, the health benefit share of compensation climbed to 7.6 percent in 2006, even higher than the average 6.9 percent recorded in the 1993–1994 period, when employers were more aggressively seeking alternatives to traditional indemnity coverage (Bureau of Labor Statistics 2004, 2006). The larger portion of employee compensation devoted to heath benefits is due to the large recent increases in health insurance premiums. According to a 2005 Kaiser/HRET survey of employer-sponsored health benefits, health insurance premiums for family coverage increased 9.2 percent in 2005, reaching an average of $10,880 annually. While the 9.2 percent increase was less than in the previous few years, health insurance premiums for family coverage have increased by 73 percent since 2000. This period of significant inflation in the prices of health-related goods and services has been attributed to a number of factors, including increases in technology, the availability of new blockbuster drugs, increased legal liability, and the aging of the population and associated prevalence of chronic diseases (Smith et al. 2006).

These large increases in the costs of health benefits have caused great concern among U.S. employers, even though the standard economic model, as discussed earlier, would suggest that employers would adapt by adjusting wages to reflect the targeted level of total compensation. Wal-Mart's benefit costs, for example, jumped to $4.2 billion in 2004 from $2.8 billion three years earlier, causing concern within the company because health benefits costs represented an increasing share of sales. In a since highly publicized internal corporate memo, Wal-Mart recommended hiring healthier employees as a way to manage the firm's increasing health costs (Greenhouse and Barbaro 2005). For some U.S. employers, large increases in health care costs have required more drastic action. General Motors CEO and chair Rick Wagoner announced that the company will eliminate twenty-five thousand hourly manufacturing jobs by 2008 and close an unspecified number of facilities, in part because of the $5.6 billion dollars that GM annually spends on health care for current and former employees and their beneficiaries (Hawkins, Boudette, and Mahe 2005).

As the economic model would predict, U.S. employers have responded to the large increases in health care costs by reducing coverage and shifting costs to employees, presumably instead of reducing wages (or the rate of wage increases). Since 2000, the percentage of firms offering health benefits coverage has dropped from 69 to 60 percent (Kaiser Family Foundation and Health Research and Education Trust 2005). Firms have also reduced their health benefits coverage to retirees (McCormack et al. 2002).[1]

Employers have also greatly increased the average employee contribution to health insurance premiums and the average out-of-pocket payments through higher copayments, deductibles, and coinsurance. According to a survey by Hewitt Associates, the average employee contribution to employer-sponsored health insurance increased from $662 in 2000 to $1,444 in 2005—143 percent. Additionally, the out-of-pocket costs for copayments, deductibles, and coinsurance increased from $708 in 2000 to $1,524 in 2005—115 percent (Block 2005).

Indeed, the move to increase employee cost sharing has fueled the "consumer-directed health care" movement (Wilensky 2006). In short, the majority of employers have responded to the recent inflationary pressure by reducing coverage/benefits, passing on more of the cost of health insurance benefits to their employees, or both—which some analysts have argued is a positive change because it makes employees understand the true costs of health insurance benefits. This response by employers, generally in line with what economic theory would predict, suggests that the trend is for employers to retreat from, rather than to increase, responsibility for health programs.

Value-Based Purchasing Efforts

While many employers have responded to recent inflationary pressures by reducing benefits and shifting costs, an alternate (though not mutually exclusive) response among the largest and most aggressive employer purchasers has been the development of programs to achieve more value from current dollars spent. This strategy, known in the health care world as value-based purchasing (VBP) (Maio et al. 2005), is similar to the industrial supply chain management approaches used regularly in business procurement (McKone-Sweet, Hamilton, and Willis 2005; Ford and Scanlon 2007).

What has fueled the VBP movement in health care is, first, evidence that the quality and safety of health care in the United States is less than ideal and, second, the assumption (for which there is isolated empirical evidence, but not broad support one way or the other) that higher quality and safer care result in lower health care expenditures. Thus, VBP approaches seek to measure the quality of care health care providers give (e.g., hospitals, doctors, integrated insurance companies) and to change the incentives in the health care system to reward providers who offer the best combination of efficiency and quality, that is, value. Admittedly this is a longer-term strategy aimed at addressing what some feel to be the underlying systemic problems in the U.S. health care system, and the payoff—in terms of reduction in health inflation and expenditures—is less certain than in the cost-shifting approaches described earlier.

Many employers active in the VBP arena have made significant investments and strides in measuring health care processes and outcomes, and this involvement is important for understanding ways employers may partner in an intersectoral public health system.

Quality and Safety in the U.S. Health Care System

Recent research estimating quality and safety deficiencies in the U.S. health care system has fueled the VBP efforts of large purchasers, including employers.

A study by McGlynn and colleagues (2003), for example, found that patients in a representative sample from twelve communities received recommended care only 55 percent of the time. Another study, using data reported by the Centers for Medicare and Medicaid Services under the Hospital Quality Alliance program, found that quality varies from hospital to hospital and within hospitals for different medical conditions (Jha et al. 2005). In *Crossing the Quality Chasm*, a highly publicized 2001 review of the quality of health care in the United States, the IOM documented similar quality problems and pointed to the need for major overhauls in the way health care is organized, financed, and delivered. The IOM's recommendations included broad suggestions for how health care purchasers, including employers, could realign incentives to reward health care providers for providing better quality of care.

Similarly, recent evidence has documented concerns about the safety of health care provided in the United States. A 1999 Institute of Medicine report, *To Err Is Human*, estimated that between 44,000 and 98,000 deaths each year are attributable to medical errors in the inpatient setting. Once again the IOM recommended that employers, particularly large employers, provide more market reinforcement for the safety of health care.

The Measurement Movement

The old cliché "You can't manage what you can't measure" has been a rallying cry for the VBP and quality improvement movement in health care. Employers have been influential in driving measurement of health care performance, beginning with the creation of the Health Employer Data Information Set (HEDIS) in 1989. Employers, HMOs, and the National Committee for Quality Assurance developed this set of standardized measures of health plan performance, which includes measures of clinical quality and appropriateness (e.g., the percentage of a health plan's members for which a test is recommended who actually receive the test), as well as measures that capture the opinions of health plan members regarding access to care, care provided by physicians, and the quality of the plan's customer service (National Committee for Quality Assurance 2005).

The Leapfrog Group and its hospital survey is another example of a coordinated effort by employers to measure the value received for health care dollars expended. A coalition of large private- and public-sector health care purchasers that provide health benefits to employees formed the Leapfrog Group in 2000 in response to the IOM's *To Err Is Human* report. In consultation with patient safety experts, the group identified four safety "leaps" that these employer purchasers now demand from urban general acute care hospitals, including the adoption of computerized physician drug order entry systems (CPOE) and the staffing of hospitals' intensive care units with physicians who are board certified in critical care medicine. The Leapfrog Group's research estimates that 65,341 deaths could be avoided annually if all targeted hospitals adopted their recommended safety practices (Leapfrog Group 2005). To establish public accountability for these safety practices and for their use by employers and consumers as purchasers, the Leapfrog Group has been surveying its targeted hospitals to determine compliance with the recommended safety practices (Galvin et al. 2005).

While HEDIS and Leapfrog are the two most well-known national efforts by employers to measure quality, safety, and value in health care, employers are involved in many others, national or regional in scope. For example, the National Business Coalition on Health's eValue8 effort is a detailed survey of health plans with a specific emphasis on the degree to which plans are developing the structure and implementing processes to better manage the care of members with chronic illnesses (Beich et al. 2006). Countless other activities operate under the purview of community-level health care or health-purchasing coalitions or other large individual employers; for example, General Motors has been using an internally developed methodology for evaluating health plans for years, and the Central Florida Health Care Coalition is developing a Regional Health Information Organization to share clinical information across providers. Thus, individual employers and employer groups have collectively played a significant role in pushing the burgeoning quality and performance measures in health care, which is likely a significant reason why the IOM's 2003 report on the future of the public's health considered employers a key partner in an intersectoral public health partnership.

Pay-for-Performance (P4P) Programs

The availability of improved performance measurement has led some employers and other purchasers, including the Medicare program led by the Centers for Medicare and Medicaid Services, to attempt to realign payment systems so that health care providers are paid according to their performance on these standardized measurements. In fact, one of the recommendations in recent IOM reports was that employers and other health care purchasers develop financial incentives to reward investments and activities that improve quality and safety.

The number of employers in the United States that have adopted pay-for-performance (P4P) mechanisms, or are pushing their contracted health plans to develop P4P programs, is growing rapidly. For example, as of November 2004, there were eighty-four P4P programs covering thirty-nine million beneficiaries, with the number of P4P programs expected to double by 2006 (Med-Advantage 2005). Perhaps the most notable P4P effort initiated by employers to date is the

Bridges to Excellence program led by General Electric Corporation, UPS, Procter & Gamble, and others (deBrantes 2003). There is little empirical evidence on P4P in health care settings, however, and on whether P4P leads to improvements in the quality of care (Petersen et al. 2006; Dudley et al. 2004; Dudley 2005). One recent study showed that P4P did improve certain quality measures in physician groups in California compared to physician groups in the Pacific Northwest receiving no incentives. The study also pointed out that paying physician groups to reach a common fixed performance target may produce a low return on investment because these programs largely reward physician groups already performing at a high level (Rosenthal et al. 2005).

Whether to reward providers according to attainment of a predetermined level of performance (i.e., an absolute performance threshold) or according to the amount of quality improvement achieved (i.e., improvement over baseline) is one issue that the design and implementation of P4P programs have yet to address. There are a number of others (Scanlon 2005). An important question is whether even the largest U.S. employers have enough market clout (i.e., market share) to seriously threaten the revenues and market share of health care providers. This is particularly true in light of the increasing consolidation of health care providers (Robinson 2004; Cueller and Gertler 2003; Scanlon et al. 2005; Scanlon, Chernew, et al. 2006; Scanlon, Swaminathanan, et al. 2006). Some have argued that without the federal (e.g., Medicare) and state government (e.g., Medicaid) purchasing programs taking the lead, VBP efforts will be less successful, a view that anecdotal evidence from some of the earliest P4P programs appears to support (Scanlon 2005).

Workplace Health Promotion and Disease Prevention Programs and Other Benefits

To improve the health of their employees, some employers have turned to disease management and health promotion programs. Disease management targets specific chronic conditions, usually those where self-management by patients is important, and has emerged as a more consumer/provider-friendly substitute to traditional utilization management methods of containing costs and improving quality (Beich et al. 2006; Felt-Lisk and Mays 2002; Villagra 2004). According to a 2005 report by Hewitt Associates, 83 percent of employers used disease management programs as part of their health insurance benefits plans in 2005, up from 73 percent in 2004. Additionally, 49 percent of companies measure the prevalence of chronic conditions in their workforce, 30 percent offer incentives to encourage employee participation in wellness programs, and 27 percent measure the health and productivity impact of disease management programs.

Like P4P, however, there is little evidence on the effectiveness of disease management programs, and the scant early reports are mixed (Beich et al. 2006; Felt-Lisk and Mays 2002; Villagra 2004). For example, one study found substantial quality improvement for adults among four disease conditions from 1996 to 2002 but not concomitant cost savings (Fireman, Bartlett, and Selby 2004). A 2004 review of the disease management research literature by the Congressional Budget Office found insufficient evidence to conclude that disease management is effective for containing costs. The review noted numerous methodological problems in the literature, including selection bias and the inability of current efforts to account for costs of the intervention itself.

In summary, our brief examination of recent trends in employer health activity suggests the modal response of employers has been either to shift costs to employees in the form of higher copremiums, copayments, and deductibles, or to adopt the so-called consumer-directed health benefits plans. Some larger employers have also responded to the latest round of health inflation and evidence about poor costs and quality by pushing for additional measures of accountability and by working to develop programs that align payment with outcomes.

Employers' Role in an Intersectoral Public Health Partnership

As the sidebar indicates, the IOM in 2003 called for employers to be an active participant in an intersectoral public health partnership, and while the report does not delineate the specific actions required of employers, it is clear the IOM is seeking participation in health-related activities beyond the current level of involvement for most employers.

The sidebar lists broad suggestions, but specific aims for improving the public's health appear in the *Healthy People 2010* public health objectives (U.S. Department of Health and Human Services 2000). The two overarching goals of this initiative—increasing the quality and years of healthy life and eliminating health disparities—are detailed in specific objectives related to twenty-eight focus areas. These areas include access to health care services; changes in health behaviors (e.g., increased physical activity and fitness and reduced tobacco and substance abuse); investments and improvements in public health infrastructure; increased primary prevention; and appropriate treatment of chronic conditions.

The key question is, What are the costs and benefits associated with employers taking an active role in these areas? As our framework identified, the benefits of participating must be measured in terms of employee recruitment, employee retention, employee productivity, or gains to firms' reputations from participating. The costs, on the other hand, are uncertain but are surely not trivial, if for no other reason than the need to plan, administer, and contract for the desired programmatic changes.

As an illustration, we examine the Healthy People 2010 goal of increased access to quality health services. Employers could contribute to this goal both by offering employer-sponsored insurance if it is not already offered, or by making insurance coverage more affordable if it is currently offered. Yet the trends in employer-sponsored insurance described earlier suggest the exact opposite is occurring: Fewer employers are offering insurance benefits, and those who do require employees to pay a larger percentage of the total costs. Employers could also contribute to this goal by measuring the quality of care provided to their employees and by providing incentives to use high-quality providers. But as we have seen, while some employers are leading these efforts, most are not actively involved in this area (Galvin and Delbanco 2005), suggesting that a major uptake by employers is unlikely.

If one considers the objective of increasing the utilization of preventive care, promoting healthy behaviors such as diet, exercise, and smoking cessation, or increasing compliance with treatment guidelines for chronic illness, it is also unlikely that employers will become involved beyond current levels unless research evidence identifies a direct payoff for doing so—again in terms of employee recruitment, retention, or enhanced productivity, or of reduced overall expenditures for health benefits. While a number of policy advocates believe that better quality is less costly, there is little evidence that broadly supports this claim, and specific studies that have examined the economic returns for better chronic illness care, for example, suggest that while quality might improve from enhanced care management, these programs tend to increase costs, at least in the short run of three to six years (Fireman, Bartlett, and Selby 2004; Selby et al. 2003). Though a time horizon of three to six years is not that long, many employers and health plans don't retain employees or members for this length of time, making the economic arguments for employer investment in better care management tenuous at best.

Thus, current evidence would suggest that if there were obvious significant benefits to employers to making the changes the IOM committee envisions, profit-maximizing employers would already have made them. Of course, it could also be the case that there are benefits to these activities that the research literature has not yet documented, suggesting that the availability of information about the return on investment (ROI) for these expenditures would generate increased voluntary involvement. If this were true, the economic model would predict that the provision of information demonstrating the value of these health-promoting activities would lead to increased employer investments in the activities desired.

While we've argued that employers currently don't have strong incentives to voluntarily join the IOM's proposed intersectoral partnership, modifying existing policy might create incentives for such partnership. One could, for example, make the existing tax exemption for employer-sponsored health insurance benefits conditional on employers' contracting with health plans or providers that demonstrate high levels of quality on standardized measures, or conditional on achieving compliance (within an employer's covered population) with recommended preventive screenings and treatment guidelines for chronic illnesses. The administration and regulation of this policy would be challenging, but linking the tax exclusion to these public health goals would be one way to change the incentives faced by employers and would generate societal benefit for what many view as the inequitable and regressive tax treatment of employer-sponsored health insurance (i.e., tax law favors workers with higher incomes) (Enthoven 2003; Reinhardt 1999). There of course are other policy options. For example, recently the Massachusetts legislature passed an individual and employer insurance mandate (Altman and Doonan 2006), and Maryland adopted the so-called Wal-Mart employer insurance mandate, requiring large employers in Maryland either to spend an amount equal to at least 8 percent of their wage payroll on employee health benefits or to make a contribution to the state's insurance program for the poor (Wagner 2006).

Since companies spend a lot of money on philanthropy for a variety of causes, another policy strategy is to make the case that businesses allocate more of these philanthropic resources to meeting public health objectives. But while it is easy to view such expenditures as altruistic, and thus easily transferred from one cause to another, those studying corporate philanthropy and community engagement know these investments are often strategically made and lead to returns for donor firms in the form of enhanced goodwill, increased community reputation, or even benefits from advertising (Stalling 1998). Kaplan and Norton (2004) suggest that companies could and should do a better job of assessing the value generated from their philanthropy, both value for the company itself and that generated by the recipient. Redirecting corporate philanthropy toward important public health objectives would likely involve a marketing campaign in which public health officials emphasize the degree to which corporate investments in health are in the best interest of the company and of society, and thus yield the largest return on investment.

While our discussion has focused on the lack of strong incentives for employers to voluntarily join an intersectoral public health partnership, it is important to consider the degree to which employed populations should be viewed as target populations for achieving public health objectives, and thus whether there is an argument for the government to encourage employer involvement by making its own investments in employer-based health activities. To pursue this argument, we must consider the potential value of employer communities contributing to the achievement of public health objectives.

In regard to the Healthy People 2010 focus areas, there is reason to believe that targeting public health efforts toward employer populations may be advantageous. Work environments offer the opportunity to identify, measure, and reach targeted employees with messages about lifestyle changes, behavior modifications, and so on. Indeed, a significant challenge in accomplishing the HP-2010 public health objectives, particularly those related to access to care and compliance with recommended treatments, is identifying a population base for accountability and for measurement, because measuring and accomplishing many of these objectives require access to personal health and medical records. Public health agencies traditionally have not had such access except for the records of those in their immediate client base.

Because employees and their families often receive health insurance benefits from the employer, and because many employers (or their agents) access and analyze medical records or claims data in aggregate for purposes of improving their health benefits programs, employers may be a natural source for obtaining this information. In addition, apart perhaps from home or school, employed individuals spend the majority of their time at work, thus again offering the advantage of reaching individuals with messages, materials, and even treatment. While other such venues exist—churches, schools, and community organizations—the workplace offers the advantage of reaching large defined populations at scheduled times.

But the thought of the public health system having entrée to employed populations seems complicated at best and unrealistic in the most likely scenario, particularly if left solely to employer volunteerism. Nevertheless, the CDC leadership has recently acknowledged the potential of employed populations and has invested in research in employer-based activities and communities in a number of ways (Gerberding 2005) for the very reasons presented here. The central hub in figure 2.1, for example, illustrates the potential of a holistic population health approach in an employment setting, although few employers link their various health programs in this way.

So while examples of partnerships do exist and there are some interesting research programs, the incentives for employers to voluntarily engage in public health partnerships are small under the current regime, despite employer populations offering certain advantages for achieving stated public health objectives, in particular the opportunity to define, target, and reach groups of individuals for purposes of measurement, care delivery, and messaging. Thus, our model predicts that additional incentives would need to be present to make wide-scale public-private partnerships more common. It seems likely that these incentives would follow one of two avenues.

The first type of incentive, public policy changes—such as reforming ERISA requirements or the IRS treatment of employer-sponsored benefits, or adopting insurance mandates, as described earlier—could change the costs and benefits to employers considering the proposed partnership. Of course, changes in public policy often result in various externalities and unintended negative consequences, so these would need to be considered and weighed as part of the policy analysis to understand their total economic and societal impact.

The second type of incentive would result in voluntary employer/employee investment due to the availability of better information regarding the ROI to employers (and employees) of engaging in specific health-related action. An example is credible research evidence that demonstrates the return on investment (e.g., reductions in trends in total health expenditures or benefits to productivity) to employers of being more actively involved in encouraging positive health behavior changes among their employees (e.g., engaging in disease management or wellness programs). Because many employer health prevention and promotion efforts may have long-term benefits for the federal Medicare program, it may make sense for the Centers for Medicare and Medicaid Services to consider incentives for these programs, such as subsidies or tax credits.

In conclusion, while there may be clear societal benefits to increased private-sector partnership in public health promotion, it is unlikely that large numbers of employers will voluntarily join in the types of partnership activities that the IOM's report recommends, given the current policy climate. The reason is simple: The private benefits gained (or the forecasted private benefits, in terms of employee recruitment and retention, etc.) are less than the private costs of those investments, even though the total benefit to society might exceed these private costs. Increasing the level of private-public partnership may depend upon the extent to which (1) the public health community identifies and is willing to invest in employed populations as an important target for addressing public health goals; (2) incentives or penalties are enacted to encourage increased participation; and (3) research provides evidence of clear benefit to employers for public health promotion activities.

Acknowledgments

We are grateful to Matthew Guldin for providing research assistance in the preparation of this chapter.

Notes

1. While many characteristics of the firm, including size, the proportion of part-time workers in the firm, average wages paid, and whether workers are unionized, affect the likelihood that a firm will offer health benefits, the most influential is size. The health insurance offer rate for the smallest employers (three to nine workers) was 47 percent in 2005 compared to 98 percent for the largest employers (two hundred or more workers) (Gabel et al. 2005).

References

Agency for Healthcare Research and Quality. 2003. *National Healthcare Disparities Report.* Rockville, Md.: Agency for Healthcare Research and Quality.

Altman, S. H., and M. Doonan. 2006. Can Massachusetts Lead the Way in Health Care Reform? *New England Journal of Medicine* 354:2093–2095.

Beich, J. J., D. P. Scanlon, J. Ulbrecht, E. W. Ford, and I. A. Ibrahim. 2006. The Role of Disease Management in Pay for Performance Programs for Improving the Care of Chronically Ill Patients. *Medical Care Research and Review* 63, 1:1–21.

Block, S. 2005. Workers May Be in for Health Plan Sticker Shock. *USA Today*, October 20.

Bureau of Labor Statistics. 2004. Employer Costs for Employee Compensation. Press release. U.S. Department of Labor. September. www.bls.gov/news.release/archives/ecec_09152004.pdf.

———. 2005. *Survey of Occupational Injuries and Illnesses: Workplace Injuries and Illnesses, 1980–2002 editions.* U.S. Department of Labor. www.bls.gov/iif/home.htm.

———. 2006. Employer Costs for Employee Compensation. Press release. Department of Labor. March. www.bls.gov/news.release/archives/ecec_06212006.pdf (accessed August 14, 2006).

Burton, W. N., C. Y. Chen, D. J. Conti, A. B. Schultz, G. Pransky, and D. W. Edington. 2005. The Association of Health Risks with On-the-Job Productivity. *Journal of Occupational and Environmental Medicine* 47, 8:769–777.

Centers for Disease Control and Prevention. 1998. *National Public Health Performance Standards Program.* www.nalboh.org/perfstds/nphpsp.htm (accessed August 14, 2006).

———. 2004. *HIV/AIDS Surveillance Report, 2003.* Atlanta: U.S. Department of Health and Human Services.

Cohen, H. W., R. M. Gould, and V. W. Sidel. 2004. The Pitfalls of Bioterrorism Preparedness: The Anthrax and Smallpox Experiences. *American Journal of Public Health* 94:1667–1671.

Collins, J. J., C. M. Baase, C. E. Sharda, R. J. Ozminkowski, S. Nicholson, G. M. Billotti, R. S. Turpin, M. Olson, and M. L. Berger. 2005. The Assessment of Chronic Health Conditions on Work Performance, Absence, and Total Economic Impact for Employers. *Journal of Occupational and Environmental Medicine* 47, 6:547–557.

Congressional Budget Office. 2004. *An Analysis of the Literature on Disease Management Programs.* Washington, D.C.: Congressional Budget Office.

Cuellar, A. E., and P. J. Gertler. 2003. Trends in Hospital Consolidation: The Formation of Local Systems. *Health Affairs* 22, 6:77–87.

Dahlgren, G., and M. Whitehead. 1991. *Policies and Strategies to Promote Social Equity in Health.* Stockholm, Sweden: Institute for Futures Studies.

Davis, K., S. R. Collins, M. M. Doty, A. Ho, and A. L. Holmgren. 2005. Health and Productivity among U.S. Workers: The Commonwealth Fund. www.cmwf.org/publications/publications.htm (accessed August 14, 2006).

deBrantes, F. 2003. Bridges to Excellence: A Program to Start Closing the Quality Chasm in Healthcare. *Journal for Healthcare Quality* 25, 2:2, 11.

Doehring, C.F.W. 1903. Factory Sanitation and Labor Protection. Bulletin. Washington, D.C.: Department of Labor.

Dudley, R. A. 2005. Pay for Performance Research: How to Learn What Clinicians and Policy Makers Need to Know. *JAMA* 294: 1821–1823.

Dudley, R. A., A. Frolich, D. L Robinowitz, J. A. Talavera, P. Broadhead, and H. S. Luft. 2004. *Strategies to Support Quality-Based Purchasing: A Review of the Evidence.* Rockville, Md.: Agency for Healthcare Research and Quality.

Employer Benefits Research Institute. 2004. Public Attitudes on the U.S. Health Care System: Findings from the Health Confidence Survey. EBRI Issue Brief 275. November. www.ebri.org/publications/ib/index.cfm?fa=ibDisp&content_id=3507.

Enthoven, A. C. 2003. Employment-Based Health Insurance Is Failing: Now What? *Health Affairs* (Millwood) Supplement Web Exclusives:W3–237–49.

Evans, R. G., and G. L. Stoddart. 1990. Producing Health, Consuming Healthcare. *Social Science and Medicine* 31:1347–1363.

Fee, E., and T. M. Brown. 2002. The Unfulfilled Promise of Public Health: Deja Vu All Over Again. *Health Affairs* (Millwood) 21, 6:31–43.

Felt-Lisk, S., and G. P. Mays. 2002. Back to the Drawing Board: New Directions in Health Plans' Care Management Strategies. *Health Affairs* (Millwood) 21, 5:210–217.

Fireman, B., J. Bartlett, and J. Selby. 2004. Can Disease Management Reduce Health Care Costs by Improving Quality? *Health Affairs* (Millwood) 23, 6:63–75.

Ford, E. W., and D. P. Scanlon. 2007. Promise and Problems with Supply Chain Management Approaches to Health Care Purchasing. *Healthcare Management Review* 32, 3:192–202.

Fox, C. E. *Remarks for the First Meeting of the Institute of Medicine's Committee on Assuring the Health of the Public in the Twenty-first Century.* 2001. newsroom.hrsa. gov/speeches/iomctte.htm (accessed August 14, 2006).

Fronstin, P. 2001. The History of Employment-Based Health Insurance: The Role of Managed Care. *Benefits Quarterly* 17:7–16.

———. 2004. Sources of Health Insurance and Characteristics of the Uninsured: Analysis of the March 2004 Current Population Survey. EBRI Issue Brief 276. December. www.ebri.org/publications/ib/index.cfm?fa=ibDisp&content_id=3508.

Gabel, J., G. Claxton, I. Gil, J. Pickreign, H. Whitmore, B. Finder, S. Hawkins, and D. Rowland. 2005. Health Benefits in 2005: Premium Increases Slow Down, Coverage Continues to Erode. *Health Affairs* (Millwood) 24, 5:1273–1280.

Galvin, R. S., and S. Delbanco. 2005. Why Employers Need to Rethink How They Buy Health Care. *Health Affairs* (Millwood) 24:1549–1553.

Galvin, R. S., S. Delbanco, A. Milstein, and G. Belden. 2005. Has the Leapfrog Group Had an Impact on the Health Care Market? *Health Affairs* (Millwood) 24:228–233.

Gerberding, J. L. 2005. Protecting Health: The New Research Enterprise. *JAMA* 294: 1403–1406.

Goetzel, R. Z., T. R. Juday, and R. J. Ozminkowski. 1999. Systematic Review of Return on Investment (ROI) Studies of Corporate Health and Productivity Management Initiatives. www.workplace.samhsa.gov/OnlineBriefings/ebriefs/rontim.aspx

Goetzel, R. Z., S. R. Long, R. J. Ozminkowski, K. Hawkins, S. Wang, and W. Lynch. 2004. Health, Absence, Disability, and Presenteeism Cost Estimates of Certain Physical and Mental Health Conditions Affecting U.S. Employers. *Journal of Occupational and Environmental Medicine* 46, 4:398–412.

Greenhouse, S., and M. Barbaro. 2005. Wal-Mart Memo Suggests Ways to Cut Employee Benefit Costs. *New York Times*, October 26.

Hawkins, L., N. E. Boudette, and K. Mahe. 2005. Wielding the Ax: GM, Amid Industry Overhaul, Cuts Health Benefits for Retirees. *Wall Street Journal*, October 18.

Hewitt Associates. 2005. Health Care Expectations: Future strategy and Direction. www.hewittassociates.com/Intl/NA/en-US/KnowledgeCenter/ArticlesReports/ArticleDetail.aspx?cid=1711 (accessed August 14, 2006).

Institute of Medicine. 1988. *The Future of Public Health*. Washington, D.C.: National Academies Press.

——. 1999. *To Err Is Human*. Washington, D.C.: National Academies Press.

——. 2000. *Promoting Health: Intervention Strategies from Social and Behavioral Research*. Washington, D.C.: National Academies Press.

——. 2001. *Crossing the Quality Chasm*. Washington, D.C.: National Academies Press.

——. 2003. *The Future of the Public's Health in the Twenty-first Century*. Washington, D.C.: National Academies Press.

Jha, A. K., Z. Li, E. J. Orav, and A. M. Epstein. 2005. Care in U.S. Hospitals: The Hospital Quality Alliance Program. *New England Journal of Medicine* 353, 3:265–274.

Jiles, R., E. Hughes, W. Murphy, N. Flowers, M. McCracken, H. Roberts, M. Ochner, L. Balluz, A. Mokdad, L. Elam-Evans, and W. Giles. 2005. Surveillance for Certain Health Behaviors among States and Selected Local Areas: Behavioral Risk Factor Surveillance System, United States, 2003. *MMWR Surveillance Summaries* 54, 8:1–116.

Kaiser Family Foundation and Health Research and Education Trust. *Employer Health Benefits 2005 Annual Survey*. 2005. www.kff.org/insurance/7315/index.cfm (accessed August 14, 2006).

Kaplan, R. S., and D. P. Norton. 2004. Keeping Score on Community Investment. *Leader to Leader*, no. 33:13–20.

Kessler, R. C., and P. E. Stang, eds. 2006. *Health and Work Productivity: Making the Business Case for Quality Health Care*. Chicago: University of Chicago Press.

Leapfrog Group. 2005. The Leapfrog Group Fact Sheet. Washington, D.C. www.leapfroggroup.org/about_us/leapfrog-factsheet (accessed August 14, 2006).

Lerner, D., B. C. Amick III, J. C. Lee, T. Rooney, W. H. Rogers, H. Chang, and E. R. Berndt. 2003. Relationship of Employee-Reported Work Limitations to Work Productivity. *Medical Care* 41, 5:649–659.

Maio, V., C. W. Hartmann, N. I. Goldfarb, A. R. Roumm, and D. B. Nash. 2005. Are Employers Pursuing Value-Based Purchasing? *Benefits Quarterly* 21, 3:20–29.

McCormack, L. A., J. R. Gabel, H. Whitmore, W. L. Anderson, and J. Pickreign. 2002. Trends in Retiree Health Benefits. *Health Affairs* (Millwood) 21, 6:169–176.

McGlynn, E. A., S. M. Asch, J. Adams, J. Keesey, J. Hicks, A. DeCristofaro, and E. A. Kerr. 2003. The Quality of Health Care Delivered to Adults in the United States. *New England Journal of Medicine* 348, 26:2635–2645.

McKone-Sweet, K. E., P. Hamilton, and S. B. Willis. 2005. The Ailing Healthcare Supply Chain: A Prescription for Change. *Journal of Supply Chain Management* 41:4–13.

Med-Advantage. 2005. Provider Pay-for-Performance Incentive Programs: 2004 National Study Results. www.medvantageinc.com/Pdf/mv_2004_P4P_National_Study_Results-Exec_Summary.pdf.

Mokdad, A. H., J. S. Marks, D. F. Stroup, and J. L. Gerberding. 2004. Actual Causes of Death in the United States, 2000. JAMA 291:1238–1245.

Moran, D. W. 2005. Whence and Whither Health Insurance? A Revisionist History. *Health Affairs* (Millwood) 24, 6:1415–1425.

National Committee for Quality Assurance (NCQA). 2005. *NCQA State of Health Care Quality 2005*. Washington, D.C.: NCQA.

Occupational Safety and Health Administration. 2002. *An Overview of Voluntary Protection Programs*. U.S. Department of Labor. www.osha.gov/oshprogs/vpp/overview.html (accessed August 14, 2006).

Pauly, M. 1999. *Health Benefits at Work: An Economic and Political Analysis of Employment-Based Health Insurance*. Ann Arbor: University of Michigan Press.

Petersen, L. A., D. W. Le Chauncy, T. Urech, C. Daw, and S. Sookanan. 2006. Does Pay-for-Performance Improve the Quality of Health Care? *Annals of Internal Medicine* 145:265–272.

Reinhardt, U. E. 1999. Employer-Based Health Insurance: A Balance Sheet. *Health Affairs* (Millwood) 18:124–132.

Robinson, J. 2004. Consolidation and the Transformation of Competition in Health Insurance. *Health Affairs* 23:11–24.

Rosenthal, M. B., R. G. Frank, Z. Li, and A. M. Epstein. 2005. Early Experience with pAy-for-Performance: From Concept to Practice. *JAMA* 294:1788–1793.

Rosner, D., and G. Markowitz. 2003. The Struggle over Employee Benefits: The Role of Labor in Influencing Modern Health Policy. *Milbank Quarterly* 81:45–73.

Salinsky, E. 2002. Will the Nation Be Ready for the Next Bioterrorism Attack? Mending Gaps in the Public Health Infrastructure. National Health Policy Forum Issue Brief 776. www.nhpf.org/pdfs_ib/IB776_Bioterror_6–12–02.pdf.

Scanlon, D. P. 2005. Evidence for Pay-for-Performance: Hope for the U.S. Health Care System? *Managed Care* 14, 12 (Supplement): 6–10.

Scanlon, D. P., M. Chernew, S. Swaminathan, and W. Lee. 2006. Competition in Health Insurance Markets: Limitations of Current Measures for Policy Analysis. *Medical Care Research and Review 63 (6 supplement): 37S–55S*.

Scanlon, D. P., S. Swaminathan, M. Chernew, J. Bost, and J Shevock. 2005. Health Plan Performance: Evidence from Managed Care Insurance Markets. *Medical Care* 43, 4:1–9.

Scanlon, D. P., S. Swaminathanan, M. Chernew, and W. Lee. 2006. Market and Plan Characteristics Related to HMO Quality and Improvement. *Medical Care Research and Review 63* (6 supplement): 56S–89S.

Schiller, J. S., P. F. Adams, and Z. C. Nelson. 2005. Summary Health Statistics for the U.S. Population: National Health Interview Survey, 2003. *Vital and Health Statistics, series* 10, no. 224.

Selby, J. V., D. P. Scanlon, J. Elston-Lafata, V. Villagra, J. Beich, and P. R. Salber. 2003. Determining the Value of Disease Management Programs. *Joint Commission Journal on Quality and Safety* 29, 9:491–499.

Short, A. C., G. P. Mays, and J. Mittler. 2003. Disease Management: A Leap of Faith to Lower-Cost, Higher-Quality Health Care. Center for Studying Health System Change, Issue Brief 69. www.hschange.org/CONTENT/607/.

Smith, C., C. Cowan, S. Heffler, and A. Catlin. 2006. National Health Spending in 2004: Recent Slowdown Led by Prescription Drug Spending. *Health Affairs* (Millwood) 25, 1:186–196.

Smith, C., C. Cowan, A. Sensenig, and A. Catlin. 2005. Health Spending Growth Slows in 2003. *Health Affairs* (Millwood) 24, 1:185–194.

Stalling, B. 1998. Volunteerism and Corporate America. *US Society and Values*, September.

Starr, P. 1982. *The Social Transformation of American Medicine*. New York: Basic Books.

Stewart, W. F., J. A. Ricci, E. Chee, S. R. Hahn, and D. Morganstein. 2003. Cost of Lost Productive Work Time among US workers with Depression. *JAMA* 289:3135–3144.

Stewart, W. F., J. A. Ricci, E. Chee, D. Morganstein, and R. Lipton. 2003. Lost Productive Time and Cost due to Common Pain Conditions in the US Workforce. *JAMA* 290:2443–2454.

United Nations Development Program. 2003. *Human Development Report 2003*. New York: Oxford University Press.

U.S. Department of Health and Human Services. 2000. *Healthy People 2010: Understanding and Improving Health*. Second ed. Washington, D.C.: U.S. Government Printing Office.

Villagra, V. 2004. Strategies to Control Costs and Quality: A Focus on Outcomes Research for Disease Management. *Medical Care* 42, 4 (Supplement): III 24–30.

Wagner, J. 2006. Maryland Legislature Overrides Veto on Wal-Mart Bill. *Washington Post, January 13*.

Wilensky, G. 2006. Consumer-Driven Health Plans: Early Evidence and Potential Impacts on Hospitals. *Health Affairs* (Millwood) 25:174–185.

Speaking for the Public

The Ambivalent Quest of Twentieth-Century Public Health

In its sobering 1988 report *The Future of Public Health,* the Institute of Medicine's Committee for the Study of the Future of Public Health cited the field's poor public image as an important facet of its contemporary "disarray." Interviews with public health workers across the United States suggested that most Americans did not appreciate or understand the importance of public health. Its services were either invisible, as in the case of clean water supplies or sewage control, or associated with stigmatized groups, such as the very poor or the dangerously ill. Public health efforts to reduce health risks through legislation and regulation, such as seat-belt laws and antismoking codes, were resented as "interference with private freedoms," while the necessity for disease surveillance often conflicted with cherished rights of personal privacy. Such misunderstandings posed a serious problem, the committee concluded, because "in a free society, public activities ultimately rest on public understanding and support, not on the technical judgment of experts." Ironically, the report noted, the "early leaders of public health" seemed better able to garner public support than did their modern counterparts (130).

The lament that the public health profession once upon a time knew how to connect with the public but has lost that skill recurs frequently in contemporary discussions of the field's precarious state. Since the disappointing aftermath of the September 11 terrorist attacks, which many hoped in vain would bring new resources to public health, the profession's sense of being misunderstood and unappreciated has only intensified. At a time when the insights of population-based sciences seem desperately needed to combat unprecedented challenges to the nation's health, from global warming and germ warfare to avian flu and obesity, that the public seems so little to value these insights is perplexing.

To explain this puzzling state of affairs, public health commentators often invoke a deep-seated conflict between popular and professional values. As Lawrence Wallack and Regina Lawrence mused in a 2005 commentary in the *American Journal of Public Health*, American culture has traditionally been dominated by a language of "individualism," centered on values of "freedom, self-determination, self-discipline, personal responsibility, and limited government." In contrast, public health professionals have traditionally spoken America's "second language," a language "rooted in egalitarianism, humanitarianism, and human interconnection," which has rendered its message "alien" to the general public, journalists, politicians, and policy makers (567, 568). Yet such an overly simplistic opposition of an "individualistic" public to a "humanitarian" profession obscures a much more complex—and interesting—history of public health's efforts to speak for the public. By surveying that complex history, this chapter seeks to contribute to the ongoing efforts to rethink public health's leadership role in the twenty-first century.

Over the past seventy-five years, as I will suggest, public health has been torn between two conceptions of its mission to speak for the public: one, a top-down, paternalistic model, influenced by laboratory ideals of scientific method and objectivity, and deliberately insulated from public irrationality and fickleness; the other, a bottom-up, populist model, grounded in social scientific methods, and engaged more directly with the people themselves. Debates over the relative value of these two models have played out against the backdrop of major changes in the nature of mass politics and the democratization of expertise.

While public health professionals in other developed nations have faced these same changes, they have presented a special challenge in the United States because the mission of public health has been defined (or perhaps "deformed" is a better word) by its embeddedness in a market-oriented, privatized health system. This system reflects the core assumptions that private enterprise is preferable to public initiative, that private rights are more important than public goods, that market thinking is the surest route to progress, and that individuals must be held accountable for their health problems (Morone and Jacobs 2005). Simply put, the scope of public health in the United States has traditionally been defined as "whatever the market won't do," as the 1988 IOM report noted (75). What seems diagnosable or fixable has become the domain of medical providers, professionals who bill by the hour or procedure; what is left over—medicine's "market failures," to use the economists' term—has been the domain of public health (Milio 2000).

This system has traditionally worked to strengthen the medical profession's warrant to speak for the patient, as opposed to public health's warrant to speak for the public. But to the extent that the private practice of medicine has repeatedly failed to meet the health needs of all Americans, its so-called market failures have formed a persistent source of discontent, among both health care professionals and the larger public. From the 1920s onward, the field of public health has sheltered, and even nurtured, critics of the existing health care system determined to press for a broader, more social definition of health. Thus public health's mission to speak for the public has inevitably become tangled up in the dangerous, complicated politics of critiquing the dysfunctional traits of the American health care system, in particular the limitations of private medicine in a market-dominated culture (Burris 1997; Brandt and Gardner 2000).

This historical account traces the ways that public health's ambivalent relationship to "the people," both real and imagined, has contributed to its current identity crisis. Speaking for the public in a privatized, market-oriented culture has required the profession to bite the hand that feeds it: to point out the defects of business as usual, while being dependent on that business for funding and authority. Yet public health's association with private medicine's market failures has resulted in opportunity as well as obstacles. It has galvanized the field to listen carefully to citizens' concerns and to forge creative alliances with reformers of many different stripes. By examining the history of these dynamics, I hope to help foster a more public-centered public health care system in the twenty-first century.[1]

The Patient/Public in a Mass Society

Questions about how public health professionals best represent the American people's health needs evolved against the backdrop of a much larger set of debates about the fate of democracy in a technocratic mass society, debates that started in the 1920s in the wake of widespread disappointment and cynicism about the outcome of World War I and have continued to this day. As political scientists have long noted, these debates grew out of the gradual transformation of nineteenth-century democracies, reliant upon certain kinds of political influence, including face-to-face negotiations, party congresses, public oratory, and the occasional election and parade, into twentieth-century democracies—large, diverse, complex, marked by declining voter turnout, and most of all, intensely mediated, that is, dominated by modern forms of mass media. Indirect forms of influence supplanted direct forms of contact between the leaders and the led; political and business elites began to use social surveys, opinion polls, and other kinds of quantitative data to discern the voice of the people. In order to claim legitimacy, as well as to get elected, politicians and parties had to learn to read the ever-changing currents of public opinion correctly, and to respond to them effectively.[2]

These same currents of change informed the politics of health care in the early twentieth century. As private and public investments in health care increased and experts on health issues proliferated, competition to speak on the public's behalf increased. In this new political climate, the professions of medicine and public health both asserted their warrants to speak authoritatively about issues of national health. Their "uneasy marriage," as Fee has described it, resulted in competing claims to be the better guardian of their "offspring," that is, the collective needs of the American people (Fee 1987, 2).

In many ways, the early twentieth-century medical profession entered the competition to articulate collective health needs with a tremendous set of advantages. Physicians' intimate relationships with their individual patients gave them enormous authority to speak on behalf of "the patient" more generally. The successful professionalization of American medicine at the turn of the last century reinforced the premise that physicians, and only physicians, had the requisite knowledge and experience to decide what was best not only for individual patients, but also for the collective benefit of patients as a group (Ludmerer 1985).

From the late 1880s onward, regular medicine's professional organizations— the local, state, and national medical societies—wielded this authority in increasingly effective ways. Using the traditional tools of political influence, such as giving speeches, writing letters, buttonholing elected officials, and getting their views into print, representatives of the regular medical profession confidently positioned themselves as the first resort when it came to questions on the patient's behalf. As Joseph N. McCormack, the mastermind behind the revitalization of the American Medical Association, wrote in 1906: "It has been found easy to demonstrate to any intelligent layman that his physician, and the profession as a whole, . . . [have] no interest which he does not share and that the daily safety and well-being of his family . . . [are] inseparable from the continued prosperity and competency of his physician and of the profession of his county, State and country as a whole" (quoted in Burrow 1977, 23).

In comparison, public health's relationship to its client base was considerably more attenuated. From its mid-nineteenth-century beginnings onward, public health leaders expressed considerable ambivalence about its popular support. The public was often lambasted as a source of political corruption and scientific irrationality. Yet public health reformers depended upon the "intelligent citizenry," that is, educated middle-class urbanites such as themselves, in order to get anything done. Without the support of middle-class citizens' groups, including women's clubs, local sanitary associations, social welfare organizations, and the like, the public health movement would have made few gains during the Progressive Era. Yet as Fee has noted, the institutionalization of public health followed "an elite vision of social reform" in which scientific experts directed change from above, rather than seeking to build alliances from below (Fee 1987, 4).

This vision reflected the close association between public health authority and the rise of an activist state. Public health powers increased dramatically in the early 1900s as a consequence of government's expanding police powers rather than as the reflection of a deepening expert-client bond. Progressive Era leaders made a persuasive argument that the laboratory-based science of bacteriology allowed them to see dangers that threatened the whole community. That far-seeing scientific authority would prove effective only if it was insulated from crass political influence. Hence the public health department was ideally set up as a civil service bastion, safe from partisan influence, a place where experts would tend to the structural determinants of health without public interference (Rosenkrantz 1972). It was a difficult position to maintain, in that looking out for the public's health involved forms of service and surveillance that were little relished or appreciated by the people themselves. Their displeasure against public health departments took many forms, from ignoring regulations to rioting against them, and even hiring lawyers to contest them (Leavitt 1982, 1997; Markel 2004).

Thus the turn-of-the-century division of labor between private medicine (individual, personal) and state medicine (collective, impersonal) gave the former a decided edge in cultivating popular support. While many Americans had a jaundiced view of organized medicine, they retained a high regard for their personal physicians (Tomes 2006b). In contrast, relatively few Americans had a personal relationship with a public health professional; those that did have such a relationship often wished they did not. As Frank Overton and Willard Denno explained in their 1920 text *The Health Officer*, doctors shirked public health work because "many persons resent interference with their personal liberties," and thus "public health workers make enemies" (50).

Yet paradoxically, the impersonal data gathering and analysis cultivated by public health experts eventually gave them a more benign way to represent the public. By developing new methods of describing and quantifying information about large populations, particularly in the fields of epidemiology and the medical social sciences, they fashioned alternate ways to represent public needs. Starting in the 1910s, vital statistics and epidemiology offered increasingly sophisticated assays of the nation's health status. The elaboration of the social science survey produced more systematic data about collective health beliefs and behaviors (Converse 1987; Winslow et al. 1952; Bloom 2002; Igo 2007). Precisely because epidemiological and sociological surveys scientifically sampled large, diverse groups of Americans, they could legitimately claim to portray a more inclusive public than just those patients under a doctor's care. Equally important, they gave public health practitioners a platform, separate from their work as state-sponsored medical police, from which to advocate for the public, as well as for their own field.

These population-based sciences were pioneered not in schools of medicine, but in departments of public health, insurance companies, universities, and nongovernmental health organizations. It was the recognition that the public health sciences required a different skill set that prompted the Rockefeller Foundation in 1916 to support the separation of schools of public health from medical schools, the "great schism" later decried by Kerr White and others. As Fee has noted, the Hopkins model eventually promoted by the foundation was the narrowest of the alternatives proposed in the 1910s. But conceptions of public health with a wider social scientific sweep flourished at other schools of public health, most notably Columbia and Yale (Fee 1987). In the context of interwar concerns about representational democracy and mass politics, the idea of creating a range of public health sciences, based on taking ever larger and more representative samples of the people's experience, appealed to many public health leaders.[3]

In Search of the People's Health: The Interwar Period

In the 1920s, as the larger debates about the problems of "mass man" and "mass culture" raged, this new conception of reading the public proved very appealing to many in the public health movement. The field's leaders eagerly asserted their own superior brand of knowledge about the public, or what interwar writings variously termed "the masses," "John Q. Public," and "the demos." Public health seemed ideally suited to produce the master planners and coordinators of health services in general. Perhaps inevitably, the new population-based approaches led some public health experts to become more critical of deficiencies in the private practice of medicine. And unlike previous critics of regular medicine, such as the medical sectarians aligned with homeopathy, osteopathy, and chiropractic, these experts spoke the language of social scientific research and claimed to have unimpeachable, objective data about the population as a whole.

Of course, this critical disposition was by no means universal; many in public health preferred to downplay their differences with the medical profession, emphasizing instead a common devotion to the scientific understanding of disease (Brandt and Gardner 2000). Yet others relished a more critical role, particularly in relation to the organization and financing of medical care; they argued that public health professionals had a special responsibility to speak for the public on these issues, as a corrective to the deficiencies of organized medicine's positions. As they emphasized, the doctor in private practice knew nothing of epidemiology or the new social sciences of economics and sociology. Medical training, while valuable in the care of individual cases of disease, did not prepare physicians to discern the broader health needs of the public. Only the interdisciplinary perspectives of public health, they suggested, allowed for an accurate reading of the nation's health needs.

This kind of argument was evident in the interwar public health movement's embrace of a risky new mission for the field, namely, critiquing the organization of personal health services. A new boldness in speaking for the public on matters of health care reform is well illustrated in the career of Harry Hascall Moore. While working for the U.S. Public Health Service, Moore earned a Ph.D. in economics from the Brookings Institute in 1926.[4] A year later, in 1927, he published *American Medicine and the People's Health,* modestly described on its title page as "an outline with statistical data on the organization of medicine in the United States with special reference to the adjustment of medical service to social and economic change." The book's frontispiece not so modestly struck a bolder note by picturing the "modern successors of the medicine man": a gallery of figures including the practicing physician, the physician in public health administration, the research physician, the epidemiologist, the sanitary engineer, the statistician, the nurse, and the dentist (see figure 3.1). While all had their contributions to make, Moore's book left no doubt that the public health expert was first among equals on this interdisciplinary team, due to his unique combination of social scientific and medical knowledge.

Significantly, Moore linked the rise of public health's authority to the growth of a more discerning public. In his preface, he suggested that the nation's rising educational attainments were inevitably going to require changes in the health care system: "The acquisition of scientific knowledge by the people has resulted in a demand that such knowledge be more effectively applied by society in both the prevention and cure of disease." Meanwhile, "the rapid development of science has resulted in an increasing participation in public health work of scientifically trained persons who are less interested in maintaining the old relationships between physician and patient than they are in preventing and curing disease in the most socially effective manner and in bringing health and prolonged life to all the people" (Moore 1927, v). Public health scientists had a critical role to play as advocates for this rising generation of educated citizens. As

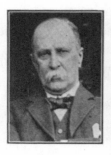

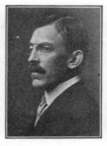

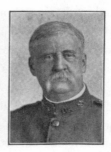

THE PRACTICING
PHYSICIAN

Willam Osler

THE PHYSICIAN IN
PUBLIC HEALTH
ADMINISTRATION

Hermann M. Biggs

THE RESEARCH
PHYSICIAN

Henry R. Carter

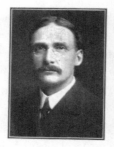

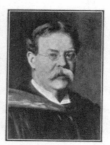

THE CHEMIST

Christian A. Herter

THE EPIDEMIOLOGIST

William P. Sedgwick

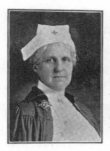

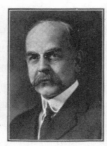

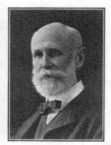

THE NURSE

Jane A. Delano

THE SANITARY ENGINEER
AND VITAL STATISTICIAN

George C. Whipple

THE DENTIST

G. V. Black

Figure 3.1 The frontispiece of Harry Moore's 1927 book *American Medicine and the People's Health* featured a diverse gallery of figures who were "modern successors of the medicine man."

the introduction, written by the Committee of Five, a group of fellow reformers, noted: "Mr. Moore is not himself a physician, but this circumstance may perhaps be considered as favorable rather than unfavorable to the task that he has undertaken. After all, it is the members of the public who purchase medical service, and Mr. Moore, as an economist, represents the fundamental interest of the public in securing the best possible medical service at the lowest possible cost" (xxi).

American Medicine and the People's Health represented only the first shot in a volley of studies and reports that would deeply involve public health leaders in the interwar critique of medicine. Moore went on to become director of the Committee on the Costs of Medical Care, which conducted the first substantive surveys of American medical practice. Moore and his associates at the CCMC published almost thirty reports between 1928 and 1933, compiling masses of data into charts and graphs. The CCMC's findings, distilled in the final report published in 1933, suggested delicately but clearly that the medical profession was not meeting its social obligations to the American people: Many areas of the country had too few doctors and hospitals, the rising cost of more technologically sophisticated medicine was proving hard for even middle-class families to bear, and the medical profession was not responding to these problems effectively, largely because of its inflexible commitment to fee-for-service practice (Falk, Rorem, and Ring 1933).

Not surprisingly, that account was immediately and vigorously disputed by the leadership of the American Medical Association, in particular Morris Fishbein, the influential editor of its journal, *JAMA*. No matter how much objective data the CCMC compiled, medical defenders responded that the evidence was biased and incomplete. Fishbein used the AMA's editorial pages to run an aggressive campaign against the CCMC and any other group that dared to suggest that all was not well with traditional fee-for-service medicine. In a famous 1933 editorial published in *JAMA*, Fishbein suggested that the CCMC's proposals constituted the first step toward "medical soviets" and that the group was "inciting" a revolution bound to end in socialism or communism.[5]

Given that many of the most visible and enthusiastic proponents of health care reform were affiliated with public health, the critique of private medicine inevitably became associated with that field. In a 1934 letter to then secretary of labor Frances Perkins, the distinguished neurosurgeon Harvey Cushing made this association explicit: "Most of the agitation regarding the high cost of medical care has been voiced by public health officials and members of foundations most of whom do not have a medical degree, much less any actual first-hand experience with what the practice of medicine and the relation of doctor to patient means" (quoted in Fishbein 1969, 199).

The AMA's vigorous attack on the CCMC was sufficient to convince the newly elected Franklin D. Roosevelt that reforming private medical care should have no place in his New Deal social programs. But although its reform initiative failed, the work of the CCMC permanently altered the terms of the debate over medical care by showcasing a new kind of policy expertise. As the physician iconoclast Hugh Cabot observed in his 1935 book *The Doctor's Bill*, the debates over medicine were no longer a "private battle" among physicians, but now involved "the economist, the statistician, [and] the social scientist," and the "reverberations of their discussions have reached to the thinking public and will shortly reach to the Halls of Congress" (vii–viii). As debates concerning national health insurance continued in the late 1930s and 1940s, public health professionals continued to play a major role in them.

The New Deal concept of the "broker state" proved hospitable to their contributions, in that it envisioned an expanded role for the "citizen consumer," along with labor and business representatives, in fashioning social policy (Cohen 1998; 2003, 28–31). As Moore had suggested earlier, social scientific experts with public health backgrounds were ideal proxies for an "enlightened public." They could reasonably assert that their superior social scientific vision allowed them to see what the public needed more clearly than did organized medicine, especially when it came to the economic side of health care. As self-appointed guardians of the people's health, public health professionals participated in a variety of health-related work sponsored by the expanding New Deal state, including the rural health programs initiated by the Farm Security Administration (Grey 1999). Similarly, they sought to represent the voice of the consumer in the long campaign to expand the regulatory power of the Food and Drug Administration, a battle that culminated in the 1938 Food, Drug, and Cosmetic Act, one of the most significant pieces of New Deal health legislation (Jackson 1970).

Yet while public health experts confidently claimed to know what the intelligent public wanted better than did organized medicine, the profession's day-to-day relations with "the people" continued to be conflict laden. The core of public health work remained in the local and state health departments, which operated according to a hierarchical power structure far more rigid than that existing between individual doctors and patients. While laypeople who disliked organized medicine still tended to have affection and respect for their own physicians, public health workers had no such well of personal affection to draw upon. The ordinary citizens expressing a fond gratitude to their local public health department for its services were few and far between.[6]

The public relations challenge faced by interwar public health departments was poignantly captured in a series of radio shows that the head of the public health department in Racine, Wisconsin, W. W. Bauer, developed in the early to mid-1930s. Modeled on a soap opera format, the shows were designed to help listeners appreciate the work of the public health department. While the story lines featured some grateful representatives of John Q. Public, far more common were portraits of difficult, unreasonable laypeople who required extensive reeducation to develop a proper appreciation of public health work.[7]

For example, in an episode aired June 10, 1931, a mother indignant that her sick child has been sent home from school threatened to call the mayor and the state board of health, saying, "I have never in my life been so insulted." Even after the public health nurse patiently explained the reasons for the quarantine, the mother grumbled, "I'm not convinced, but I suppose I'm helpless, if you have the law on your side." (She did come around, grudgingly, at the end.) "Not many mothers greet the nurses with such a torrent of unfriendly criticism," the commentator concluded, and once they understand what the nurse is trying to do, "they are likely to be friendly and cooperative." Yet few episodes featured the friendly and cooperative; the grumblers had a clear majority, expressing views obviously drawn from life, such as the mother who complained that "no one has any right" to take her child's temperature without her permission, or the one who responded to a nurse's visit, "We have always preferred to handle our own affairs ourselves." The very fact that the radio scripts worked so earnestly to justify the health department's "interference" suggests the entrenched resentment that the medical police continued to engender.

To some extent, public health leaders compensated for their often hostile client base by forging alliances with what today are called "nongovernmental organizations." Public health professionals joined, and often led, the many coalitions of academics, social workers, journalists, union leaders, and other lay groups advocating for various health measures. They developed strong ties with the voluntary health associations, such as the Child Health Association, the National Tuberculosis Association, the American Cancer Society, and the National Foundation for Infantile Paralysis. On the whole, the public health profession had far denser, more positive ties with the many voluntary health associations than did their medical counterparts (Carter 1992).

Yet these connections were little match for the increasing effort and money invested in the public relations campaigns of the American Medical Association and its state affiliates in the 1940s and 1950s. Motivated by survey evidence that suggested widespread public dissatisfaction with organized medicine, the AMA introduced a variety of measures to repair the image of private medicine. Among the best known was the public relations campaign developed by the Whitaker Baxter agency to derail efforts to pass a national health insurance program.

Bankrolled by an unprecedented public relations tax on physician member-
ship, this aggressive counterpoint to the attack on private medicine seemed, at
least in the short run, to be spectacularly successful. As a more conservative
political climate followed the turbulent years of the New Deal, the medical profession's bid to speak for the patient appeared far sturdier than public health's
bid to speak for the public (Tomes 2006b).

Postwar Public Health Statesmanship and the Push from Below

Interwar public health's uneasy conception of its popular mission, which combined lofty rhetoric about representing the thinking public with an uneasy
awareness of the unpopular functions of medical policing, persisted in the
post–World War II period. Starting in the 1940s, a massive expansion of public
and private investment in biomedical research, hospital infrastructure, and
private workplace–based medical insurance rapidly increased the disparity in
resources between medicine and public health. In retrospect, the direction of
post-1940 policy choices seems to represent a decisive triumph for the biomedical model of disease: Taxpayer dollars were invested in basic science, hospital construction, and aggressive cure over prevention, while an expanding
system of voluntary insurance subsidized the private practice of medicine (Starr
1982). Yet despite these trends, public health leaders in the 1950s were no less
confident of their discipline's centrality to the making of postwar health care
policy. Indeed, America's ascent to Cold War leadership and growing involvement in international health issues lent an even more grandiose cast to their
rhetoric. American public health experts now asserted their abilities to discern
not only what the American people required, but what the rest of the world
needed as well.

This postwar vision of public health statesmanship was beautifully illustrated in a 1952 lecture by then surgeon general Leonard A. Scheele, delivered
at Yale University as the first in a series to honor Charles-Edward Amory
Winslow. "History shows that great economic and social forces flow like a tide
over communities only half conscious of that which is befalling them," Scheele
began. "Wise statesmen"—by implication, people like himself—"foresee what
time is bringing and try to shape institutions and mold men's thoughts and purposes in accordance with the change that is silently coming." In public health,
"the same bits and pieces of modern society present themselves to us in an endless variety of patterns and problems"; like a kaleidoscope, public health's mission was to pull those bits and pieces into focus. At a time of unprecedented
growth in scientific knowledge and technological capacities, the integrative perspectives of public health were all the more critical. In terms strikingly similar

to those in the 1988 IOM report, Scheele noted that "public health progress depends more upon the quality of our statesmanship than upon the specificity of our techniques" (3).

Buried within the surgeon general's explication of public health statesmanship was an interesting commentary on the field's relationship to the public. Whereas the interwar generation represented by Harry Moore had seen public health experts as proxies for enlightened public opinion, Scheele acknowledged a different scenario, in which representatives of the public forced public health experts to take a particular issue more seriously. As a case in point, he mentioned growing public concerns about harmful chemicals in the environment. In the Progressive Era, citizens' groups had been the ones who pressured public health departments to look into the dangers of air pollution. Likewise, he noted: "In 1949, it was a local labor union that requested the Public Health Service to make a thorough study of the 'smog' in Donora, Pennsylvania." Scheele warned: "If public health workers do not see beyond the performance of their prescribed routines; if they do not recognize the health implications of the new environment nor bestir themselves to interpret the problems to society, then we can say that their statesmanship in environmental health does not measure up" (8).[8]

As Scheele's remarks suggest, no matter how top-down its conception of expertise, the field of public health retained a special obligation to heed popular health discontents. Like the proverbial canary in the mines, concerned citizens might spot health harms before they registered at a more general level of scientific and statistical certainty. To be sure, this mechanism of bottom-up influence had no institutionalized place in public health; in the 1950s and 1960s, public health departments remained embedded in an institutional milieu that reinforced a very narrow conception of their mission. So long as the core of public health work remained its state medicine functions, supported by tax dollars and dependent on the support of elected officials, any moves to take that work in controversial directions were liable to be met with resistance not only from business and industry groups, but also from other branches of the government. Industrial hygiene was a case in point: The relationships among public health researchers, government agencies, employers, and labor unions were a study in resistance and complexity (see, for example, Markowitz and Rosner 2002; Sellers 1997).

But starting in the 1950s, a more rambunctious kind of lay health activism began to challenge this inertia. Even before the well-publicized eruption of health activism in the late 1960s, public health professionals sensed rumblings of popular discontent with medicine. In their 1965 textbook *Preventive Medicine*, Herman Hilleboe and Granville Larimore noted that health professionals had to contend with a more educated, prevention-minded public: "This generation has seen the emergence of a lay public that is well aware of the wonders modern medical science offers. Mass communications have created, as never before, an urgent and persisting demand by patients for a brand of medical care that promises continued health" (3).

Similarly, in an influential 1963 article on the idea of community medicine, William H. Stewart stressed the push from below as a motivation for rethinking the boundaries between medicine and public health. "More than once in the past," he wrote, "public health has been saved as a social institution because some of its leaders were willing to respond affirmatively to long-neglected demands from the people" (97). By combining "the methodologies of the social sciences, epidemiology, behavioral science, and perhaps other methods not yet devised," he proclaimed, "we physicians who are engaged in preventive medicine careers today can be crusaders for community medicine, as our professional ancestors were crusaders for sanitary reform and care of the sick. To do so we must recapture their eagerness to innovate, to create and test new ideas for service to our communities 'in sickness and in health'" (99).[9]

The "Hidden Enemies of Health":
Public Health in the 1960s and 1970s

With the advent of the various rights revolutions of the late 1960s and 1970s, lay activists became increasingly radical in their questioning of authority, including deference to scientific experts. In general, respect for authority declined precipitously starting in the 1960s, and the resulting democratization of expertise inspired a particularly fierce attack on medical authority. These attacks came from many quarters, including popular movements for women's rights, disability rights, gay rights, welfare rights, and environmental protection. Most activists involved in these causes were openly suspicious of the scientific authority claimed by public health, as well as by medicine.[10] In the wake of highly publicized revelations about the role of the U.S. Public Health Service with the Tuskegee syphilis experiment, governmental health agencies aroused new and intense suspicion (Reverby 2000). Yet compared to the wrath directed at the medical profession, and in particular organized medicine, public health had more potential to redeem itself in the eyes of its advocates. As young activists themselves began to enter the medical and public health professions, they proved more than willing to explore the redemptive qualities of public health analysis (Rogers 2001).

By the early 1970s, it seemed as if public health was poised for a dramatic reversal of fortunes and might at long last reemerge as the authentic champion of the people's health. Many public health workers looked to alliances with groups of angry patient/consumers as a way to leverage their own influence within the health care system. While the medical profession remained at best wary and at worst contemptuous of the new health activism, public health leaders quickly moved the category of health consumers to the center of the field's vision, as evident in the cover illustration for the 1969 American Public Health Association meeting (see figure 3.2).

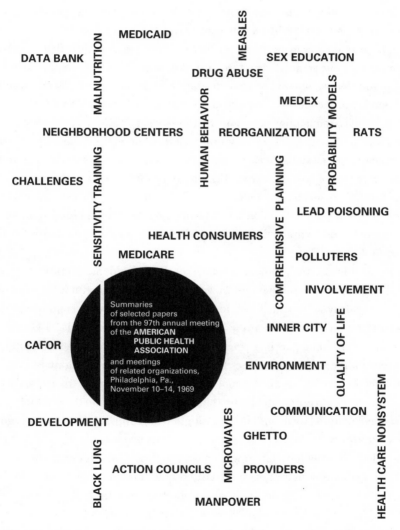

Figure 3.2 The cover illustration of the program for the American Public Health Association's 1969 annual meeting reflected the growing importance of the category "health consumer."

This new populist tone of public health was evident in Paul Cornely's fiery presidential address to the APHA in 1971. The first African American to receive a doctorate in public health, and a longtime professor of community health at Howard University, Cornely titled his lecture "The Hidden Enemies of Health and the American Public Health Association." He began by wondering why a nation that prided itself on "efficiency, managerial expertise, organizational abilities, and mass production" had produced a health care system noted for its inefficiency and inequity. It was not, he pointed out, for lack of concrete plans to correct those deficiencies; dating back to the 1930s, public health workers had been suggesting ways to correct them. "Why have we not moved?" Cornely asked (7, 8).

The answer, he suggested, lay in "hidden enemies of health" that "permeate the matrix of our societal structure and, therefore, are all too often extremely subtle and deeply imbedded so as to defy easy recognition." The core of the problem lay in the nature of American life itself. Since World War II, the expansion of a mass consumer economy had created a "national addiction to the abundant life," which was deeply implicated in the nation's health problems. "The health professional was no exception," Cornely observed, for "like the others, he wants a greater share of the abundant life," from a high return on his stock portfolio to an energy-dependent lifestyle complete with a suburban home, air conditioning, and television set. "Like the Pharisees, he is eloquent in telling others what to do" while pursuing this addiction to consumer comforts, Cornely noted (8, 9).

From this central problem flowed the other "hidden enemies" of public health. Powerful economic interests were invested in the maintenance not only of an unhealthy American lifestyle, but also of a medical system oriented to repairing rather than preventing its physical consequences. Health care, he warned, had become part of a "mega economy" dominated by a small group of large corporations who exercised their considerable clout to maintain not only a military-industrial but also a "medical-industrial" complex. In a "perversion of democracy," governmental bodies charged with protecting the public interest had been corrupted by economic special interest groups. Health care was going the same direction as the rest of the American economy, and thus, Cornely concluded: "It is not too soon to warn health professionals and recipients of care that the medical-industrial octopus will become influential in policy and decision making in the health field." Finally, Cornely located the pathogenic qualities of American culture in mass media and advertising, or what he described as the "pollution of the mind" by television and radio. Funds devoted to prevention, he noted, paled in comparison to the immense advertising budgets devoted to convincing the American people to eat unhealthy food, smoke cigarettes, and indulge in other health risks. He also pointed to the racial discrimination and segregation that accompanied the post–World War II economic boom as the root cause of the urban crisis threatening to tear apart American cities (9, 10).

Having identified these "hidden enemies," Cornely went on to describe the needed solutions: replacing the national addiction to prosperity with a new sense of social responsibility, and replacing special interest influence with community participation and control. The time had come, he argued, to go beyond reliance on indirect political action: For too long, "professional health and welfare agencies of this country have been content . . . to develop standards, to prepare position papers, to hold forums, to plan resolutions, and to write letters to the legislative and executive branches of government." But these kinds of activities no longer sufficed. Significantly, in urging the public health field to become more advocacy oriented, Cornely suggested that his colleagues consider emulating the American Medical Association. "Ever since the Whitaker and Baxter era, that association has used the political process to achieve its ends which quite often have not been in the best interest of the American public." It was time, he concluded, for public health organizations to use similar techniques to connect with the communities they served, so as to force health care policy in a more progressive direction (13, 14).

Thus the late 1960s and early 1970s ushered in a very different era in the public health field's relations with the public. With a host of advocacy groups arguing for radical change, public health seemed well positioned to voice the needs of ordinary people left unmet by the "American health empire" described in a 1970 book by John and Barbara Ehrenreich. The public health profession embraced the cause of the empowered patient/health consumer in many different ways. For example, the APHA voted in 1970 for a new set of bylaws designed "to move this organization into the arena of advocacy for the consumer," as Cornely noted approvingly in his 1971 speech (16). The association also supported the work of the Citizen's Board of Inquiry into Health Services for Americans, which culminated in the 1972 report *Heal Your Self*, an anecdote- and data-laden account of the frustrated "voice of the consumer." In place of the more abstract conception of the public, public health advocates now focused more specifically on the community as the power base for reform. That trend was reflected not only in the new community medicine departments being set up in many medical schools, but also in the proliferation of community health centers being founded in poor urban neighborhoods.

As in the interwar period, public health activism in the 1970s influenced the research agenda, as a new generation of epidemiologists and social scientists sought to document the health needs of groups long neglected or mistreated by private medicine, such as women, industrial workers, the poor, and racial minorities. As is evident in the pages of the *American Journal of Public Health* (*AJPH*) and other professional journals, the 1970s saw an avalanche of studies seeking to support public health measures, from antismoking labels and group health clinics to environmental health protection and feminist health reform. Simply by applying the standard tools of scientific research to groups likely to be poorly served by the "medical-industrial complex," such as Medicaid patients and poor pregnant women, they pursued subversive agendas, for example, to provide hard evidence that the penny for prevention was more cost effective than the pound for cure, and to show that health care delivered in ways other than traditional fee-for-service medicine was as good as if not better than private medicine.[11]

In a more direct break with the past, public health activists championed the cause of citizen/consumer involvement in health policy planning and implementation. Instead of studying and representing the needs of the masses, this approach required letting consumers speak directly for themselves. The concept of consumer representation first implemented in the New Deal broker state took on new life as the Great Society programs attempted to use federal funding and regulation as tools for change. Starting in the 1960s, federal laws began to require citizen representation on review boards and planning commissions as a means to check the power of special interest groups, especially as federal spending on health increased dramatically. Citizen involvement was a cornerstone of the National Health Planning and Resources Development Act as passed in 1974 and revised in 1979. Bringing consumer representatives into policy planning and implementation offered public health specialists a seemingly golden opportunity to build alliances with community groups, patient activists, and others dissatisfied with the existing health care system (Checkoway 1981).

The public health generation of the 1970s hoped that by restoring power to the people, change would bubble up from below; an army of motivated citizen/patients would discipline the medical industrial complex, and in the process, public health would enjoy new prestige and authority. Yet they realized that harnessing this power required a profound reorientation of public health leadership. In his 1969 APHA presidential address, Lester Breslow acknowledged that the public health professional's "world is being shaken." The "inner-directed health agency, where the consumer had little voice, is threatened by the community forces recently set in motion." In this new era of consumer empowerment, public health experts could no longer expect to be deferred to by virtue of their technical competence. Again invoking the golden age of public health, he concluded optimistically: "Exciting days lie ahead—in recapturing the spirit of the founders of public health, in the rejoining of technical endeavor with social action" (16).

Yet it was quickly evident that citizen groups were no match for the institutional forces arrayed against them. As a 1981 study of citizen participation in health planning concluded, simply including consumers on planning boards did not result in noticeable improvements in planning rationality or in lower health care costs. A defect in the 1974 law required planning boards to have a majority of consumer representatives but did not specify how they should be chosen, a problem that led immediately to lawsuits. But even more important, contributors to the volume concluded, was the overall imbalance in power. Consumer boards tended to end up serving as rubber stamps for better-organized interest groups, particularly those dominated by physicians. When they did try to act more assertively, consumers ran into enormous resistance, also from physician-dominated groups. As Barry Checkoway summed up the problems in his article "The Empire Strikes Back" (a reference to the Ehrenreichs' 1970 title, *The American Health Empire*): "Health planning operates in an imbalanced political arena." As he observed: "We formed an organization as a way to overcome the customary pattern of provider dominance and consumer subservience. In time, however, providers—who have the advantages of disproportionate resources, unequal interest, and ongoing organizations—became aroused; they united to defeat the common consumer threat and to capture the local health planning board" (xx). Under these circumstances, the move to centralized planning gave consumers the worst of both worlds, in that it enhanced the power of the better-organized and better-financed interest groups while providing a fig leaf of democratic participation.

Proponents of citizen/consumer representation hastened to emphasize that the experience had not been a complete loss: They had learned valuable political lessons by participating in planning boards (see, for example, Sparer, Dines, and Smith 1970). The experience helped them identify areas where they could more effectively make a difference, for example, by lodging complaints about the restricted access of low-income citizens to the local hospital, creating a community health hotline for complaints about local doctors and hospitals, and setting up a women's self-help group. But the overall lesson was not an uplifting one. Even before Ronald Reagan won election in 1980, bringing a new era into being, the limits of the 1970s approach to community organizing had already started to become evident (Checkoway 1981).

Not the least of the problems involved in the community action model of public health was the landscape of racial, ethnic, and class divisions in which it operated. Public health professionals in the 1970s soon found that their attempts to coordinate community health issues met with stiff resistance from community members themselves. In these encounters, the gulf between public health science and community opinion loomed large. That sense of division was evident in a 1979 *AJPH* article titled "How to Keep Your Mandated Citizen Board out of Your Hair and off Your Back," which offered tongue-in-cheek advice about how to "contain and render ineffective" their citizen boards. "It requires great understanding and patience for the human service professional to continue to provide impartial scientific guidance to community programs in these days of conflict and chaos," the authors, Allen Steckler and William Herzog, noted. Describing mandated citizen boards as "the latest in a series of fads," they argued that citizen participation "poses a serious threat to efficient and professional operations" (809). The article provided many practical tips—holding meetings during the workday to "limit attendance of blue collar workers or women with small children," setting up meaningless committees, and using "technical terminology and jargon, especially bureaucratic alphabet soup (HMO, PSRO, CHP, HEW, etc.) to keep the consumers confused and quiet" (811).

In the turbulent decades of the 1960s and 1970s, many public health professionals tried to broaden the field's angle of vision and to embrace a more expansive notion of the public. Responding to the challenges posed by the civil rights movement, second-wave feminism, and the environmental movement, they gladly took on the responsibility for exposing the "hidden enemies of health" and advocating on behalf of those underserved by the new "medical-industrial complex." But these reform initiatives met stiff resistance. No matter how statistically significant their findings, public health reformers faced better-organized and better-funded interest groups that advanced opposing agendas. In addition, they often encountered suspicion from the very groups they wanted better to represent, that is, neighborhood activists who wanted to speak for themselves rather than have public health professionals do it for them. Thus, once the federal funding for Office of Economic Opportunity programs, community health centers, and other 1970s innovations dried up, their potential as laboratories for change weakened as well.

A Difficult Challenge: Public Health and
the "Marketization" of Health Care

In the wake of the 1980 Reagan revolution, a more conservative conception of health promotion came to the fore. Rather than acting collectively in political or policy domains, enlightened consumers were to make their wishes known by the exercise of individual choice: to discipline the marketplace by choosing to enroll in an HMO or to abstain from risky behaviors such as smoking or unprotected sex. Of course, the more expansive conception of public health advocacy by no means disappeared; public health workers continued to try to work out creative alliances with activists, as in the AIDS epidemic, and aligned with state governments concerned about health care costs to broker the tobacco settlement. Yet the strategies that succeeded tended to be those most compatible with the theme of individual responsibility. Public health professionals continued to be hammered by the activists on the Left and the Right for their role in creating what Charles Edgley and Dennis Brissett described as a "nation of meddlers." As the IOM report ruefully observed in 1988: "People tend to be positive about public health values, but negative about the present public health agency" (41).

As this chapter suggests, the image problems identified in the 1988 IOM report are but the latest installment in a series of long-running debates about how the profession of public health should represent the people. From the late nineteenth century to the present, these debates have reflected a deep sense of ambivalence about public health's popular constituency, played out against the backdrop of a new era of mass politics and democratization of expertise. Unresolved tensions between public as enemy and public as ally have been reflected in the two very different tacks that public health professionals have pursued in search of the authentic health needs of the nation: first, the refinement of population-based sciences capable of providing objective, collective, data-driven measures of the public's health status, and second, the articulation and organization of popular discontent with health care institutions in order to foment basic change. These competing formulations of public as enemy versus ally, and of population science versus political advocacy, have persisted from the paternalistic era of the Progressive period through the post-1970 explosion of consumer health movements.

Speaking for the public has often resulted in public health critiques of a health care system dominated by a preference for market mechanisms and private medicine. While many in public health have preferred to avoid this critical tendency, a visible and vocal group repeatedly took an alternate course, pointing out the defects of health business as usual, whether in political or economic terms. Small wonder, then, that the field of public health has led an increasingly precarious existence since the 1930s, hostage to the ups and downs of the activist state. Dependent on the funding mechanisms and regulatory scope associated with big government, locked in an ambivalent relationship with the medical profession, vulnerable to red-baiting and taxpayers' revolts, and with an unstable client base to depend on, the strategy of simply accumulating data and writing reports has proven the safest route to follow. Forays into social action have often been unsuccessful and exposed public health to the wrath of political conservatives. While these problems certainly intensified with the Reagan revolution, they clearly existed well before 1980.

Nancy Milio suggests in her 2000 book, *Public Health in the Market*, that in the face of "managed care, lean markets, and health disparities," the "marketization" of health care has left the public health community an unenviable set of choices: Adopt the values of the market and try to identify "marketable packages of personal and environmental services" that public health professionals can offer to individuals, or try to alter the current system by intervening more effectively in political and policy decision making. She clearly favors the latter policy and believes that data-driven methods (including traditional ones such as epidemiology and biostatistics and newer ones associated with quality assessment and outcomes research) can be better used to that end. Milio admits that this strategy clearly poses serious political risks, but she believes they can be offset by "fram[ing] public health policy at the growing edge of public opinion and lead[ing] from that point forward" (275).

While it sounds good in theory, I anticipate that finding the leading edge of public opinion will be a challenge. Briefly, in the aftermath of September 11, it seemed the task might be easier. But all too quickly, the concept of preparedness devolved into haphazard purchases of equipment. (My favorite was the crash cart purchased by one town to be kept at the local high school, to revive football fans overcome by the game.) Now we have the post-Katrina rush equivalent: frenzied efforts with seemingly little cohesion that will bring further dubious purchases in their wake, while leaving untouched the underlying problems. Meanwhile, conservative criticisms of the nanny state, of which public health serves as a favorite exemplar, continue as vitriolic as ever.

Still, with the growing recognition that the American health care system is like the Titanic headed for its iceberg, there undoubtedly lies opportunity as well. Today we are faced with sharply divergent models of what a consumer-driven health care system should look like. Some equate such a system with universal health insurance and controls on prescription drug prices, while others advocate for medical savings accounts and direct-to-consumer advertising of prescription drugs. In the complex world of policy making today, sorting out all these competing claims to speak on behalf of the great patient/public is a daunting task, but one for which public health professionals would seem to be uniquely qualified. Like the patient in patient-centered medicine, or the consumer in consumer-driven health care, the publics of public health are not easy to pin down. But despite the uncertainties and hazards the mission entails, the field of public health has no choice but to continue trying to speak for them.

Notes

1. This is a good example of the kind of professional regression described in Abbott 1988, in that the problematic areas created by one professional group become the opportunity of its competitors.

2. This evolution has been a primary concern of political science since the 1920s. A classic articulation of the problem is Almond and Verba 1963. For particularly good recent reviews of these debates, see Herbst 1998 and Morone 1998. For a superb historical account of survey research, see Igo 2007.

3. Note that market research developed in this same time period, and modern methodologies of sampling and statistical analysis were traded among academic and commercial researchers (see Converse 1987). Yet market research was essentially private research, a kind of corporate trade secret that was not meant directly to shape public debate. In contrast, social scientific research had direct relevance to the political quest to uncover the authentic voice of the patient/public.

4. *Who Was Who in America*, vol. 2 (1943–1950), s.v. "Moore, Harry Hascall."

5. There is an extensive historical literature on the CCMC. For a recent, detailed review of the CCMC's history, see Engel 2002.

6. Public opinion polls in the 1950s first documented the dichotomy between the public's attitudes toward organized medicine and toward its own personal physicians, and likely it existed in the 1930s and 1940s as well. See Tomes 2006b.

7. Bauer, W. W. Racine Scripts. Box 2, Bauer Papers. Wisconsin Historical Society, Madison.

8. On the Donora smog incident and its impact, see Snyder 1994.

9. Stewart explicitly promoted the term "community medicine" as a less controversial substitute for the term "social medicine," which "for cultural and political reasons well known to all of us . . . could not be employed" in the United States (1963, x).

10. This questioning of scientific authority was part of a larger revolt against expertise in general. See for example Lipset and Schneider 1987 and Maasen and Weingart 2005. For a good review of its manifestations in medicine, see Schlesinger 2002.

11. These generalizations are based on my reading of the *AJPH* and *Public Health Reports*. See for example Sellers 1970, Birch 1976, and Galiher and Costa 1975.

References

Abbott, A. 1988. *The System of Professions*. Chicago: University of Chicago Press.

Almond, G. A., and S. Verba. 1963. *The Civic Culture: Political Attitudes and Democracy in Five Nations*. Princeton: Princeton University Press.

Birch, J. S. 1976. New and Traditional Sources of Care Evaluated by Recently Pregnant Women. *Public Health Reports* 91, 5:412–422.

Bloom, S. 2002. *The Word As Scalpel: A History of Medical Sociology*. New York: Oxford University Press.

Brandt, A. M., and M. Gardner. 2000. Antagonism and Accommodation: Interpreting the Relationship between Public Health and Medicine in the United States during the Twentieth Century. *American Journal of Public Health* 90, 5:707–714.

Breslow, L. 1970. The Urgency of Social Action for Health. *American Journal of Public Health* 60, 1:10–16.

Burris, S. 1997. The Invisibility of Public Health: Population-Level Measures in a Politics of Market Individualism. *American Journal of Public Health* 87, 10:1607–1610.

Burrow, J. 1977. *Organized Medicine in the Progressive Era*. Baltimore: Johns Hopkins University Press.

Cabot, H. 1935. *The Doctor's Bill*. New York: Columbia University Press.

Carter, R. 1992. *The Gentle Legions: National Voluntary Health Organizations in America*. New Brunswick: Transaction Publishers. (Orig. pub. Doubleday, 1961.)

Checkoway, B., ed. 1981. *Citizens and Health Care: Participation and Planning for Social Change*. New York: Pergamon.

———. 1982. The Empire Strikes Back. *Journal of Health Politics, Policy, and Law* 7:111–124.

Citizens Board of Inquiry into Health Services for Americans. 1972. *Heal Your Self*. Washington, D.C.: American Public Health Association. (Repr., 1971.)

Cohen, L. 1998. The New Deal State and the Making of Citizen Consumers. In *Getting and Spending: European and American Consumer Societies in the Twentieth Century*, ed. S. Strasser, 111–125. New York: Cambridge University Press.

———. 2003. *A Consumers' Republic: The Politics of Mass Consumption in Postwar America*. New York: Knopf.

Converse, J. M. 1987. *Survey Research in the United States: Roots and Emergence, 1890–1960*. Berkeley: University of California Press.

Cornely, P. B. 1971. The Hidden Enemies of Health and the American Public Health Association. *American Journal of Public Health* 61, 1:7–18.

Edgley, C., and D. Brissett. 1999. *A Nation of Meddlers*. Boulder, Colo.: Westview.

Ehrenreich, J., and B. Ehrenreich. 1970. *The American Health Empire: Power, Profits, and Politics*. New York: Random House.

Engel, J. 2002. *Doctors and Reformers: Discussion and Debate over Health Policy, 1925–1950*. Columbia: University of South Carolina Press.

Falk, I. S., C. R. Rorem, and M. D. Ring. 1933. *The Costs of Medical Care*. Chicago: University of Chicago Press.

Fee, E. 1987. *Disease and Discovery: A History of the Johns Hopkins School of Hygiene and Public Health*. Baltimore: Johns Hopkins University Press.

Fishbein, M. 1969. *Morris Fishbein, M.D.: An Autobiography*. Garden City: Doubleday.

Galiher, C. B., and M. A. Costa. 1975. Consumer Acceptance of HMOs. *Public Health Reports* 90, 2:106–112.

Grey, M. R. 1999. *New Deal Medicine: The Rural Health Programs of the Farm Security Administration*. Baltimore: Johns Hopkins University Press.

Herbst, S. 1998. *Reading Public Opinion: How Political Actors View the Democratic Process*. Chicago: University of Chicago Press.

Hilleboe, H. E., and G. W. Larimore. 1965. *Preventive Medicine: Principles of Prevention in the Occurrence and Progression of Disease*. Philadelphia: W. B. Saunders.

Igo, S. E. 2007. *The Averaged American: Surveys, Citizens, and the Making of a Mass Public*. Cambridge, Mass.: Harvard University Press.

Institute of Medicine. 1988. *The Future of Public Health*. Washington, D.C.: National Academies Press.

Jackson, C. O. 1970. *Food and Drug Legislation in the New Deal*. Princeton: Princeton University Press.

Leavitt, J. W. 1982. *The Healthiest City: Milwaukee and the Politics of Health Reform*. Princeton: Princeton University Press.

———. 1997. *Typhoid Mary: Captive to the People's Health*. Boston: Beacon.

Lipset, S. M., and W. Schneider. 1987. *The Confidence Gap: Business, Labor, and Government in the Public Mind*. Rev. ed. Baltimore: Johns Hopkins University Press.

Ludmerer, K. M. 1985. *Learning to Heal: The Development of American Medical Education*. New York: Basic Books.

Maasen, S., and P. Weingart, eds. 2005. *Democratization of Expertise?* Dordrecht: Springer.

Markel, H. 2004. *When Germs Travel*. New York: Pantheon.

Markowitz, G., and D. Rosner. 2002. *Deceit and Denial: The Deadly Politics of Industrial Pollution*. Berkeley: University of California Press.

Milio, N. 2000. *Public Health in the Market*. Ann Arbor: University of Michigan Press.

Moore, H. H. 1927. *American Medicine and the People's Health*. New York: D. Appleton.

Morone, J. A. 1998. *The Democratic Wish: Popular Participation and the Limits of American Government*. Rev. ed. New Haven: Yale University Press.

Morone, J. A., and L. R. Jacobs. 2005. *Healthy, Wealthy, and Fair: Health Care and the Good Society*. New York: Oxford University Press.

Overton, F., and W. J. Denno. 1920. *The Health Officer*. Philadelphia: W.B. Saunders.

Reverby, S. M., ed. 2000. *Tuskegee's Truths: Rethinking the Tuskegee Syphilis Study*. Chapel Hill: University of North Carolina Press.

Rogers, N. 2001. Caution: The AMA May Be Dangerous to Your Health. *Radical History Review* 80:5–34.

Rosenkrantz, B. G. 1972. *Public Health and the State: Changing Views in Massachusetts, 1842–1936*. Cambridge, Mass.: Harvard University Press.

Scheele, L. A. 1952. Public Health Statesmanship. First Annual Charles-Edward Amory Winslow Lecture. Typescript. Yale University School of Medicine Library. New Haven.

Schlesinger, M. 2002. A Loss of Faith: The Sources of Reduced Political Legitimacy for the American Medical Profession. *Milbank Quarterly* 80, 2:185–235.

Sellers, C. C. 1997. *Hazards of the Job: From Industrial Disease to Environmental Health Science*. Chapel Hill: University of North Carolina Press.

Sellers, R. V. 1970. The Black Health Worker and the Black Health Consumer: New Roles for Both. *American Journal of Public Health* 60, 11:2154–2170.

Snyder, L. P. 1994. The Death-Dealing Smog over Donora, Pennsylvania. *Environmental History Review* 18, 1:117–139.

Sparer, G., G. B. Dines, and D. Smith. 1970. Consumer Participation in OEO-Assisted Neighborhood Health Centers. *American Journal of Public Health 60*, 6:1091–1102.

Starr, P. 1982. *The Social Transformation of American Medicine*. New York: Basic Books.

Steckler, A. B., and W. T. Herzog. 1979. How to Keep Your Mandated Citizen Board out of Your Hair and off Your Back: A Guide for Executive Directors. *American Journal of Public Health* 69, 8:809–812.

Stewart, W. H. 1963. Community Medicine: An American Concept of Comprehensive Care. *Public Health Reports* 78, 2:93–100.

Tomes, N. J. 2006a. Patients or Health Care Consumers? Why the History of Contested Terms Matters. In *Public Health and Public Policy*, ed. R. Stevens, C. Rosenberg, and C. Burns, 83–110. New Brunswick: Rutgers University Press.

———. 2006b. Who Speaks for the Patient? Historical Reflections and Contemporary Challenges. Typescript. Author files.

Wallack, L., and R. Lawrence. 2005. Talking about Public Health: Developing America's "Second Language." *American Journal of Public Health* 95, 4:567–570.

White, K. L. 1991. *Healing the Schism: Epidemiology, Medicine, and the Public's Health*. New York: Springer-Verlag.

Winslow, C-E. A., et al. 1952. *The History of American Epidemiology*. St. Louis: Mosby.

Part II

Contested Boundaries

This section presents five case studies of instances in which the scope of public health—what the profession can or should do—has been the subject of debate. Phil Brown examines the extent to which environmental health should be considered a core component of public health. Although the genesis of public health in the nineteenth century was a response to environmental hazards such as contaminated water and slum housing, these venerable antecedents have not translated into modern-day support for public health involvement, as the extended controversies over lead paint abatement and regulation of workplace toxins illustrates. Citing the ways that disciplines such as toxicology and molecular biology can advance the cause of social justice, Brown argues for the centrality of environmental health to a public health practice that is both technically rigorous and politically engaged.

Marian Moser Jones and Ronald Bayer examine the public health experience with a behavior—riding a motorcycle without a helmet—that imposes no third-party harms and endangers only those who engage in it. Once considered a public health success story, laws requiring the use of motorcycle helmets have been repealed around the country in recent years by citizen groups who objected to what they saw as unacceptable paternalism and infringement on individual liberty.

William McAllister, Mary Clare Lennon, and Işıl Çelimli make the case that the population-level perspective of the public health profession makes it the ideal analytic framework for addressing the problem of homelessness, a notoriously intractable social problem with multiple determinants. Their analysis, which indicates the value of bringing issues of social and economic well-being firmly into the purview of public health, has profound implications for prevention more generally.

Amy Fairchild examines efforts to locate the fine line where public health *practice* turns into *research.* Many routinely performed activities, including collection and analysis of statistics and outbreak investigation, produce generalizable knowledge, which makes them—according to most standard definitions—a form of research. If health agencies are truly engaged in research, as some have claimed, then must they be subject to the regulatory oversight of institutional review boards in order to protect members of the public who are the subject of such inquiries?

Finally, Alvin Tarlov addresses one of the most enduring and consequential points of contention in the field of health in America: the conceptual and institutional split between public health and clinical medicine. In a fresh and forward-looking approach to the topic, he proposes a new conceptual framework that could synthesize preventive and curative approaches for the ultimate betterment of both individuals and populations.

Environmental Health as a Core Public Health Component

A well-rounded and comprehensive public health approach must incorporate many components of environmental health. Indeed, environmental health has always been central to public health. That is why it is no accident that John Snow's classic cholera study, the stepping-stone of scientific epidemiology, concerns environmental contamination of the public water supply. If we think back to some of the most elemental public health principles and accomplishments, we note that central elements of reduction in mortality—sewage, sanitation, and clean water supply—are environmental health actions. When we move forward to the present day, we find that environmental health still plays a major role: Scientists searching for environmental factors in disease and symptoms have opened innovative channels for research in epidemiology, toxicology, biomonitoring, molecular biology, toxicogenomics, and GIS modeling. As well, environmental health is integrally based on a population health model, making it congruent to public health in general.

Environmental health represents an arena where public health concerns link up with social activism to improve health status, while increasing democratic participation in public life. The environmental justice movement, initially focused on hazards in communities of color, is a prime example. Environmental justice activism, in tandem with the community-based participatory research that often accompanies it, has shown the importance of lay-professional collaboration to research, remediate, and prevent environmental degradation from air particulates, military toxics, oilfield wastes, abandoned industrial facilities, incinerators, refineries, and vehicle traffic.

In addition, environmental justice projects demonstrate the intersecting nature of advanced public health, linking health and environment to other social sectors, such as transportation, urban development, housing, the built environment, school siting and environmental hazards in schools, sustainable development, and food security features such as farmers markets, community gardens, and healthy food in schools. This definition mirrors the World Health Organization's broad definition of health that has so powerfully influenced public health practitioners and supporters.

A broader environmental health movement has also developed, overlapping with environmental justice and involving many types of organizations, from local to state to national levels. Environmental health has been crucial in the expansion of community-based participatory research. Its advocates often challenge the corporate world by arguing for a safe and precautionary approach to chemicals, radiation, and other hazards, and by placing such safety over the primacy of profit. These advocates also push government regulatory systems toward more precautionary regulations and greater enforcement (Brown 2007).

Presently, environmental health is a battleground for many key public health concerns. There have been purges in federal agencies of environmental health scientists and officials, and on advisory panels on asthma and second-hand tobacco smoke of members who lean toward a rational, scientific approach rather than an ideological one. Despite excellent environmental health departments in some public health schools, the field is under siege from antiregulatory government agencies and from the business world. Even without government antagonism, environmental health faces other challenges. It has often been separated from public health, in that much regulation and research has come from state and federal environment agencies rather than public health agencies. Environmental health is hardly touched on in medical education, and physicians are typically unfamiliar with environmental factors that cause illness.

Yet, in the areas I have mentioned, environmental health is a beacon for broader public health theory, policy, and practice. This chapter will examine how environmental health poses valuable directions for public health, using specific examples of environmental health organizing and practice, and developing a theoretical framework in which environmental health is a microcosm of the entire public health outlook.

One Starting Point: An Environmental Justice Framework for Asthma and Its Social Correlates

While not all environmental health advocates, scientists, and educators are activists who see themselves as part of a social movement, a substantial number have such a movement-centered perspective. Even for those who do not, the environmental health movement has helped them to go beyond routine science by mobilizing many people and groups and by creating a broader perspective. Environmental justice activism around asthma offers an example of how an environmental health concern gets amplified into a broader social justice frame, while involving increasingly more sectors of society.

Two groups provide good vehicles for understanding this development. The first, Alternatives for Community and Environment (ACE), began in 1993 as an environmental justice organization based in the Roxbury-Dorchester area of Boston. One of its earliest actions was a successful mobilization to prevent the permitting of an asphalt plant. ACE had initially expected to focus on issues such as vacant lots, but in a year of talking with the community, ACE learned that residents identified asthma as their number one priority.

The second group, West Harlem Environmental Action (WE ACT), was founded in 1988 in response to environmental threats to that community created by the mismanagement of the North River Sewage Treatment Plant and the construction of the sixth bus depot in northern Manhattan. WE ACT quickly evolved into an environmental justice organization with the goal of improving environmental protection and public health in the predominantly African American and Latino communities of northern Manhattan. They identified a wide range of environmental threats, including air pollution, lead poisoning, pesticides, and unsustainable development (Loh et al. 2002).

Both groups frame the unequal burden of asthma in their communities in terms of inequality, rights, and social justice. For ACE and WE ACT, the environmental justice frame is a useful tool for addressing social and environmental causes of asthma.

By linking present conditions to a historical political-economic approach, they incorporate in their focus the full range of social structural inequalities, including housing, transportation, employment, municipal services, land use, and education (Loh et al. 2002).

ACE encourages communities to take ownership of the asthma issue and to push for proactive, empowered solutions. Central to this effort are direct action and education, such as a campaign in which residents identified idling trucks and buses as a major source of particulate irritants. They organized an anti-idling march and began giving informational parking tickets to idling buses and trucks that explained the health effects of diesel exhaust (Brown et al. 2004).

Since ACE identified diesel buses as an air pollution problem, the group has taken up transportation issues more broadly. ACE ran a major campaign targeting local and state government over the allocation of transit resources. Charging "transit racism," ACE argued that the estimated 366,000 daily bus riders in Boston were being discriminated against: While more than $12 billion of federal and state money was being spent on the Big Dig highway project, the Massachusetts Bay Transit Authority (MBTA) refused to spend $105 million to purchase newer, cleaner buses and bus shelters. In tying dirty buses to higher asthma rates, ACE successfully framed an issue of transit spending priorities into one of health, justice, and racism. In 2000 the Transit Riders' Union, largely created by ACE, got the MBTA to allow free transfers between buses, since the many inner-city residents who relied on two buses for transportation had to pay more than subway riders, who had free transfers. ACE's pressure also helped propel the purchase of more compressed natural gas buses (Brown et al. 2004).

Similarly, WE ACT identified diesel exhaust as a major factor behind the disparate burden of asthma experienced in the group's community. Using publicity campaigns such as informative advertisements placed in bus shelters, public service announcements on cable television, and a direct mailing, WE ACT has let a vast number of community residents and public officials know that diesel buses could trigger asthma attacks. Though their efforts increased public awareness of WE ACT and its efforts to reduce asthma, the media campaign did not lead to a shift in New York's Metropolitan Transit Authority's (MTA) policy toward diesel buses. So in November 2000, WE ACT filed a lawsuit against the MTA with the federal Department of Transportation, claiming that the MTA advances a racist and discriminatory policy by disproportionately siting diesel bus depots and parking lots in neighborhoods whose primary residents are people of color (Shepard et al. 2002).

A key component of ACE's education and empowerment efforts is its Roxbury Environmental Empowerment Project (REEP). REEP teaches classes in local schools, hosts environmental justice conferences, and through its intern program trains high school students to teach environmental health in schools. Classes educate students about environmental justice, using asthma as a focal issue. For example, REEP teachers discuss a process for siting a hazardous facility in a neighborhood and ask the students why it might be sited there and what they would do about the siting decision. They teach students how to locate on local maps the potentially dangerous locations in their area. ACE has helped some of its high school interns get into college as a result of the education they received in the REEP program and participates in job fairs to help students explore good employment prospects (Brown et al. 2004).

WE ACT's Healthy Home Healthy Child campaign reflects a similar community empowerment approach. Developed in partnership with the Columbia Center for Children's Environmental Health, the campaign educates the community on a variety of risk factors, including cigarettes, lead poisoning, drugs and alcohol, air pollution, garbage, pesticides, and poor nutrition. Educational materials, translated into Spanish and written in accessible language, inform residents about the effects of risk factors and actions they can take to alleviate or minimize those effects. As with ACE's experience in identifying community issues, WE ACT's Healthy Home Healthy Child campaign began by focusing on specific asthma triggers but soon expanded to include residents' key concerns, such as drugs, alcohol, and garbage (Shepard et al. 2002).

The broad public health perspective these groups take in part developed alongside the collaborative work of air particulate researchers and other scientists, mainly located in public health schools. As I will discuss later on, this community-based participatory research approach to science and public health marks a powerful democratic impulse reminiscent of the nation's earliest public health campaigns.

Expansion of the Environmental Justice Framework

From these examples, we can see quite a breadth of issues that stem from what was initially a limited focus. Environmental justice activists, originally concentrated on toxic waste and other noxious sites and on unequal exposure to toxics, now work for better communities through intersecting approaches that touch on virtually all sectors of society. Concern for air particulates led logically to mass transit equity issues (Bullard, Johnson, and Torres 2004). Concerns about transportation called into question the manner in which decisions about urban and economic development issues were made, leading activists to press for more community-oriented development, rather than schemes that primarily benefited real estate developers (Shutkin 2001). A focus on unhealthy housing conditions involved in asthma triggers led to a deeper emphasis on housing and the built environment (Hynes and Brugge 2000). Activists have sought more and improved parklands and have sought to reclaim abandoned sites and rundown watersheds (Woonasquatucket River Watershed Council 2007). Activists have sought to make schools healthier places, alert to the dangers of carpeting, allergenic building materials, and toxic cleaning supplies. They have fought against building schools on brownfields that have been improperly, or not at all, cleaned up (Center for Health, Environment, and Justice 2006). Environmental justice organizers have taken up the issue of food security, pressuring for healthy school food, running community gardens and farmers markets, and supporting local sustainable agriculture. Food security organizers point to the inadequate diets of many poor people and people of color, often due to the lack of supermarkets and fresh produce in their neighborhoods, to poor school lunches, and to an excess of fast-food meals. They point to the higher obesity in those populations, often resulting in extremely high diabetes rates. Extending their critique to the ever-more-monopolized food industry and the federal agencies that support it, these activists make an issue of the problem that a major part of the overall economy goes toward producing poor food, poor diets, and poor health outcomes (Gottlieb 2002).

For another example of such an expanded environmental justice framework, we can observe how Alaska Natives and their allies have integrated a broad array of concerns. Through Alaska Community Action on Toxics and the Aleutian-Pribilof Islands Association, as well as a host of local and tribal organizations, they work for the cleanup of approximately seven hundred former military sites. They study the dangers of PCBs and other chemicals in the subsistence fish and marine mammals that are core parts of their diet. Their efforts advance the study of global climate change, ocean currents, and air transport of toxics. They point to the presence of chemicals in breast milk as a result of such contamination and pursue research in that area. They work to prevent improper development of their lands, such as the proposal to drill in the Arctic National Wildlife Refuge. In the process, they protect natural beauty and religious and traditional settings (Alaska Community Action on Toxics 1998; Aleutian Pribilof Islands Association 2007). This vast assortment of concerns points to the complexity of issues that make up environmental health in the largest sense.

Another Avenue: Environmental Breast Cancer Activism

The environmental breast cancer movement is another example of an ever-broadening environmental health approach. The movement has reframed the successes of the broader breast cancer movement in order to focus on potential environmental causes and to change how breast cancer is researched and publicly perceived (McCormick, Brown, and Zavestoski 2003). For example, for years people accepted the position of the American Cancer Society, National Cancer Institute, and other parts of the cancer establishment that mammography is the best way to prevent breast cancer. But environmental breast cancer activists argue that once a tumor is detected, prevention has failed, since the tumor now exists. The growing scientific awareness that mammography is not very effective in women under fifty lends support to this stance.

Activists also challenge the corporate control of Breast Cancer Awareness Month. They point out that Imperial Chemical Industries, the parent company of Zeneca (later merged with Astra to become Astra-Zeneca), invented Breast Cancer Awareness Month and retains authority to approve or disapprove all printed materials used by participating groups. Tying the political economy critique to their belief in environmental causation, activists point out that Astra-Zeneca at the same time produces pesticides and herbicides that may be causing breast cancer (Zones 2000). They have additionally mounted a campaign to have breast cancer stamp revenues shifted from the National Cancer Institute, where research on environmental factors is not supported, to the National Institute of Environmental Health Sciences.

In 1995, Breast Cancer Action became a founding member of the Toxics Link Coalition and helped organize the first Cancer Industry Tour, a toxic tour of the type that has become a hallmark of environmental justice activities. Breast Cancer Action has collaborated with the San Francisco Department of Public Health Breast and Cervical Cancer Services and various community and health organizations to organize Town Halls on breast cancer in low-income communities of color. There is crossover in leadership between breast cancer and environmental organizations. Environmental breast cancer groups have been key founders of precautionary principle-based organizing and have been centrally involved with the campaign for safe cosmetics. Groups like Breast Cancer Action have started a "Think before You Pink" coalition of organizations that point out the flaws and biases in the many mainstream/corporate pink campaigns (promotions in which companies promise to support breast cancer projects, using very small portions of products bought by supporters). These activists also claim that pharmaceutical producers and doctors often downplay side effects, including uterine cancer from Tamoxifen. Marin Breast Cancer Watch in the San Francisco Bay Area, for example, emphasizes environmental causes of breast cancer, highlights community-based participatory research approaches, and features speakers from environmental justice and environmental health activist groups like West County Toxics Coalition and Commonweal.

In the Boston area, Silent Spring Institute (SSI) has been a major player in extending the scientific study of environmental factors in breast cancer. In an air, dust, and urine sampling of many chemicals, SSI researchers characterized for the first time many toxic substances, leading the way for other studies of household and body burden contaminants (Rudel et al. 2003). SSI engages in outreach via educational sessions and provides extensive scientific information to the general public. Their *Cape Cod Breast Cancer and Environment Study Atlas* contains Cape-specific information on breast cancer incidence; pesticide historically used for agricultural land and tree pests; drinking water quality; census data, such as income and education; and land use, including the location of waste disposal sites and the dramatic transition from forested land to residential housing.[1] SSI believes that scientific data should be circulated widely to provide the fullest possible access to information to people actually and potentially affected by breast cancer. The Massachusetts Breast Cancer

Coalition, which founded the Silent Spring Institute, was one of the four founding members of the Precautionary Principle Project, later the Alliance for a
Healthy Tomorrow, which was a core vehicle for expanding the precautionary
principle throughout the United States (Mayer, Brown, and Linder 2002). (In
the context of the impact of human actions on human health, the precautionary
principle supports taking preventive action, even in the face of uncertainty
about the scope and extent of adverse events associated with exposures; shifting the burden of proof to the proponents of an activity; widening the range of
alternatives assessed; and increasing public participation in decision making.)

More specific connections between breast cancer activism and environmental justice have developed in the last several years. One of the nation's best-
known environmental justice groups, West Harlem Environmental Action, held
the first conference combining the two issues on October 23, 2004, in New
York. At the conference, titled "Breast Cancer, the Environment, and
Communities of Color," the group linked some of their traditional environmental justice issues with the concerns of many of their constituents facing breast
cancer. Prominent members from the breast cancer movement attended, providing input on environmental factors. Elsewhere, Sistahs United, an African
American–led breast cancer group in Tillery, North Carolina, is affiliated with
the environmental justice group Concerned Citizens of Tillery, which has pioneered in the struggle to protect people from hog farm contamination.

In 2004, an environmental justice grant from the National Institute of
Environmental Health Sciences (NIEHS), the first in that program to include
breast cancer, went to the Silent Spring Institute, along with Communities for a
Better Environment, one of the nation's oldest environmental justice groups,
and researchers at Brown University. In 2005 a complementary grant from the
National Science Foundation contributed more support for this project. The
team extended SSI's innovative work on environmental factors in breast cancer
to a community populated by women of color that was already the site of environmental justice organizing around the many oil refineries in the area. The
partners have organized residents of these neighborhoods and help them build
their own capacity to research and challenge environmental contaminants. The
project conducted home environmental exposure assessments, collecting air
and dust samples to assess indoor levels of pollutants, especially endocrine
disruptors, that are potentially linked to breast cancer, reproductive disorders,
neurological development, and other health outcomes.

Data collection, analysis, community education, and organizational linkages
occurred in two locations in Cape Cod, Massachusetts, and Richmond, California,
that are largely composed of people of color and impacted by industrial facilities,

especially oil refineries. Study results have been shared both as aggregate information presented through community meetings, news media, and online, and as individual report-back information to study participants. The goal is to maximize understanding of exposure data and their limitations, as well as to address the ethical issues of ensuring community and individual autonomy, right to know, and ultimately the right to act on scientific information by reducing exposures. The project's focus on individual report-back meshes with a growing effort to do such report-back in studies arising both out of institutional settings and out of environmental activist groups. This research right-to-know is a new direction that is rapidly gaining attention.

Contributions from the Broader Environmental Health Movement

The growth of a broader environmental health movement offers public health a stimulus for reenergizing its activist focus. As with all scientific and health-related endeavors, public health has become increasingly specialized and bureaucratized. Public health schools are mainly staffed with soft-money academics dependent on foundation and federal grants, who are hence less able to take chances on highly innovative projects. A more specialized and scientized mindset has often put advanced research interests above the needs of applied practice. Due to pressure from governors and legislatures, state public health departments are less likely to stand up for communities that believe they are the victims of environmental contamination, and increasingly they have seen their resources transferred to bioterrorism preparedness.

In such a milieu, alternative visions from environmental health movement activists provide a forum for the necessary revisioning. We can see a good example in the work of Commonweal, a California organization involved in environmental health research and activism, as well as in direct service to people with cancer, which recently initiated the Collaborative on Health and the Environment (CHE). CHE has been a powerful force for bringing together many groups and individuals. CHE's task forces conduct frequent telephone conference calls, often with a hundred participants, including an impressive range of government officials, scientists, educators, scholars, and activists on topics such as biomonitoring, asthma, endocrine disrupters, and the health effects of Hurricane Katrina. CHE's work groups on diverse areas of environmental health provide ongoing forums and have prepared major review articles on environmental health effects. It is apparent from such organizing efforts that only the progressives have the vision that can attract others to a comprehensive public health frame.

The toxics movement has been important in directing attention to disease clusters and to hazard exposure. At the national level, the Center for Health,

Environment, and Justice, directed by Lois Gibbs, the leader of the Love Canal community that sparked the toxics movement, has aided thousands of local groups to deal with the issues. Statewide and regional groups like the Toxics Action Center in New England have done so too, with specialized focus on their regions. This kind of toxics action has triggered much new research that has advanced science, which in the absence of such pressure would not necessarily have a spur to examine new areas.

The precautionary approach has been a powerful force in this new environmental health movement. The Alliance for a Healthy Tomorrow (a Massachusetts statewide organization that grew out of the Precautionary Principle Project and now connects over a hundred groups) has played a central role in spreading the precautionary principle, which has been widely accepted in Europe. The alliance does educational work with the public and among labor, health, and environment organizations and has a strong legislative program that has introduced bills on child health, safer chemical alternatives, mercury, and cleaning products. Coalitions in other parts of the country, starting with the San Francisco Bay Area, have succeeded in passing legislation to have municipalities adopt the precautionary principle approach (Mayer, Brown, and Linder 2002; Tickner 1999).

Environmental health activists have been able to convince some manufacturers to change production practices to use safer substances. This has been especially noticeable in the action of Massachusetts's Toxics Use Reduction Institute (TURI), initiated by the state through the influence of environmentalists. In one decade TURI reduced toxic emissions in the state by more than half, without any damage to business (Mayer, Brown, and Linder 2002). Sustainable-production scientists and green chemists at the University of Massachusetts, Lowell, have pioneered alternative production and disposal processes that hold much promise for corporations seeking to limit liability issues, insurance costs, disposal costs, and more regulation (Geiser 2001). The Safe Cosmetics Campaign has convinced some large firms to remove phthalates from their products, while also pointing to the racial targeting of many cosmetic product ads.

Citizen-Science Alliances and Community-Based Participatory Research

The environmental health field has pioneered unique approaches to lay-professional collaboration and to democratic forms of participation. It is useful to transfer this model to public health practice on a wider scale, since public health has its roots in such a worldview.

Citizen-science alliances are lay-professional collaborations in which citizens and scientists work together on issues identified by laypeople (Brown et al. 2001). These citizen-science alliances challenge, and sometimes change, scientific norms by valuing the embodied knowledge of illness sufferers. These alliances between researchers and community groups may be formal or informal. Formal alliances often occur in university-based "science shops" (most well-known in the Netherlands), in research consulting organizations (such as the Loka Institute in Amherst, Massachusetts, or John Snow, Inc., in Boston), or through government-funded programs that set research agendas based on lay demands (such as Silent Spring Institute, initially funded by the Massachusetts legislature, which studies potential environmental factors in breast cancer). More informal citizen-science alliances have arisen in response to contaminated communities, most notably in Love Canal (Gibbs 1981) and Woburn (Brown and Mikkelsen 1990).

Citizen involvement in public health programs began in the 1960s with community mental health centers, neighborhood health centers, and rural health centers. Since the 1990s there has been a resurgence of lay involvement, increasingly aimed at participation in health research. Foundations and government agencies have responded positively to national reports such as *Healthy People 2000* (U.S. Department of Health and Human Services 1990) and *Healthy People 2010* (U.S. Department of Health and Human Services 2001), both of which set community-based programs as priority areas by funding health research that incorporates public involvement. Furthermore, there has been an increase in federal funding for environmental health research with community participation components, though some of it is merely participation in review panels rather than full-scale community-based participatory research. The National Institute of Environmental Health Science, the Department of Defense, the Environmental Protection Agency, the Centers for Disease Control, the Department of Housing and Urban Development, and the Agency for Toxic Substances and Disease Registry have at various times supported programs with a range of public involvement. In the early 1990s, NIEHS initiated a Translational Research Program to encourage collaboration between community members and scientists through "a methodology that promotes active community involvement in the processes that shape research and intervention strategies, as well as in the conduct of research studies" (Green et al. 2002).

Community-based participatory research (CBPR) goes beyond the traditional models of public involvement by requiring active community participation at every stage in the research process. Put simply, it is research that is done with and for communities, not on communities, involving community partners in all phases of the research process: defining the problem; designing the study; gathering, interpreting, and analyzing the data; disseminating the results; and creating and evaluating plans of action. The purpose is to enhance community understanding of issues affecting community partners, to provide interventions that benefit the community, to enhance the capacity of community partners, and to provide findings in accessible language that will be useful for the community. There is a strong ethical component, in that these collaborations are based on mutual respect; recognition of knowledge, expertise, and resource capacities of all partners; open communication; community ownership of data and control of access to data; and research protections for individuals and communities (Minkler and Wallerstein 2003).

NIEHS has continued to be the primary federal agency supporting community-based participatory research, especially in the environmental justice area. By legitimizing such work, the program has paved the way for other collaborative projects. In 2002 the National Institute of Occupational Safety and Health began partnering with NIEHS to coordinate joint reviews of CBPR projects in environmental justice, a logical development given the many similarities in how occupational and environmental health deal with hazards and with corporate resistance and problems with governmental regulation. Some CBPR funding has gone toward setting up ongoing centers; for example, NIEHS, the Environmental Protection Agency (EPA), and the Centers for Disease Control and Prevention teamed up in 1998 to develop the Centers for Children's Environmental Health and Disease Prevention Research program. The goal of this program was to support research efforts that would translate basic research on children's environmentally related diseases into community-based prevention and intervention applications. Respiratory disease was one of two foci for the initial round of funding. Five centers currently focus on asthma, respiratory disease, and/or air pollution. Their activities include monitoring air pollution, tracking community trends in respiratory health, decreasing pollution, doing educational outreach, encouraging community participation, and increasing community capacity to conduct future research. One of these centers, the Columbia Center for Children's Environmental Health, works in collaboration with the activist group West Harlem Environmental Action, as we have seen.

The most egalitarian community-academic collaboration occurs when there is a grassroots movement, since this makes it more likely that community groups will initiate or play key roles in the process rather than merely sit on advisory boards. More comprehensive citizen involvement in research often occurs as a social problem becomes more public and a social movement gains strength and momentum. This is because the increasingly public nature of discussion on the problem, amplified by a cogent critique of how science has failed to address local concerns, has the potential to highlight the constraints of traditional scientific approaches. In this process activists become increasingly knowledgeable about a disease and begin to push for involvement in defining and researching it.

New Approaches to Population Health

Public health has often pointed to its population health focus as one factor that differentiates it from clinical medicine. That distinction needs upgrading, and environmental health offers some necessary elements. Health inequality has become a key area of research in the last decade and has contributed much to public health. Yet that area mainly examines social determinants of health and differential access to care. It is striking that one could read the burgeoning literature on health inequalities and find nothing on environmental health, especially environmental justice. Here, I take up some of the valuable biomonitoring issues that environmental health scientists and advocates are pursuing.

Improved Monitoring and Surveillance

In a time when biomonitoring has become so important, it is worth noting that environmental health scientists have long sought disease registries and health-tracking programs that could demonstrate environmental factors in disease.

Much contestation over environmental factors stems from lack of information. One way to deal with that lack is health tracking and monitoring, which have been generally absent in public health. However, there have been some promising moves in this direction. In March 2001, the Centers for Disease Control and Prevention (CDC) released the first-ever report on toxic chemicals present in our bodies. For chemicals with known toxicity levels, CDC can show the number of people who exceed currently accepted toxic levels. For all chemicals, the project can show differential exposure by age, sex, and racial/ethnic group. CDC can use these data to track exposure over time and to set research agendas for health effects.

The tests measured 27 substances, including mercury, organophosphates (found in pesticides), and phthalates (plasticizers found in children's toys, cosmetics, and medical devices). While some of these chemicals had been tested in soil, air, and water, levels in humans had never been directly measured. CDC continued testing, adding 89 chemicals to the screen, as shown in their 2003 report. CDC points out that the data detail exposure of the U.S. population to toxins; it does not present new data on health risks caused by different exposure levels (CDC 2003). CDC's third report, released in 2005, included blood and urine levels for 148 chemicals, with the notable addition of several PCBs, certain phthalate metabolites, the pyrethroid insecticide permethrin, and the organochlorine pesticides aldrin, endrin, and dieldrin. Although CDC hopes to get several sets of data before addressing trends in chemical exposures, these data are useful not only in establishing the effectiveness of current public health efforts and identifying which chemicals need to be further addressed, but also, divided into groups by age, gender, and race, in identifying disparities in these exposures. CDC will continue to increase the number of chemicals monitored, including 309 and 473 chemicals in 2007 and 2009 respectively (CDC 2005). These reports serve as tools for other researchers to begin to assess environmental health threats and, as trends become increasingly clear, will help to guide public health decisions.

This screening process is a step in the right direction, and the information collected should be used to promote more research into environmental links to diseases, as proposed by the Trust for America's Health (TFAH, previously Health-Track). The TFAH mission, supported by the Pew Charitable Trusts, is to identify and track the links between environmental hazards and illnesses and to provide researchers and public health officials with the necessary tools to prevent disease. Beyond the process of health tracking, of course, is the application of its findings toward reducing or eliminating toxic substances.

The National Children's Study (NCS), authorized by Congress in 2000 and launched in 2004, offers another longitudinal approach to monitoring. Led by a collaboration of federal agencies including the Department of Health and Human Services, EPA, CDC, and NIEHS, the study examines the influences of environmental factors on the health of children by following more than 100,000 children from before birth to the age of twenty-one by enrolling pregnant women, couples planning pregnancy, and women of child-bearing age not planning pregnancy to participate in a minimum of fifteen visits with a local research team. Several factors differentiate NCS from other studies being done in the United States, one of the most influential being its definition of "environment," which includes genetics, cultural influences, physical surroundings, diet, and biological, chemical and social factors (National Children's Study 2005a). NCS expects its first results to be available in 2009. Furthermore, the study is aimed at examining a variety of different issues that arise during childhood, from the development of attention deficit disorder, schizophrenia, autism, asthma, obesity, and heart disease, to injuries resulting from poor neighborhood planning and violent behavior in teenagers (National Children's Study 2005b; Nesmith 2005). However, despite indications that the results of the study could lead to annual reductions of health care costs that would amount to be greater than the costs of the study, the federal budget for NCS was cut from $27 million to $12 million in the fiscal year 2005 (Nesmith 2005).

In 2002 members of Congress introduced the Nationwide Health Tracking Act, largely tied to antiterrorist biomonitoring, which appropriated $17.5 million toward building a health-tracking network, adding another $28 million in 2003 to expand the program (Trust for America's Health 2005a). As a result, CDC was able to award health-tracking grants to several states in order to build environmental public health capacity, improve collaborations between environmental health agencies, evaluate existing tracking systems, build community partnerships, and develop model systems (Trust for America's Health 2005b).

Grassroots Body Burden Testing

One kind of new science that derives from the citizen-science alliance is what I term "grassroots body burden testing." This is at the intersection of three of my areas of concern: the new forms of population health I have addressed here, citizen-science alliances and community-based participatory research, and social activism. In light of CDC's study mentioned earlier, the Environmental Working Group (EWG), an activist organization, decided to publicize the need for human monitoring. Working with Mount Sinai School of Medicine in New York and Commonweal, a California environmental group, researchers examined a far larger number of chemicals than did CDC. They found an average of 91 industrial compounds, pollutants, and other chemicals in the blood and urine of their nine volunteers, and a total of 167 chemicals; of these, 76 cause cancer in humans or animals, 94 are toxic to the brain and nervous system, and 79 cause birth defects or abnormal development. As with most chemicals, the dangers of exposure to these chemicals in combination have never been studied (Environmental Working Group 2003).

EWG's small-scale body burden study included nine well-known environmental activists and other public figures, who permitted themselves to be publicly identified in order to show people what it was like to discover the toxic substances inside one's body. Besides producing a grassroots version of the CDC study, EWG also had impetus from seeing the increase in many diseases, from realizing that chemicals are usually studied only after they are associated with known harm, and from understanding that federal regulations, especially the Toxic Substances Control Act, were failing to regulate chemicals. EWG also wanted to promote awareness that many effects are now found below "safe doses" set by regulatory bodies. On the EWG Web site, the viewer can click on the thumbnail photo of each person to see what contaminants are in that person's body. A graphic resembling the periodic table of the elements shows up, and those chemicals in that person's body are highlighted. Clicking on any chemical box brings up information on that chemical (Environmental Working Group 2003).

By advising participants of their personal burden and having them go public, EWG was pursuing a radical path. The typical epidemiological study informs people only that their population (e.g. people in their census tract, or town, or county) had a lower, similar, or higher rate than the general population. People do not usually learn their own body burden or household contaminant level, except for certain well-known testing protocols for chemicals with well-established health effects, such as blood lead levels. Not giving people their personal data violates their right to know what is in their bodies. This process of informing people of their personal data, the "research right-to-know," is a major step forward.

Several decades of activism concerning democratization of science have led to major changes in conceptions of who has the legal and ethical right to be involved in scientific research on people. Informed consent is increasingly understood as much more than a clinical treatment or research subject protection. Rather, it incorporates many concerns about the rights of people and communities to decide if they should indeed be the focus of research, about the right to own their own data, and about reciprocal relationships between researchers and those being studied. The growing movement of community-based participatory research has been key in this transformation of informed consent from a largely bureaucratic process to a major democratic right (Israel et al. 1998; Minkler and Wallerstein 2003). African American, Latino, and Native American populations have been among the greatest critics of academic research that is exclusively controlled by scientists who develop research questions without community input, and that has little or no benefit to the community. In some community-academic partnerships, the community partner requires the researchers to inform the community before they disseminate research results or give presentations on these results (Akwesasne Research Advisory Committee 1996).

The CDC's body burden study was a great advance, yet it is only the first step. As the Environmental Working Group study showed, it was important to go beyond individual chemicals in a multitude of people to individual people for a multitude of chemicals. And it was important to let people know their individual burdens. Many more such studies, with larger samples, are necessary in order to understand what levels of toxics are in our bodies and, one hopes, to correlate that burden with actual health status. Some researchers are increasingly turning their attention to breast milk monitoring, given the high concentrations of toxics in breast milk. This is a fruitful avenue for advocates to press, since human breast milk has many toxins, often at levels that surpass EPA limits on manufactured food products (Steingraber 2001).

EWG went further in its grassroots body burden direction with a breast milk–monitoring study in 2003, examining the flame retardant PBDE. The average level in the milk of twenty first-time mothers was seventy-five times the average found in recent European studies that led the EU to ban a number of the substances. Milk from two women contained the highest levels of fire retardants ever reported in the United States, and milk from other mothers in the study had among the highest levels ever detected worldwide. EWG is aware that the beneficial aspects of breast-feeding may outweigh the risks of PBDEs and other toxins in breast milk and did not try to convince mothers to stop breast-feeding. Some environmental health groups are reluctant to support breast milk monitoring because of the problematic nature of such research. Nevertheless, this kind of publicity can be helpful, since it resulted in the Great Lakes Chemical Corporation ceasing production of the penta-PBDE mixture that is the largest source of PBDE exposure (Sharp and Lunder 2004).

Continuing its biomonitoring work, EWG announced in July 2005 results from its study of toxins in umbilical cord blood, in which 287 different chemicals were detected in the umbilical cord blood of ten babies born in August and September of 2004 in U.S. hospitals (averaging 200 chemicals and pollutants per infant). Of the 287 chemicals, 212 of which the federal government had already banned or severely restricted and many of which are found in consumer products such as stain repellants, fast-food packaging, clothes, and textiles, 180 are known carcinogens, 217 are toxic to the brain and nervous system, and 208 cause birth defects and abnormal development in animal tests (Houlihan et al. 2005). The study results led EWG to argue for more rigorous federal policies regarding industrial chemicals.

Another interesting approach to grassroots body burden testing occurred October 20, 2004, at the annual meeting of the Society of Environmental Journalists in Pittsburgh. Guest speaker Jack Spengler, one of the best-known specialists in air pollution and other environmental health effects, suggested that the journalists might learn a lot if he took hair samples at the beginning of the conference, tested them for mercury, and returned the results by the end of the conference. Spengler's staff took 199 samples, flew back to Boston to analyze them, and brought the results back in two days. Aggregate data were presented, and each individual could receive his or her personal burden data. The tests found high levels of mercury in many people, mostly correlated with older age and greater fish consumption; combined, those two factors accounted for 45 percent of the variance, with fish consumption being the stronger predictor. EPA's reference dose is one part per million for pregnant women, and one-fourth of the sample exceeded that. A Greenpeace survey of 1,149 people found similar data, with 21 percent of women between sixteen and forty-nine exceeding that level. Projecting from that data, we would expect 300,000–630,000 births per year of children at risk of mercury effect, mostly developmental (Spengler 2004). One might argue that Spengler's study is not grassroots because it was conducted solely by a researcher. But even if a community group did not do the study, its approach was based on supporting grassroots groups, and individual notification and rapid attention to personal data are hallmarks of a grassroots approach.

In addition to pushing for government policy and scientific research, one objective of these sorts of grassroots body burden studies is to personalize environmental issues. When people can examine their own burden of dangerous chemicals, they may be more likely to take both personal preventive action and broader social action for changes in corporate practices and public policy. Another objective is to show physicians the need to test people for dangerous chemicals.

But there is a caution necessary when dealing with this level of information. Unlike Spengler's study of mercury, a substance that has many clearly understood health effects, we do not always have clear evidence of the health effects associated with PBDEs and some other toxins. Hence, even some longstanding environmental health advocacy groups are concerned that providing much information may scare people. In the case of breast milk monitoring for PBDEs, they worry that some women will choose to not breastfeed as a result. In fact, strong advocates of such monitoring do make public statements about the relative benefits of breastfeeding. But for this and other body burden testing, it is crucial to understand that we don't always know how to use all the information we can get. Still, that is not necessarily a reason to hold off on such efforts. It's most likely that community-based environmental health groups will be the most prepared to grapple with the implications of such imperfect and potentially disturbing data.

Good Science, Bad Science, Censored Science

All the wonderful advances discussed here have come up against large barriers. Environmental health issues have been at the forefront of the recent government assault on science. Vigorous responses by environmental health scientists and advocates have offered the larger public health community an example of how important it is to counter such attacks.

Air quality research has been among the major targets. The antiregulatory stance of the Bush administration makes it unlikely that further air quality regulation will be produced during his term of office, based on the executive branch's claim that this science is far from conclusive. Instead, the administration has promised to study regulations broken by polluting industry, has weakened health standards and air pollution regulation, and has delayed the deadlines for removing fine particles from the air (Ledford 2004). Further, the Shelby Amendment of 1999 required researchers to turn over primary data to any party, a practice that gives corporations a major weapon in opposing environmental health research and also threatens the confidentiality of health data. Many have viewed this move as intended to quash critical research that can affect clean air regulation, and as a clear message from a conservative Congress that EPA's research and regulatory approach to air pollution was not going to be tolerated. The 2002 Federal Data Quality Act allows actors such as corporations or industry groups to force the government to halt regulation if a minor error is found anywhere in the volumes of research documents used in support of regulatory processes (Michaels et al. 2002).

Also in 2002, the Bush administration had the secretary of health and human services disband the National Human Research Protections Advisory Committee and the Advisory Committee on Genetic Testing, since religious right organizations considered those committees' advice on genetic testing and research threatening. In addition, the administration replaced fifteen of eighteen members of the Advisory Committee to the director of the National Center for Environmental Health (NCEH) at CDC at once, mostly with scientists long associated with chemical and oil industries and with records of opposition to environmental protection. Within the federal government, the NCEH has been one of the strongest forces for environmental health research and stronger regulation (Michaels et al. 2002). Then the administration removed NCEH director Richard Jackson. Similar purges have occurred on the President's Council on Bioethics and on NIH study sections (Steinbrook 2004). Similarly, the administration placed proindustry scientists on the Department of Health and Human Services Advisory Committee on Childhood Lead Poisoning Prevention, in order to oppose a planned review on what should constitute elevated blood levels of lead (Ferber 2002). Donald Kennedy (2003), the editor of *Science* and FDA commissioner in the Carter administration, has suggested that "loyalty tests" instead of scientific expertise are now required for members of federal science advisory panels.

Current practice on air pollution resembles the Bush administration's approach to global warming and climate change: Deny the reality of scientific consensus, express concern about economic costs, and stall by calling for more research. In 2003 when the EPA published a report on the state of the environment, the administration directed the agency to remove any discussion of climate change, another area that the overwhelming body of scientific evidence agrees on, claiming that the report would not address the complexities of the issue (Environmental Protection Agency 2003). Advisors to the president even demanded the removal of references to a National Research Council report previously cited by the president that indicated human contributions to global warming (Revkin and Seelye 2003). Eventually, even a conservative Republican EPA administrator, Christine Whitman, felt compelled to resign her office in the face of White House demands to tailor periodic mandated air quality reports to political ends, such as by deleting any mention of global warming. Federal Web sites have been stripped of data that can help contaminated communities locate pollution sources. The new director of NIEHS, who took office in 2005 (and who has since stepped down temporarily), has sought to cut out the environmental justice/community-based participatory research programs and to privatize *Environmental Health Perspectives*, a well-respected journal.

This conservative onslaught has pressed for opposition to class-action lawsuits on environmental matters (as well as on other health issues) and called into question much evidence for routine environmental regulation. Furthermore, it has expanded Daubert challenges—challenges to the legitimacy of scientific evidence presented in court based on the 1993 Supreme Court decision in *Daubert v. Merrell Dow*, a case regarding side effects of medication, which effectively made judges the gatekeepers of science. The *Daubert* ruling, which states that judges should allow only evidence that is relevant and reliable in the scientific community and that uses "generally accepted" scientific methods, has effectively barred many scientific experts from the courtroom and been viewed as an attack on science by allowing such experts to be rejected under allegations that their work was nothing more than "junk science" (Project on Scientific Knowledge and Public Policy 2003).

The routine process of evaluating hazard levels is a major public health task, and so in 2002 CDC's lead advisory committee prepared to review whether it was time to revise the recommended blood level as science gave us better information to act on. A few weeks before the deliberations, Health and Human Services secretary Tommy Thompson personally rejected new members of the advisory panel, the first time a secretary had ever done so. At the same time, Thompson filled the panel with people who had consulted for and testified for the lead paint industry, including one who argued that no health effects were found below 70 µg/dl (the current danger level is 10 µg/dl). Similar removals have occurred in countless other federal health panels. As for the panel members who are considered acceptable, one appointment to the FDA's reproductive health panel is an ob-gyn who refuses to prescribe contraceptives to unmarried women, and who recommends using Bible passages to treat PMS.

A further example of Bush administration interference concerned James Huff, a key scientist at the National Toxicology Program, responsible for testing chemicals that might otherwise never have been studied for their harmful effects. Apparently he was too diligent, and because the National Toxicology Program published much data on toxics, he was told that he could not publish anything without prior censorship and approval by NIH officials. Many scientists voiced their protest, and Huff's gag order was rescinded.

Early in this decade the Bush administration successfully gagged the EPA, preventing agency staff from publicly discussing the extent of perchlorate pollution, although research shows high levels of the rocket fuel component in water and food and the agency had recently recommended more stringent regulation in the face of widespread concern that concentrations over one part per billion were harmful to infants. Yet fears of liability for cleanups by the Pentagon and defense contractors triumphed, as industry and military leaders argued that perchlorate is safe in drinking water at levels as much as two hundred times higher than EPA recommendations. The White House went so far as to propose a bill in Congress that would exempt the Pentagon and defense industry from most potential liability on the ground of military necessity. The White House Office of Management and Budget, which has increasingly stepped in to halt scientific research, halted regulatory action, pending further review by the National Academy of Sciences. In the interim the EPA told staff not to speak about perchlorate, despite the clarity of the recent studies (Waldman 2003).

This assault on science has been so extensive that the Union of Concerned Scientists (UCS) published a widely cited report in February 2004 signed by twenty Nobel laureates and by former directors of the National Science Foundation, the National Institutes of Health, and some of the NIH Institutes. *Scientific Integrity in Policymaking* documents a long legacy of the Bush administration's assaults on science, and UCS members have traveled around the country discussing that problem.

These assaults on science and public health are so largely focused on environmental health that the field bears a special responsibility to lead the country in opposing them. Through their leadership in such defenses, environmental health scientists and advocates have shown many public health professionals how to act in similar circumstances.

Elements of a Theory and Framework

The issues I have discussed in this chapter provide us with a way to invigorate public health with concepts and applications from environmental health. Indeed, all this can work to bring public health full circle to its earliest years, when it was integrally connected with environmental concerns such as clean water, sanitation, and factory working conditions.

We require a *theory* that entails a holistic approach to health/environmental health, bringing a focus on all social sectors: health care, environmental regulation, transportation, occupational safety and health, urban development, housing, the built environment, school siting and environmental hazards in schools, sustainable development, and food security. Such a theory must begin with strong ethical components that respect both individuals and communities and make them a part of the whole public health enterprise.

We need a *policy* that is inclusive and precautionary, bringing stricter regulation that puts health above corporate profit and government ideology, greater enforcement of existing laws and regulations, disease registries, and health tracking. Precautionary approaches, such as those embodied in many European countries and the EU, need to play a larger role, from the municipal to the federal level. We need long-range planning to avoid the pitfalls of short-term advantage only to select actors.

We need a *practice* that not only brings the public into deep levels of participation but also is receptive to innovative methods and approaches by citizen-science alliances, such as air monitoring at peak traffic times and at children's heights. Scientists can continue to expand air monitoring in different settings, such as in the vicinity of large emitters that are escaping monitoring and adequate regulation. (For example, there are many endocrine disrupters and other chemicals that had not been tested until Silent Spring Institute did so, and there remains a lot to be done in this area.) Geographical information systems (GIS) have become one of the hottest new techniques, and because GIS is so useful for identifying multiple hazards in a community, along with land use and demographics, many activist groups have pioneered this technique. Scientists can learn a lot from these applications, especially in terms of characterizing hazards that are not part of routine regulatory observation. Environmental health activists have also pursued ecological levels of analysis, which use aggregate characteristics of communities, rather than solely individual exposures, to estimate health effects. Such measurements are often easier to obtain, since they do not require individual sampling, and they are sensible since they refer to community-level problems. Epidemiologists and other public health scientists have much to learn from this way of looking at environmental health.

So, across a variety of areas, environmental health scientists and activists have carried on classical traditions of a community-centered, hands-on, applied public health. They have updated such approaches when public health lost a good deal of its pioneering capacity, and they have added new elements to the public health toolkit. In this way environmental health offers a powerful vision for a democratic, precautionary public health.

Notes

1. For the Silent Spring Institute's *Cape Cod Breast Cancer and Environment Study Atlas*, see www.silentspring.org/newweb/atlas/index.html.

References

Akwesasne Research Advisory Committee. 1996. Akwesasne Good Mind Research Protocol. *Akwesasne Notes*, no. 21:94–110.

Alaska Community Action on Toxics. 1998. *Preventing Toxics in Alaska.* Anchorage: Alaska Community Action on Toxics. www.akaction.org/metadata/guide3.html.

Aleutian Pribilof Islands Association. 2007. About Us. www.apiai.com/about.asp? page=about.

Brown, P. 2007. *Toxic Exposures: Contested Illnesses and the Environmental Health Movement.* New York: Columbia University Press.

Brown, P., and E. J. Mikkelsen. 1990. *No Safe Place: Toxic Waste, Leukemia, and Community Action.* Berkeley: University of California Press.

Brown, P., S. Zavestoski, S. McCormick, J. Mandelbaum, T. Luebke, and M. Linder. 2001. A Gulf of Difference: Disputes over Gulf War-Related Illnesses. *Journal of Health and Social Behavior* 42:235–257.

Brown, P., S. Zavestoski, T. Luebke, J. Mandelbaum, S. McCormick, and B. Mayer. 2004. Clearing the Air and Breathing Freely: Disputes over Air Pollution and Asthma. *International Journal of Health Services* 34:39–63.

Bullard, R., G. S. Johnson, and A. O. Torres, eds. 2004. *Highway Robbery: Transportation Racism and New Routes to Equity.* Boston: South End Press.

Center for Health, Environment, and Justice. 2006. *Building Safe Schools: Invisible Threats, Visible Actions.* Falls Church, Va.: Center for Health, Environment, and Justice.

Centers for Disease Control and Prevention. 2003. Second National Report on Human Exposure to Environmental Chemicals. Atlanta: Centers for Disease Control and Prevention, National Center for Environmental Health.

———. 2005. Third National Report on Human Exposure to Environmental Chemicals. Atlanta: Centers for Disease Control and Prevention, National Center for Environmental Health.

Environmental Protection Agency. 2003. *Draft Report on the Environment.* www.epa. gov/indicators/roe/html/roeAirGlo.htm.

Environmental Working Group. 2003. *Body Burden: The Pollution in People.* Oakland, Calif.: Environmental Working Group.

Ferber, D. 2002. Overhaul of CDC Panel Revives Lead Safety Debate. *Science*, October 25.

Geiser, K. 2001. *Materials Matter: Toward a Sustainable Materials Policy.* Cambridge, Mass.: MIT Press.

Gibbs, L. 1981. *Love Canal: My Story.* Albany: State University of New York Press.

Gottlieb, R. 2002. *Environmentalism Unbound: Exploring New Pathways for Change.* Cambridge, Mass.: MIT Press.

Green, L., M. Fullilove, D. Evans, and P. Shepard. 2002. "Hey, Mom, thanks!" Use of Focus Groups in the Development of Place-Specific Materials for a Community Environmental Action Campaign. *Environmental Health Perspectives* 110 (Supplement. 2): 265–269.

Houlihan, J., T. Kropp, R. Wiles, S. Gray, and C. Campbell. 2005. *Body Burden—The Pollution in Newborns: A Benchmark Investigation of Industrial Chemicals, Pollutants, and Pesticides in Umbilical Cord Blood.* Oakland, Calif.: Environmental Working Group.

Hynes, H. P., and D. Brugge. 2000. Public Health and the Physical Environment in Boston Public Housing: A Community-Based Survey and Action Agenda. *Planning Research and Practice* 15:31–49.

Israel, B. A., A. J. Schulz, E. A. Parker, and A. B. Becker. 1998. Review of Community-Based Research: Assessing Partnership Approaches to Improve Public Health. *Annual Review of Public Health* 19:173–202.

Kennedy, D. 2003. An Epidemic of Politics. *Science*, January 31, 625.

Ledford, A. 2004. Foreword: The Dirty Secret behind Dirty Air. In *Dirty Air, Dirty Power: Mortality and Health Damage due to Pollution from Power Plants*, ed. C. Schneider. Boston: Clean Air Task Force.

Loh, P., J. Sugerman-Brozan, S. Wiggins, D. Noiles, and C. Archibald. 2002. From Asthma to AirBeat: Community-Driven Monitoring of Fine Particles and Black Carbon in Roxbury, Massachusetts. *Environmental Health Perspectives* 110 (Supplement 2): 297–301.

Mayer, B., P. Brown, and L. Linder. 2002. Moving Further Upstream: From Toxics Reduction to the Precautionary Principle. *Public Health Reports* 117:574–586.

McCormick, S., P. Brown, and S. Zavestoski. 2003. The Personal Is Scientific, the Scientific Is Political: The Environmental Breast Cancer Movement. *Sociological Forum* 18:545–576.

Michaels, D., E. Bingham, L. Boden, R. Clapp, L. R., Goldman, P. Hoppin, S. Krimsky, C. Monforton, D. Ozonoff, and A. Robbins. 2002. Advice without Dissent. *Science*, October 25.

Minkler, M., and N. Wallerstein, eds. 2003. *Community-Based Participatory Research for Health*. San Francisco: Jossey-Bass.

National Children's Study. 2005a. What Is the National Children's Study? Rockville, Md.: National Children's Study. nationalchildrensstudy.gov/about/mission/overview.cfm.

———. 2005b. What Makes This Study Different from Other U.S. Health Studies? Rockville, Md.: National Children's Study. nationalchildrensstudy.gov/about/mission/unique.cfm.

Nesmith, J. 2005. Children's Health Study in Need of Money. *Atlanta Journal-Constitution*, May 11.

Project on Scientific Knowledge and Public Policy. 2003. Daubert: The Most Influential Supreme Court Ruling You've Never Heard Of. Boston: Tellus Institute. www.defending science.org.

Revkin, A., and K. Seelye. 2003. Report by EPA Leaves Out Data on Climate Change. *New York Times*, June 19.

Rudel, R. A., D. E. Camann, J. D. Spengler, L. R. Korn, and J. G. Brody. 2003. Phthalates, Alkylphenols, Pesticides, Polybrominated Diphenyl Ethers, and Other Endocrine-Disrupting Compounds in Indoor Air and Dust. *Environmental Science and Technology* 37:4543–4553.

Sharp, R., and S. Lunder. 2004. *High Levels of Toxic Fire Retardants Contaminate American Homes*. Oakland, Calif.: Environmental Working Group.

Shepard, P. M., M. E. Northridge, S. Prakash, and G. Stover. 2002. Preface: Advancing Environmental Justice through Community-Based Participatory Action Research. *Environmental Health Perspectives* 110:139–144.

Shutkin, W. 2001. *The Land That Could Be: Environmentalism and Democracy in the Twenty-first Century*. Cambridge, Mass.: MIT Press.

Spengler, Jack. 2004. Persistent Organic Pollutants. Presentation. Silent Spring Institute, Newton, Mass. November 30.

Steinbrook, R. 2004. Science, Politics, and Federal Advisory Committees. *New England Journal of Medicine*, April 13, 1454–1460.

Steingraber, S. 2001. *Having Faith: An Ecologist's Journey to Motherhood*. New York: Perseus.

Tickner, J. 1999. A Map toward Precautionary Decision Making. In *Protecting Public Health and the Environment: Implementing the Precautionary Principle*, ed. C. Raffensperger and J. Tickner, 162–186. Washington, D.C.: Island Press.

Trust for America's Health. 2005a. Health Tracking Network. Washington, D.C.: Trust for America's Health. healthyamericans.org/topics/index.php?TopicID=28.

———. 2005b. Nationwide Health Tracking: Investigating Life-Saving Discoveries. Washington, D.C.: Trust for America's Health. healthyamericans.org/reports/files/HealthTrackingBackgrounder.pdf.

U.S. Department of Health and Human Services. 1990. *Healthy People 2000: Understanding and Improving Health*. Washington, D.C.: Department of Health and Human Services.

———. 2001. *Healthy People 2010: Understanding and Improving Health*. Washington, D.C.: Department of Health and Human Services.

Waldman, P. 2003. EPA Bans Staff from Discussing Issue of Perchlorate Pollution. *Wall Street Journal*, April 28.

Woonasquatucket River Watershed Council. 2007. About Us. www.woonasquatucket.org/aboutus.htm.

Zones, J. S. 2000. Profits from Pain: The Political Economy of Breast Cancer. In *Breast Cancer: Society Shapes an Epidemic*, ed. A. S. Kasper and S. J. Ferguson, 119–152. New York: St. Martin's.

Paternalism and Its Discontents

Motorcycle Helmet Laws, Libertarian Values, and Public Health

In the face of overwhelming epidemiological evidence that motorcycle helmets reduce accident deaths and injuries, state legislatures in the United States have rolled back motorcycle helmet regulations during the past thirty years. From the jaws of public health victory, the states have snatched defeat. There are many ways to account for the historical arc; we focus here on the enduring impact libertarian and antipaternalistic values may have on U.S. public health policy.

Currently, only twenty states, the District of Columbia, and Puerto Rico require all motorcycle riders to wear helmets. In another twenty-seven states, mandatory helmet laws apply only to minors (aged younger than eighteen years or twenty-one years depending on the state), and three states—Colorado, Illinois, and Iowa—have no motorcycle helmet laws. Additionally, six of the twenty-seven states with minor-only helmet laws require that adult riders have $10,000 of insurance coverage or that helmets be worn during the first year of riding (National Highway Traffic Safety Administration 2006). This uneven patchwork of state regulations on motorcycle helmet use contrasts dramatically with the picture thirty years ago, when forty-seven states, the District of Columbia, and Puerto Rico had passed mandatory helmet laws that applied to all riders (de Wolf 1986; Preusser, Hedlund, and Ulmer 2000).[1] The repeal of motorcycle helmet laws has occurred as the United States has moved toward greater statutory regulation of automobile safety. During the past twenty years, every state except New Hampshire has enacted a mandatory seatbelt law, and since 1998, the National Highway Traffic Safety Administration (NHTSA) has required that all new cars sold in the United States be equipped with dual air bags (National Highway Traffic Safety Administration 2004; Kahane 1996).

The repeal of motorcycle helmet laws in the United States contradicts a global movement toward enacting mandatory helmet laws; as of 2003, at least twenty-nine countries—including most European Union countries, the Russian Federation, Iceland, and Israel—had passed mandatory helmet laws for motorcycles. Developing countries, including Thailand and Nepal, also have passed helmet laws in recent years. Varying levels of enforcement and other factors, such as the general safety and quality of the roads, influence the effectiveness of these laws in different countries (World Health Organization 2005).[2] In 1991, the World Health Organization launched a global helmet initiative to encourage motorcycle and bicycle helmet usage worldwide (World Health Organization 2003). Why then have things taken such a different turn in the United States? We conducted a historical examination of the debates on motorcycle helmet laws in the United States to answer this question. In reporting the results, we address tensions between paternalism and libertarian values in the public health arena—tensions that have come to the fore recently with developments in tobacco policy. As efforts to articulate an ethics of public health advance, it is crucial to address the question of paternalism. The history of motorcycle helmet legislation provides a unique vantage point on that issue.

The Origin of Motorcycle Helmet Laws

Motorcycle racers used crash helmets as early as the 1920s. Helmets were more widely used during World War II, when Hugh Cairns, a consulting neurosurgeon to the British army, recommended mandatory helmet use for British service dispatch riders, who carried instructions and battle reports between commanders and the front lines via motorcycles (Cairns 1952). Cairns first became concerned about helmet use after treating the war hero T. E. Lawrence—Lawrence of Arabia—for a fatal head injury suffered during a 1935 motorcycle accident. Cairns later published several landmark articles that used clinical case reports to show that motorcycle crash helmets mitigated the severity of head injuries suffered by military motorcyclists during crashes (Maartens, Wills, and Adams 2002; Cairns 1941, 1946; Cairns and Holbourn 1943).

After World War II, the British government's Ministry of Transport became the first regulatory agency in the world to establish research-based motorcycle helmet performance standards. During the early 1950s, the ministry offered the British Standards Institute "kite mark" (a diamond-shaped seal) as an indicator of helmet quality and performance (Becker 1998). In the United States, however, no such standard existed, and ads for American motorcycles invariably showed riders without helmets or goggles. The initial market for these bikes included returning veterans who had learned to ride military-issue Harley-Davidsons while overseas (Fuglsang 1997; Krens and Drutt 1998). During the late 1940s and early 1950s, motorcycle clubs created an outlaw masculine social identity around motorbikes—part of an emerging cultural reaction to the social confines of 1950s suburbia. At the same time, the motorcycle took its place amid the variety of new postwar consumer culture offerings, and many young men took up riding motorcycles as a weekend hobby (Fuglsang 1997).

The 1966 National Highway Safety Act introduced drastic and unwelcome changes to U.S. motorcycle culture. The law, which was introduced after the 1965 publication of *Unsafe at Any Speed*, Ralph Nader's scathing indictment of the U.S. auto industry's vehicle safety standards, included a provision that withheld federal funding for highway safety programs to states that did not enact mandatory motorcycle helmet laws within a specified time frame. This provision was added after a study showed that helmet laws would significantly decrease the rate of fatal accidents. The National Highway Safety Act passed without debate on the helmet law provision (House Committee on Public Works and Transportation 1975). Adoption of this measure drew upon a broader movement within public health to expand its purview beyond infectious disease to "prevention of disability and postponement of untimely death" (Rutstein 1965). Several years later, this shift sparked debate on the role of both individual and collective behaviors in contemporary patterns of morbidity and mortality, which led to Marc Lalonde's *New Perspective on the Health of Canadians* (1974), the U.S. government's *Healthy People* report (1979), and, most famously, John H. Knowles's controversial but agenda-setting article, "The Responsibility of the Individual," which asserted that individual lifestyle choices determined the major health risks for Western society (Knowles 1977).

As of 1966, only three states—New York, Massachusetts, and Michigan—and Puerto Rico had passed motorcycle helmet laws, but between 1967 and 1975, nearly every state passed statutes to avoid penalties under the National Highway Safety Act. By September 1975, California was the only state that had not passed a mandatory helmet law of any kind. This resistance carried weight, because California had both the highest number of registered motorcyclists and the highest number of fatal motorcycle crashes (Kraus, Peek, and Williams 1995). Additionally, motorcycle groups in the state had developed into a powerful antihelmet lobby. State legislators made eight attempts between 1968 and 1975 to introduce helmet legislation, but they were thwarted by vocal opposition from the motorcycle groups (Pullen 1975). In September 1973, when a Burbank councilman proposed a mandatory motorcycle helmet ordinance after the death of a fifteen-year-old motorcyclist, more than a hundred motorcyclists came to the council's chamber to protest during hearings on the ordinance. The *Los*

Angeles Times reported that the Hells Angels planned to bring "at least 500 members" on the day of the scheduled vote. The councilman then withdrew his proposed ordinance (Quinn 1973a,b).

Constitutional Challenges to Mandatory Helmet Laws

As soon as states began to pass mandatory helmet laws, opponents mounted constitutional challenges to them. Some challenges involved appeals in criminal cases against motorcyclists who had been arrested for failing to wear helmets; others were civil suits brought by motorcyclists who alleged that the laws deprived them of their rights. Between 1968 and 1970, high courts in Colorado, Hawaii, Louisiana, Missouri, Massachusetts, New Jersey, North Carolina, North Dakota, Ohio, Oregon, Tennessee, Texas, Vermont, Washington, and Wisconsin and lower courts in New York all rejected challenges to the constitutionality of their state motorcycle helmet laws.[3] In June 1972, a U.S. district court in Massachusetts similarly rejected a challenge to the state's helmet law that was brought on federal constitutional grounds, and in November of that year, the U.S. Supreme Court affirmed this decision on appeal without opinion (*Simon v. Sargent* 1972).

The constitutional challenges focused principally on two arguments: (1) helmet statutes violated the equal protection clause of the Fourteenth Amendment or state constitutional equivalents by discriminating against motorcycle riders as a class; and (2) helmet statutes constituted an infringement of the motorcyclist's liberty and an excessive use of the state's police power under the due process clause of the Fourteenth Amendment or similar state provisions. Only the Illinois Supreme Court and the Michigan Appeals Court accepted these arguments. The Illinois Supreme Court ruled that the helmet laws constituted an infringement on motorcyclists' rights.

> If the evil sought to be remedied by the statute affects public health, safety, morals or welfare, a means reasonably directed toward the achievement of those ends will be held to be a proper exercise of the police power [citations omitted]. However, [t]he legislature may not, of course, under the guise of protecting the public interest, interfere with private rights [citations omitted]. . . . The manifest function of the headgear requirement in issue is to safeguard the person wearing it—whether it is the operator or a passenger—from head injuries. Such a laudable purpose, however, cannot justify the regulation of what is essentially a matter of personal safety. (*People v. Fries* 1969, 450)

The Michigan Appeals Court heard a case brought by the American Motorcycle Association, then the country's largest organization for motorcyclists, which argued that the state's motorcycle law violated the due process, equal protection, and right to privacy provisions of the federal Constitution. The association cited the U.S. Supreme Court's birth control decision in *Griswold v. Connecticut* as authority for establishing a right to privacy. The state attorney general contended that the law did not just concern individual rights and was intended to promote public health, safety, and welfare. Furthermore, the state argued that it had an interest in the "viability" of its citizens and could pass legislation "to keep them healthy and self-supporting." The appeals court, however, countered that "this logic could lead to unlimited paternalism" and found the statute unconstitutional. The court also rejected the claim that the state's power to regulate the highways provided the basis for imposing helmet use. "There can be no doubt that the State has a substantial interest in highway safety . . . but the difficulty with adopting this as a basis for decision is that it would also justify a requirement that automobile drivers wear helmets or buckle their seatbelts for their own protection!" (*American Motorcycle Association v. Department of State Police* 1968, 357).

The plaintiff in the Massachusetts District Court case used an argument nearly identical to those that had been successful in Illinois and Michigan: A helmet law was designed solely to protect the motorcyclist (*Simon v. Sargent* 1972, 278). The plaintiff's argument cited John Stuart Mill's assertion that "the only part of the conduct of anyone, for which he is amenable to society, is that which concerns others." The district court rejected this line of reasoning. Although it relied on Mill's distinction between self-regarding and other-regarding behavior, the court clearly found injuries that resulted from motorcycle riders failing to wear a helmet to be other-regarding harms. Even more striking was that the court found the psychological burden on caregivers to be an other-regarding basis for intervention.

> For while we agree with plaintiff that the act's only realistic purpose is the prevention of head injuries incurred in motorcycle mishaps, we cannot agree that the consequences of such injuries are limited to the individual who sustains the injury. In view of the evidence warranting a finding that motorcyclists are especially prone to serious head injuries . . . the public has an interest in minimizing the resources directly involved. From the moment of the injury, society picks the person up off the highway; delivers him to a municipal hospital and municipal doctors; provides him with unemployment compensation if, after recovery, he cannot replace his lost job; and, if the injury causes permanent disability, may assume the responsibility for his and his family's continued subsistence. We do not

understand a state of mind that permits plaintiff to think that only he himself is concerned. (*Simon v. Sargent* 1972, 279)

Although others echoed the Massachusetts decision by using economic—utilitarian—arguments to reject constitutional challenges to helmet laws, some courts upheld motorcycle statutes on the basis of the narrow ground that helmet use affects the safety of other motorists. A Florida U.S. district court held that a requirement for motorcyclists to wear both helmets and eye protection was not an unreasonable exercise of state police power because "[a] flying object could easily strike the bareheaded cyclist and cause him to lose control of his vehicle," and "the wind or an insect flying into the cyclist's eyes could create a hazard to others on the highway" (*Bogue v. Faircloth* 1970, 489).

The Biker Lobby Roars into Action

Motorcyclists had long been organized—whether they belonged to informal clubs, racing associations under the aegis of the American Motorcycle Association, or outlaw biker gangs, such as the Hells Angels—and the passage of motorcycle helmet laws galvanized the groups to become political. During the 1970s, the American Motorcycle Association, which was founded in 1924 as a hobbyist group, organized a lobbying arm to "coordinate national legal activity against unconstitutional and discriminatory laws against motorcyclists, to serve as a sentinel on federal and state legislation affecting motorcyclists, and to be instrumental as a lobbying force for motorcyclists and motorcycling interests" (American Motorcyclist Association n.d.). Additionally, those who identified with the biker culture, including members of outlaw motorcycle gangs and thousands of other men who rode choppers (modified motorcycles with high handlebars and custom detailing), became involved in state-level and national-level groups that advocated the repeal of helmet laws and other limitations to riding motorcycles (Fuglsang 1997). In its October 1971 issue, *Easyriders*, a glossy magazine for chopper riders, underscored the need for a national effort.

> You, as an individual, can stand on your roof-top shouting to the world about how unjust, how stupid, and how unconstitutional some of the recently passed, or pending, bike laws are—but all you will accomplish is to get yourself arrested for disturbing the peace. Individual bike clubs can go before city councils, state legislatures, and congressional committees, but as single clubs, and unprofessional at the game of politics, their efforts are usually futile. . . . We need a national organization of bikers. An organization united together in a common endeavor, and in

sufficient numbers to be heard in Washington, DC, in the state legislatures, and even down to the city councils.[4]

The article went on to ask for three-dollar donations to the National Custom Cycle Association, a nonprofit organization established by the magazine. By the following February, the organization had members in forty-four states and had changed its name to ABATE (A Brotherhood Against Totalitarian Enactments).

Other state-level groups, which called themselves motorcyclists' rights organizations, also began to form around the country. The Modified Motorcycle Association, a group of chopper riders founded in 1973 that eschewed the outlaw behavior of Hells Angels, engaged in both antihelmet law political activity and local campaigns against police harassment of bikers (Modified Motorcycle Organization of California n.d.; Dodson 1981).

In 1975, these groups began to turn the tide against proponents of mandatory helmet laws. Motorcyclists, who had only thus far been successful in the appellate courts of two states and in stopping helmet bills in California, had evolved into an organized and powerful national lobby. In June and again in September 1975, hundreds of bikers descended on Washington, D.C., where they rode their choppers around the U.S. Capitol to protest mandatory helmet laws. In the post-Watergate environment, motorcyclists found a newly receptive ear in Congress (Cronin 1980). Representatives of ABATE, the American Motorcycle Association, the Modified Motorcycle Association, and other motorcyclists' rights organizations were invited to hearings held in July 1975 by the House Committee on Public Works and Transportation to discuss revisions to the National Highway Safety Act.

Recognizing that proponents of motorcycle helmet laws, in the tradition of public health, had used statistical evidence of injury and death to make their case, the first motorcyclist to speak at these hearings, Bruce Davey of the Virginia chapter of ABATE, opened with a frontal attack on such data. He charged that NHTSA had manipulated evidence about the effectiveness of motorcycle helmets. Furthermore, he asserted that helmets actually increased the likelihood of neck injuries (House Committee on Public Works and Transportation 1975, 401). Davey then advanced a series of constitutional claims that were rooted in an antipaternalistic ethic enshrined a concept of personal liberty and that bore a striking similarity to those that had failed in the judicial arena. In an argument more reflective of cultural attitudes than of legal precision, he stated: "The Ninth Amendment [to the U.S. Constitution] says no law shall be enacted that regulates the individual's freedom to choose his personal actions and mode of dress so long as it does not in any way affect the life, liberty, and happiness of others. We are being forced to wear a particular type of apparel because we choose to ride motorcycles" (House Committee on Public Works and Transportation 1975, 373).

Not surprisingly, the issue of choice emerged as the central theme in the arguments of those opposed to helmet laws, similar to the arguments of women's reproductive rights advocates. Just as proponents of legalized abortion had argued that they were not pro-abortion but were in favor of a woman's right to choose whether to terminate a pregnancy, ABATE chapter literature from Washington, like that in other states, declared that "ABATE does not advocate that you ride without a helmet when the law is repealed, only that you have the right to decide."

At the end of the hearings, Representatives James Howard (D-NJ) and Bud Schuster (R-PA) said they would support revisions to the National Highway Safety Act that removed the tie between federal funding and state helmet laws. Stewart McKinney (R-CT), an avid motorcyclist who had already introduced a bill in the House that included these revisions, remarked: "My personal philosophy concerning helmets can be summed up in three words. It's my head. Personally, I would not get on a 55-mile-per-hour highway without my helmet. But the fact of the matter is that if I did, I wouldn't be jeopardizing anyone but myself, and I feel that being required to wear a helmet is an infringement on my personal liberties" (House Committee on Public Works and Transportation, 387).

The prospect of ending a threat to withdraw highway funds attracted the notice of liberal senator Alan Cranston (D-CA), who signed on as a cosponsor of a Senate bill introduced by archconservative senators Jesse Helms (R-NC) and James Abourezk (R-SD). On December 13, 1975, the Senate voted 52 to 37 to approve a bill that revised the National Highway Safety Act. The House passed a similar measure. The revisions were incorporated into a massive $17.5 billion bill for increasing highway funds to the states, and President Gerald Ford signed the bill on May 5, 1976 (Young 1975; *Los Angeles Times* 1975, 1976; Cookro 1979).

Helmetless Riders: An Unplanned Public Health Experiment

During the next four years, twenty-eight states repealed their mandatory helmet laws. The consequences of these repeals were most succinctly expressed in the September 7, 1978, *Chicago Tribune* headline "Laws Eased, Cycle Deaths Soar." Overall, deaths from motorcycle accidents increased 20 percent, from 3,312 in 1976 to 4,062 in 1977 (Peterson 1978). In 1978, NHTSA administrator Joan Claybrook wrote to the governors of states that had repealed their laws and urged them to reinstate the enactments. She cited studies that showed motorcycle fatalities were three to nine times higher among helmetless riders compared with helmeted riders and that head injury rates had increased steeply in states where helmet laws had been repealed (*Wall Street Journal* 1979; Holsendolph 1979; Preusser, Hedlund, and Ulmer 2000). "Now that some states have repealed such legislation we have control and experimental groups which when compared show that one of the rights enhanced by repeal is the right to die in motorcycle deaths," opined an editorialist in the June 1979 issue of the *North Carolina Medical Journal*.

Those concerned about public health viewed the unfolding events with alarm. In the June 1980 issue of the *American Journal of Public Health*, Susan Baker, an epidemiologist and director of the Johns Hopkins Injury Prevention Center, compared the situation to one where "scientists, having found a successful treatment for a disease, were impelled to further prove its efficacy by stopping the treatment and allowing the disease to recur" (Baker 1980, 573). Invoking the 1905 U.S. Supreme Court decision in *Jacobson v. Massachusetts* that upheld compulsory immunization statutes, Baker asserted that the state had the authority to limit individual liberty to protect the public's health and the rights of others. In a reprise of arguments made a decade earlier when helmet laws were under constitutional attack, Baker emphasized the social burden created by motorcycle accidents and fatalities.

In 1981, the *American Journal of Public Health* published a counterpoint to Baker's editorial, which was unusual in that it came from a public health official. Richard Perkins of New Mexico's Health and Environment Department attacked the argument that the motorcyclist was reducing the freedom of others by not wearing a helmet as "so ridiculous as to be ammunition for the anti-helmet law forces." Noting that there were no helmet laws for rodeo contestants and rock climbers, he argued that laws should consider not only safety but also "such intangible consequences as potential loss of opportunity for individual fulfillment and loss of social vitality" (Perkins 1981, 294, 295).

Baker and Stephen Teret's rebuttal to Perkins stated that his argument "implies that if policy is not applied at the outer limits of a continuum of circumstances, it would be unreasonable to apply that policy at any point along the continuum" (Baker and Teret 1981, 295). They defended their reliance on *Jacobson v. Massachusetts* by pointing out that the decision has been used as a precedent for decisions that cover "manifold" restraints on liberty for the common good beyond the scope of contagious disease.

During the next decade, evidence of the human and social costs of repeal continued to mount. Medical costs among helmetless riders increased 200 percent compared with helmeted riders, and in some states, helmetless riders were more likely to be uninsured (Watson, Zador, and Wilks 1980; McSwain and

Petrucelli 1987; Scholten and Glober 1984; Chenier and Evans 1987; Lloyd, Lauderdale, and Betz 1987; Evans and Frick 1988). The April 1987 issue of *Texas Medicine* published an editorial entitled "How Many Deaths Will It Take?" The editorial exemplified the growing frustration among physicians, epidemiologists, and public health officials with legislatures that failed to act on evidence that showed helmet law repeals increased fatalities and serious injuries. "I invite our legislators and those opposed to helmet laws to spend a few nights in our busy emergency rooms," wrote the author, who was the chief of neurosurgery at Ben Taub General Hospital in Houston. "Let them talk to a few devastated mothers and fathers of sons with severe head injuries—many of whom will needlessly die or remain severely disabled." Posing a challenge to the antipaternalism that had inspired the repeal of laws, he contended that "[a] civilized society makes laws not only to protect a person from his fellowman, but also sometimes from himself as well" (Nayaran 1987, 5).

Other studies adopted a more narrowly economic perspective on the impact of helmet law repeals. In a 1983 article, researchers sponsored by the Insurance Institute for Highway Safety used mathematical models to estimate the number of excess deaths—those that would not have occurred had the motorcyclist been wearing a helmet—in the twenty-eight states that had repealed their helmet laws by 1980. They then conducted an economic analysis of the costs to society as a result of these deaths. This cost calculation incorporated direct costs (emergency services, hospital and medical expenses, legal and funeral expenses, and insurance and government administrative costs) and indirect costs (the value of the lost earnings and services due to the death of the person). The researchers found that the costs totaled at least $176.6 million (Hartunian et al. 1983).

In Europe, meanwhile, where helmet laws were being enacted for the first time, studies were showing an opposite trend. In Italy, where a compulsory motorcycle helmet law went into effect in 1986, a group of researchers compared the accidents in one district (Cagliari) during the five months before and the five months after the law's enactment. They found a 30 percent reduction in motorcycle accidents and an overall reduction in head injuries and deaths (Nurchi et al. 1987).

Helmet Laws in the Congress Once Again

In May 1989, against a backdrop of thirty-four states adopting mandatory automobile seatbelt laws, Senator John Chafee (R-RI) held a news conference to announce he was introducing a bill—the National Highway Fatality and Injury Reduction Act of 1989—that would empower the U.S. Department of Transportation to withhold up to 10 percent of federal highway aid from any state that did not require motorcyclists to wear helmets and front-seat automobile passengers to wear seatbelts (Senate Committee on Environment and Public Works 1989; Dosa 1989; Greene 1989). The conference was strategically held during a meeting of the American Trauma Society.

A hearing on the bill that was held by the Senate Committee on Environment and Public Works in October 1989 provided yet one more opportunity to engage (in a federal forum) the argument about the potential benefits that would result from the enactment of mandatory helmet laws and the deep philosophical issues such laws raised. As had others before him, Senator Daniel Patrick Moynihan (D-NY) sought to compare the imposition of helmet requirements with the public health justification for compulsory immunization. Senator James Jeffords (R-VT) responded with an invocation of the antipaternalistic argument so resonant in American political culture.

> Would you urge us then, at the Federal level, to mandate diets and to investigate homes as far as diets are concerned? We would save a lot more money if we had good nutrition in this country. Do you think that is a proper role of the government? . . . I think there is a vast difference in vaccination, where you are subjecting others to a health problem, . . . where you are trying to protect the individual health of someone who is in a sense endangering himself and not the public. I grant the arguments are there on cost, but the arguments are there on cost in nutrition, as well. I have a hard time, philosophically, accepting that the role of the government is to tell us how to lead our lives. Why don't we have motorcycle riders wear armored suits? Where do you draw the line? It is my understanding that the largest percentage of injuries are not by head, but are injuries to the chest and the abdominal areas and things like that. So where do you stop? (Senate Committee on Environment and Public Works 1989, 18–19)

Senator Jeffords's comments were echoed by Robert Ford, chair of Massachusetts Freedom First, an auto group that had led a successful campaign to repeal the state's seatbelt law. Ford did not quibble with statistics that showed seatbelts make people safer. Instead, he argued that the issue was about fundamental individual liberty.

> We do not want to be told how to behave in matters of personal safety. We do not want to be forced to wear seatbelts or helmets because others think that it is good for us. We do not want to be forced to eat certain diets because some think that it too may be good for us, reduce deaths and medical costs, and make us more productive citizens. We do not

want to be forced to give up certain pastimes simply because some may
feel they entail any amount of unnecessary risk. (Senate Committee on
Environment and Public Works 1989, 70–71)

Instead of confronting the moral arguments made by opponents of helmet
laws, proponents of such measures sought once again to marshal the compelling
force of evidence. In 1991, at the request of Senator Moynihan, the General
Accounting Office issued a comprehensive report that documented the toll. The
report reviewed forty-six studies and found that they overwhelmingly showed
helmet use rose and fatalities and serious injuries plummeted after enactment of
mandatory universal helmet laws (General Accounting Office 1991).

Despite the fierce opposition of motorcycle groups, Senator Chafee ultimately succeeded in getting the motorcycle helmet law and seatbelt law provisions added to a major highway funding bill that was passed in December 1991.
Under the law—which was far less punitive than the one Senator Chafee had
originally proposed—states that failed to pass helmet laws would have 3 percent
of their highway funds withheld (Curtin 1996).

Reenactment and Repeal

In 1991, the momentum seemed to be turning in favor of state motorcycle
helmet laws. For the first time in its history, California enacted a universal
mandatory helmet law, which took effect on January 1, 1992 (Bishop 1992).
However, this brief moment of public health optimism was short-lived. In 1995,
after the "Gingrich revolution" in which conservative Republicans took control
of Congress, the national motorcycle lobby succeeded in getting the federal
3 percent highway safety fund penalties repealed (Hess 1995). In 1997, after
pressure from state-level motorcycle activists, Arkansas and Texas repealed
their universal helmet laws and instead required helmets only for riders aged
younger than twenty-one years. These repeals were followed by similar actions
in Kentucky (1998), Louisiana (1999), Florida (2000), and Pennsylvania (2003).
In a move that gave credence to the well-worn claim about the social costs of
private choice, several of the new laws required riders to have $10,000 of med-
ical insurance coverage policy before they could ride helmetless.

This new round of repeals of motorcycle helmet laws produced a predictable series of studies, with all too predictable results: In Arkansas and
Texas, helmet use decreased significantly, head injuries increased, and fatalities
rose by 21 percent and 31 percent, respectively (Preusser, Hedlund, and Ulmer
2000). In 2003, a study of Louisiana and Kentucky fatalities found that after
repeal of helmet laws, there was a 50 percent increase in fatalities in Kentucky

and a 100 percent increase in fatalities in Louisiana. In 2005, the Insurance Institute for Highway Safety released a study that showed Florida's helmet law repeal had led to a 25 percent increase in fatalities in 2001 and 2002 compared with the two years before the repeal (Associated Press 2005).

Embracing Paternalism

Over the past thirty years, helmet law advocates have gathered a mountain of evidence to support their claims that helmet laws reduce motorcycle accident fatalities and severe injuries. Thanks to the rounds of helmet law repeals, advocates have been able to conclusively prove the converse as well: helmet law repeals increase fatalities and the severity of injuries. But the antihelmet law activists have had three decades of experience fighting helmet laws, and they have learned that their strategy of tirelessly lobbying state legislators can work. As one activist wrote: "I learned that the world is run by those who bother to show up to run it" (Ray 1998). More important, they have learned a lesson about how persuasive unadorned appeals to libertarian values can be.

This history of motorcycle helmet laws in the United States illustrates the profound impact of individualism on American culture and the manner in which this ideological perspective can have a crippling impact on the practice of public health. Although the opponents of motorcycle helmet laws seek to shape evidence to buttress their claims, abundant data make it clear—and have done so for almost three decades—that in the absence of mandatory motorcycle helmet laws, preventable deaths and great suffering will continue to occur. The NHTSA estimated that 10,838 additional lives could have been saved between 1984 and 2004 had all riders and passengers worn helmets (National Highway Traffic Safety Administration 2006). The success of those who oppose such statutes shows the limits of evidence in shaping policy when strongly held ideological commitments are at stake.

Early on in the battles over helmet laws, advocates for mandatory measures placed great stress on the social costs of riding helmetless. The courts, too, have often adopted claims about such costs as they upheld the constitutionality of statutes that impose helmet requirements. Whatever the merit of such a perspective, it involved a transparent attempt to mask the extent to which concerns for the welfare of cyclists themselves were the central motivation for helmet laws. The inability to successfully and consistently defend these measures for what they were—acts of public health paternalism—was an all but fatal limitation.

The recent trend toward motorcycle helmet laws that cover minors, however, shows that legislators and some antihelmet law forces have accepted a role for paternalism in this debate. The need for a law that governs minors shows a tacit acknowledgment that (1) motorcycle helmets reduce deaths and injuries and (2) the state has a role in protecting vulnerable members of society from misjudgments about motorcycle safety. Ironically, then, it is the states within which the motorcycle lobby has been most effective that have most directly engaged paternalist concerns.

The challenge for public health is to expand on this base of justified paternalism and to forthrightly argue in the legislative arena that adults and adolescents need to be protected from their poor judgments about motorcycle helmet use. In doing so, public health officials might well point to the fact that paternalistic protective legislation is part of the warp and woof of public health practice in America. Certainly, a host of legislation—from seatbelt laws to increasingly restrictive tobacco measures—is aimed at protecting the people from self-imposed injuries and avoidable harm.

With the latest round of helmet law repeals, motorcycle helmet use has dropped precipitately to 58 percent nationwide, and fatalities have risen (National Highway Traffic Safety Administration 2006). Need anything more be said to show that motorcyclists have not been able to make sound safety decisions on their own and that mandatory helmet laws are needed to ensure their safety?

Notes

1. The forty-seven state statutes marked the high water point for mandatory helmet legislation, reached between September 1, 1975, and May 1, 1976. They do not include Utah, which in the 1970s required helmets only on roads with a speed limit of thirty-five miles per hour or higher.

2. The article reports a study showing that Thailand's helmet law has failed to reduce fatalities by motorcycle accidents partly because helmet quality is unregulated and proper helmet usage is not enforced.

3. State appeals or supreme courts have found mandatory motorcycle helmet laws to be a constitutional exercise of police power in: *Love v. Bell*, 171 Colo. 27, 465 P. 2d 118 (Colo. 1970); *Hawaii v. Lee*, 51 Haw. 516, 465 P. 2d 573 (Hawaii 1970); *Missouri v. Cushman*, 451 S.W. 2d 17 (Mo. 1970); *North Carolina v. Anderson*, 275 N.C. 168, 166 S.E. 2d 49 (1969); *New Jersey v. Krammes*, 105 N.J. Super. 345, 252 A. 2d 223 (1969); *North Dakota v. Odegaard*, 165 N.W. 2d 677 (N.D. 1969); *Ohio v. Craig*, 19 Ohio App. 2d 29, 249 N.E. 2d 75 (1969); *Oregon v. Fetterly*, 254 Ore. 47, 456 P. 2d 996 (Ore. 1969); *Arutanoff v. Metro Government of Nashville and Davidson County*, 223 Tenn. 535, 448 S.W. 2d 408 (Tenn. 1969); *Ex parte Smith*, 441 S.W. 2d 544 (Tex. Cr. App. 1969); *Vermont v. Solomon*, 128 Vt. 197, 260 A. 2d 377 (Vt. 1969); *Washington v. Laitinen*, 77 Wash. 2d 130, 459 P. 2d 789 (Wash. 1969); *Bisenius v. Karns*, 42 Wis. 2d 42, 165 N.W. 2d 377 (1969); *Overheard v. City of New Orleans*, 253 La. 285, 217 So. 2d 400 (1969); *Com. v. Howie*, 354 Mass. 769, 238 N.E. 2d 373 (Mass. 1968). State appeals or high courts have found mandatory motorcycle helmet laws to be unconstitutional in *People v. Fries*, 42 Ill. 2d 446, 250 N.E. 2d 149 (1969), and *American Motorcycle Association v. Department of State Police*, Docket No. 4,445, Court of Appeals of Michigan, 11 Mich. App. 351; 158 N.W. 2d 72.

4. From "Street Legal Chopper: Circa 1973?" reprinted from *Easyriders*, October 1971; *www.bikerrogue.com/articles/biker_rights/history_of_abate/history_of_abate.htm* (accessed December 17, 2006).

References

American Motorcycle Association v. Department of State Police. 1968. 11 Mich. App. 351.

American Motorcylist Association. N.d. The History of the AMA. *www.amadirectlink.com/whatis/history.asp* (accessed December 17, 2006).

Baker, Susan P. 1980. On Lobbies, Liberty, and the Public Good. *American Journal of Public Health* 70:573.

Associated Press. Deaths Up since Florida Helmet Law Repealed. 2005. August 10. *www.msnbc.msn.com/id/1341966* (accessed October 20, 2006).

Baker, Susan P. 1980. On Lobbies, Liberty, and the Public Good. *American Journal of Public Health* 70:573–575.

Baker, Susan P., and Stephen P. Teret. 1981. Freedom and Protection: A Balancing of Interests. *American Journal of Public Health* 71:295–296.

Becker, Edward B. 1998. Helmet Development and Standards. In *Frontiers in Head and Neck Trauma: Clinical and Biomedical*, ed. N. Yoganandan, F. A. Pintar, S. J. Larson, and A. Sances Jr. Burke, Va.: IOS Press.

Bishop, Katherine. 1992. California's Helmetless Ride Is Over, but Not the Debate. *New York Times*, January 1.

Bogue v. Faircloth. 1970. 316 F. Supp. 486.

Cairns, Hugh William Bell. 1952. Obituary. *Lancet*, July 26, 202.

Cairns, R. F. Hugh. 1941. Head Injuries in Motorcyclists: The Importance of the Crash Helmet. *British Medical Journal* 2:465–483.

———. 1946. Crash Helmets. *British Medical Journal* 2:322–324.

Cairns, R. F. Hugh, and A.H.S. Holbourn. 1943. Head Injuries in Motorcyclists, with Special Reference to Crash Helmets. *British Medical Journal* 1:592–598.

Chenier, Thomas C., and Leonard Evans. 1987. Motorcyclist Fatalities and the Repeal of Mandatory Helmet Wearing Laws. *Accident Analysis and Prevention* 19:133–139.

Chicago Tribune. 1978. Law Eased, Cycle Deaths Soar. September 7.

Cookro, Dennis V. 1979. Motorcycle Safety: An Epidemiologic View. *Arizona Medicine*, August, 605.

Cronin, Thomas E. 1980. A Resurgent Congress and the Imperial Presidency. *Political Science Quarterly* 95:209–237.

Curtin, Wayne T. 1996. *Focus + Unity = Repeal of Federal Helmet Law*. Motorcycle Riders Foundation White Paper. September. *www.mrf.org/pdf/whitepapers/volume4–1996/repealoffederalhelmetla.pdf* (accessed October 20, 2006).

de Wolf, V. A. 1986. *The Effect of Helmet Law Repeal on Motorcycle Fatalities*. NHTSA Technical Report, DOT HS 065. December. Washington, D.C.: National Highway Traffic Safety Administration.

Dodson, Marcida. 1981. Bikers Find No Vroom to Be Alone. *Los Angeles Times*, May 21.

Dosa, Laszlo. 1989. Worried about Dying? Worry about Accidents. *Washington Post*, June 13.

Evans, Leonard, and Michael C. Frick. 1988. Helmet Effectiveness in Preventing Motorcycle Driver and Passenger Fatalities. *Accident Analysis and Prevention* 20:447–458.

Fuglsang, Ross. 1997. *Motorcycle Menace: Media Genres and the Construction of a Deviant Culture*. Ph.D. diss., University of Iowa.

General Accounting Office. 1991. *Highway Safety: Motorcycle Helmet Laws Save Lives and Reduce Costs to Society.* GAO/RCED-91–170. Washington, D.C.: U.S. General Accounting Office.

Greene, Robert. 1989. Cyclists, Officials Oppose Bill Tying Road Aid to Helmet, Belt Laws. Associated Press, October 17.

Hartunian, Nelson S., Charles N. Smart, Thomas R. Willemain, and P. L. Zador. 1983. The Economics of Safety Deregulation: Lives and Dollars Lost due to Repeal of Motorcycle Helmet Laws. *Journal of Health Politics, Policy, and Law* 8:76–98.

Hess, David. 1995. Leverage on Budget Goes to Republicans; Clinton's Concessions Frustrate Dems. *Houston Chronicle*, December 2.

Holsendolph, Ernest. 1979. U.S. Safety Chief Urges Helmets to Cut Deaths of Motorcyclists. *New York Times*, January 12.

Institute of Medicine. 1979. *Healthy People: The Surgeon General's Report on Health Promotion and Disease Prevention.* DHEW (PHS) publication no. 79–55071A. Washington, D.C.: U.S. Government Printing Office.

Kahane, C. J. 1996. *Fatality Reduction by Air Bags: Analyses of Accident Data through Early 1996.* NHTSA Report No. DOT HS 808 470. *www.nhtsa.dot.gov/cars/rules/regrev/evaluate/808470.html* (accessed October 20, 2006).

Knowles, John H. 1977. The Responsibility of the Individual. *Daedalus*, Winter, 57–80.

Kraus, F. F., C. Peek, and A. Williams. 1995. Compliance with the 1992 California Motorcycle Helmet Use Law. *American Journal of Public Health* 85:96–99.

Krens, Thomas, and Matthew Drutt, eds. *The Art of the Motorcycle.* 1998. New York: Solomon R. Guggenheim Foundation.

Lalonde, Marc. 1974. *A New Perspective on the Health of Canadians: A Working Document.* Ottawa, Can.: Department of National Health and Welfare.

Lloyd, Linda E., Mary Lauderdale, and Thomas G. Betz. 1987. Motorcycle Deaths and Injuries in Texas: Helmets Make a Difference. *Texas Medicine* 83:30–35.

Los Angeles Times. 1975. Senate Votes Reprieve for States Lacking Motorcycle Helmet Law. December 13.

———. 1976. Ford Signs Extension of Highway Aid. May 6.

Maartens, Nicholas F., Andrew D. Wills, and Christopher B. T. Adams. 2002. Lawrence of Arabia, Sir Hugh Cairns, and the Origin of Motorcycle Helmets. *Neurosurgery* 50:177.

McSwain, Norman E., and Elaine Petrucelli. 1987. Medical Consequences of Motorcycle Helmet Nonusage. *Journal of Trauma* 19:233–236.

Modified Motorcycle Organization of California. *www.mma-ca.org.* Accessed November 22, 2006.

Narayan, Raj K. 1987. How Many Deaths Will It Take? *Texas Medicine* 83:5–6.

National Highway Traffic Safety Administration. 2004. States with Primary Safety Belt Laws. www.nhtsa.dot.gov/people/outreach/state_laws-belts04/safeylaws-states.htm (accessed October 20, 2006).

———. 2006. Traffic Safety Facts Laws: Motorcycle Helmet Use Laws. January. *www.nhtsa. dot.gov/staticfiles/DOT/NHTSA/Rulemaking/Articles/Associatedpercent20Files/03 percent20Motorcycle percent20Helmet percent20Use.pdf* (accessed November 22, 2006).

North Carolina Medical Journal. 1979. The Motorcyclist as Gladiator. Editorial. *North Carolina Medical Journal*, June, 362–364.

Nurchi, G. C., P. Golino, F. Floris, V. Meleddu, and M. Coraddu. 1987. Effect of the Law on Compulsory Helmets in the Incidence of Head Injuries among Motorcyclists. *Journal of Neurosurgical Science* 31:141–143.

People v. Fries. 1969. 42 Ill. 2d 446.

Perkins, Richard J. 1981. Perspective on the Public Good. *American Journal of Public Health* 71:294–295.

Peterson, Iver. 1978. Motorcyclists, Helmeted or Not, Fight Restriction. *New York Times*, July 31.

Preusser, D. F., J. H. Hedlund, and R. G. Ulmer. 2000. Evaluation of Motorcycle Helmet Law Repeal in Arkansas and Texas. National Highway Traffic Safety Administration. September.

Pullen, Emma E. 1975. State Faces Loss of U.S. Road Funds. *Los Angeles Times*, August 5.

Quinn, James. 1973a. Cyclists Take Aim at Proposed Helmet Law. *Los Angeles Times*, September 16.

———. 1973b. Motorcycle Helmet Proposal Withdrawn by Councilman. *Los Angeles Times*, September 23.

Ray, Ken. 1998. *The Giant Sucking Sound*. Motorcycle Riders Foundation. September. www.mrf.org/pdf/WhitePapers/Volume5–1998/TheGiantSuckingSound.pdf (accessed October 20, 2006).

Rutstein, David D. 1965. At the Turn of the Next Century. In *Hospitals, Doctors, and the Public Interest*, ed. John H. Knowles. Cambridge, Mass: Harvard University Press.

Scholten, Donald J., and John L. Glober. 1984. Increased Mortality Following Repeal of Mandatory Motorcycle Helmet Law. *Indiana Medicine* 1984:252–255.

Simon v. Sargent. 1972. 346 F. Supp. 277; Appeal, 409 U.S. 1020; 93 S. Ct. 463.

U.S. Congress. House. Committee on Public Works and Transportation. 1975. *Surface Transportation, Part 1, Hearing of the House Committee on Public Works and Transportation.* July 9–31, H 641–5.

U.S. Congress. Senate. Committee on Environment and Public Works. 1989. *National Highway Fatality and Injury Reduction Act of 1989: Hearing before the Subcommittee on Water Resources, Transportation, and Infrastructure of the Committee on Environment and Public Works.* 101st Cong., 1st sess., October 17.

Wall Street Journal. 1979. Highway Panel Seeks Required Helmet Use by Motorcycle Riders. January 12.

Watson, Geoffrey, Paul Zador, and Alan Wilks. 1980. The Repeal of Helmet Use Laws and Increased Motorcyclist Mortality in the United States, 1975–1978. *American Journal of Public Health* 70:579–584.

World Health Organization. 2003. *Worldwide Motorcycle Safety Helmet Laws.* UNESC Working Party on Road Traffic Safety; TRANS/WP. 1.80/Rev 28 January 2003, Table 9. *www.whohelmets.org/helmetlaws.htm* (accessed November 22, 2006).

———. 2005. Thailand: Effect of a Mandatory Helmet Law on Fatalities. *World Health Organization Helmet Initiative Headlines Newsletter. www.whohelmets.org/headlines/05-summer-thailandlaws.htm* (accessed October 20, 2006).

Young, David. 1975. State to Present Case on Cycle Helmet Ruling. *Chicago Tribune*, September 29.

William McAllister, Mary Clare Lennon,
and Işıl Çelimli

Chapter 6

Prevention Strategies and Public Health

Individual and Structural Prevention in Homelessness

In the roughly thirty years since homelessness has resurfaced in the United States, it has affected or threatens to affect tens of millions of people living in this country.[1] Even restricting homelessness to only those living in shelters or on streets yields an estimate of 7.4 percent of U.S. adults becoming homeless during their lives—16 million people. A more expansive definition that includes doubling and tripling up with friends and relatives suggests as many as 30 million people (14 percent) have been homeless over their lives.[2] Although useful trend data to estimate future homelessness are not available, increasing absolute housing costs, declining low-income wages, and the reduced value and availability of transfer benefits—among other features of poor people's lives—suggest we might expect increased homelessness.

Public health research in the United States has played a role in trying to understand and address the problem. By the end of the 1980s, analysts saw public health as an important site for addressing homelessness (e.g., Stoner 1989; Sclar 1990). In particular, the role of mental health policy making in producing homelessness (Torrey 1988; Jencks 1994) fits with public health's role in addressing the mental health of the U.S. population. Partly as a result, public health researchers have carried out much research concerning homelessness (e.g., Saegert et al. 2003; Robertson et al. 2004; Caton et al. 2005), and there is a history of public health research linking housing and health, and of public health practice trying to improve housing to improve health (Rosen 1958; Krieger and Higgins 2002; Saegert et al. 2003). In this context, a center for generating research and practice to help prevent homelessness has recently been set up at a leading school of public health.[3]

One of the core concepts in the research and practice of public health is prevention (Breslow 1998). To reduce disease, public health research has tried to identify social and economic as well as biological causal relationships with disease, and public health practice has sought initiatives that address these relationships.[4] Research suggests, for example, that the built environment of our cities and suburbs affects rates of obesity and of coronary heart disease by encouraging people to be sedentary (e.g., Cervero and Duncan 2003; Mobley et al. 2006).[5] Based on these findings, one set of disease prevention strategies could be to promote exercise (through advertising, physician advice, and so forth) to everyone, to those in the problematic locales, or to people with high rates of obesity or heart disease. Another set of prevention strategies could be to (re)design the built environment to reduce its sedentary features or to change certain features of the environment only for those either with heart disease or more likely to contract it. The first set of strategies exemplifies individual-level prevention— efforts aimed at addressing the causes of who experiences a problem. The second exemplifies structural-level prevention—efforts aimed at affecting the causes of the problem itself. Both types characterize public health research and practice. In this chapter, we analyze each kind of prevention in the context of homelessness to understand how, in addressing problems like homelessness, the results public health can expect are bounded by its choice of prevention strategies.[6] We argue that if public health seeks to end or reduce the amount of homelessness in a society, it should focus on structural-level rather than individual-level prevention.[7]

Individual-Level Prevention

Homeless prevention is commonly conceived as a problem of individuals. That is, our usual analytic and policy strategies to prevent new or renewed homelessness seek to identify persons with certain traits that put them at risk of becoming or remaining homeless and then to provide assistance to prevent that homelessness.[8] Efforts aimed at such persons have to know three things: who has a strong likelihood of becoming homeless, what services work to prevent it among the identified, and how to make sure those identified use such services. We know little about the first two conditions and assume the third (McAllister and Berlin 1994; Shinn and Baumohl 1999; Shinn, Baumohl, and Hopper 2001).

Identification

Identifying who is likely to become homeless is not easy. Poverty seems intu- itively a likely identifier, for example. But even if all homeless people in the United States, including children, come from households in poverty, only about one in sixteen poor people become homeless (Burt, Aron, and Lee 2001).[9]

Four studies explicitly attempting to identify those likely to enter home-less shelters show how difficult identification is.[10] Knickman and Weitzman (1989) used survey data from families requesting shelter and an ordinary least squares model that included demographic, housing, drug, and family history variables and current familial circumstances to predict homelessness. They found targeting 3 percent of the Aid to Families with Dependent Children pop-ulation (AFDC) would find 30 percent of AFDC families requesting shelter. (At that time, about 90 percent of shelter-entering families used AFDC.) Over the course of a year, this would mean providing homeless prevention services to about 8,100 families to reach 2,700 who would request shelter. Thus, 70 per-cent of entering families would remain unidentified, and almost 70 percent of families identified as shelter requesters would not request shelter.[11]

In a more recent analysis using the same data, Shinn and colleagues (1998) found a best model that identified 66 percent of actual shelter requesters and that misidentified only 10 percent of the population as shelter requesters. This has some of the same problems as the prior analysis, and from a policy per-spective, as Shinn, Baumohl, and Hopper (2001) point out, employing this model would mean providing prevention services to 27,000 nonrequesting families (10 percent of the then annual AFDC caseload) to reach the 6,000 requesting families (66 percent of annual shelter requesters at that time). Thus, over 80 percent of families receiving services would not be in danger of entering a shelter, though such services might be otherwise useful to these families.

In a third study, using data from New York City's social service records, Towber and Flemming (1989) found that families who had moved at least twice in the previous year before entering a shelter and whose welfare eligibility had ended (and been reinstated) at least twice since inception were more likely than other AFDC families to enter a shelter. These criteria fit 12 percent of New York's AFDC population, among whom were 42 percent of families entering shelters—that is, almost 60 percent of families entering shelters would be missed, and almost 90 percent of families expected to enter a shelter would not do so. We note that for this and the previous two studies, families not in danger of entering a shelter at the time of the study might have been in danger of entering at some future time. Thus the cited rates underestimate the chance for successful prevention, although we do not know by how much.

Finally, a very recent study (Phinney et al. 2007) followed welfare recipi-ents in an urban county in Michigan from 1997 to 2003. Incorporating measures of education, criminal conviction, substance abuse, work skills and experience, mental and physical health and extensive sociodemographic variables into a multivariate logistic regression model, the study calculated sensitivity and specificity curves for becoming homeless.[12] For people in this population with a predicted probability of becoming homeless greater than 0.11, the model correctly identified 75 percent of those who actually became homeless and correctly excluded from homelessness 67 percent of those who did not become homeless. As in the study by Shinn and colleagues, these estimates are social scientifically strong, but perhaps not strong enough for making policy or creating programs. Policy makers and intervention programs are likely to fear they would spend too many resources on people not becoming homeless while failing to direct resources to many of the people who needed them.

These four studies focused on families, not on would-be homeless individuals. Because homeless families are generally less mobile than homeless individuals and because they tend to come from the population of families known to local welfare agencies, identifying and finding them is likely much easier than identifying and finding similarly fated single individuals. But individuals make up about 85 percent of households that become homeless (Burt, Aron, and Lee 2001). Thus, the overwhelming majority of the would-be homeless are much harder to distinguish than these family-based studies imply.[13]

Different efforts have been made to deal with the identification problem. Some try to reduce the problem by using late intervention models, which help a family or person when the loss of housing is imminent or has recently occurred. But this may not make identification much easier. Evicted people, for example, are more likely to double up or move to cheaper or other housing than to enter a shelter. Towber and Flemming (1989) reported that 75 percent of the New York City households in their sample who lost housing did not enter a shelter but stayed with friends and relatives until finding their own permanent housing. More generally, homelessness may be only weakly associated with formal acts such as eviction (New York State Department of Social Services 1990; Shinn and Baumohl 1999; White et al. 2005). One innovative approach uses geographic targeting. New York City created an initiative that utilizes local knowledge of neighborhood nonprofits to identify families in "high-risk" neighborhoods likely to enter shelters. This improves on the more blunt at-risk measures typical of statistical modeling efforts, but early evidence suggests it does not work to identify the would-be homeless (White et al. 2005).

Services

Assuming we can identify those likely to become homeless, what can we do to prevent that outcome? Individual-level prevention programs try to address particular problems thought specific to generating homelessness, but evidence that these services work to prevent homelessness among those assisted is weak or nonexistent (Shinn and Baumohl 1999; Shinn, Baumohl, and Hopper 2001; McAllister, Berlin, and Lennon 2004).[14] Reviewing forty-two prevention programs, the U.S. Government Accounting Office (1990) identified only eight that followed up, but found these studies were not done well enough to support programmatic claims of success. And there's little evidence, as Shinn and Baumohl (1999) explicitly note, that the situation had improved over the subsequent decade.

One common approach is to address specific fiscal housing problems, particularly the threat of eviction for nonpayment of monthly charges, and prevent homelessness by providing one-time rent, utility, or mortgage payments, financial counseling, or landlord-tenant mediation. However, such programs or studies of them do not provide comparative data specifying what proportion of those helped would have become or stayed housed absent the program (e.g., Schwartz, Devance-Manzini, and Fagan 1991; Feins, Fosburg, and Locke 1994; New York City Family Homelessness Special Master Panel 2003; White et al. 2005). Further, these claims usually do not distinguish between being evicted and becoming homeless by, say, entering a shelter, sleeping in public, and so forth.[15]

One study of late-intervention prevention programs across New York State made this distinction and projected 12 to 16 percent of those assisted would have entered a shelter (New York State Department of Social Services 1990), although errors in calculation may make this an overestimate (see Shinn and Baumohl 1999). But the estimated proportion of evictions that would have been averted absent prevention programs is not based on experimental data. Rather, service providers supplied the data, and since programs were not fully operational, the numbers are projections of what service providers expected would happen. Typically, service providers are likely to overestimate their abilities, do not track their efforts very well, and have incentives to present an optimistic picture.

Evidence for the effectiveness of other kinds of individual-level initiatives is also in short supply. Studies of intensive case management, for instance, either found no effect (Zlotnick, Robertson, and Lahiff 1999) or could not distinguish an effect (Weitzman and Berry 1994). Treatment for mental health problems was not effective in preventing homelessness among a sample of domiciled individuals with histories of psychiatric hospitalization (Sosin and Grossman 1991). And although various kinds of domestic violence are associated with homelessness, efforts to prevent homelessness by addressing such violence do not exist and are unlikely to be effective even if they did (Shinn and Baumohl 1999).

In addition, most prevention services seem to address the potential homelessness of families, not of individuals, and the latter comprise the bulk of those who become homeless (Burt, Aron, and Lee 2001). And they may not address the problems of families or individuals likely to be longer-term homeless. Rather, prevention services typically address the short-term housing problems of families with incomes far above those of the average homeless person or family, a circumstance that makes them unlikely to stay homeless a long time (e.g., Schwartz, Devance-Manzini, and Fagan 1991; New York City Family Homelessness Special Master Panel 2003; White et al. 2005). We note that we do not know enough about how people become homeless to say conclusively that those with seemingly short-term problems would not become long-term homeless if the short-term problems were not resolved. Redburn and Buss (1986) suggest that short-term adult shelter users might have been evicted or suffered a singular disaster or personal crisis, whereas long-term users may have serious mental or physical disabilities or other dysfunctions (see also Kuhn and Culhane 1998).

Absent direct empirical evidence, we might try to assess services' impact indirectly. Available data allow only rough, but perhaps not unrealistic, estimates of possible effects. Focusing on the sheltered homeless, for example, we optimistically assume programs can identify 40 percent of entering families and 30 percent of entering singles. Assume further that services keep 45 percent of assisted families or singles in their current housing, move them into other permanent housing, or get them help that works to prevent their entering a shelter.[16] Using the estimate in Burt, Aron, and Lee (2001) that 85 percent of homeless households are single adults and that 15 percent are families, we estimate 14 percent of adults and families who enter shelters would not do so.[17] While arguably helpful, this is not the major impact on homelessness usually expected from prevention efforts (e.g., New York City Family Homelessness Special Master Panel 2003), and this effect is likely to be lower, perhaps much lower, for the nonsheltered homeless. Further, since this estimates the reduction in the overall number of entrants to shelters (dominated by shorter-term users), the impact would be smaller on the prevalence of shelter use (dominated by longer-term users).

Service Use

A final limit on individual-level prevention is the ability or willingness of the would-be homeless to use services (in general, see Rose 1985). Insofar as services require overt action by the individual or family, their effectiveness relies on would-be homeless people taking that action, and such action can be very hard to achieve. That this is a concern of homelessness service providers is evidenced by the existence of outreach programs and of low-threshold initiatives that make few demands on would-be service users. Aside from those not using services for reasons linked to the severity of their mental illness, would-be homeless people may not be aware of services or may not think of themselves as would-be homeless. The experience of a community-based initiative in New York City suggests both of these as possible explanations for the inability of nonprofits to attract enough would-be homeless clients (White et al. 2005).

Individual-Level Prevention More Generally

This cumulative combination of empirical uncertainties in identifying the would-be homeless, knowing what services work to deter their becoming homeless, and ensuring service use makes it difficult to have much confidence that, at present, individual-level prevention efforts can effectively stop would-be homeless people from becoming homeless. The logic and evidence just discussed focused on issues in individual-level homeless prevention for what is commonly called secondary prevention—addressing causes of who becomes homeless among those at-risk of becoming homeless. But our argument generally holds for two other kinds of individual-level prevention that are commonly differentiated: primary prevention, which addresses causes of who becomes homeless among an entire population; and tertiary prevention, which addresses causes of who remains homeless among those already homeless.

In primary prevention, the identification issue is muted, since the entire population is "treated" and services are universally applied, for example, in dealing with homelessness, teaching money management skills in school (to combat nonpayment of rent as a cause of homelessness), broadly advertising the importance of intact marriages (to combat divorced males or single-motherhood as causes), and so forth. But in dealing with homelessness, primary prevention will be problematic exactly because it treats the entire population, resulting in extremely low specificity rates, and because services are likely to be too general to have much impact on those for whom they may be most useful. More deeply, we suspect such services may misapprehend causes. Teaching money management skills, for example, argues that people miss their housing payment because they do not spend their income appropriately rather than because their income is too low.

In tertiary prevention, identification may also not be thought a problem, since those targeted are already homeless. Because longer-term homeless may disproportionately use resources (Culhane, Metraux, and Hadley 2002), however, we may want to spend scarce resources on people likely to be longer-term homeless, as in the federal government's current interest in ending "chronic" homelessness (U.S. Department of Health and Human Services 2003). But most people seem to be homeless relatively briefly (McAllister and Berlin 1994; Kuhn and Culhane 1998), requiring us to differentiate likely longer-term homeless among those already homeless. At present, we simply do not know how well we can identify such homelessness. (A 2005 study by Caton and colleagues identified some risk factors for longer-term homelessness from a population of those already homeless, but did not estimate how well these factors differentiated the longer-term from the shorter-term homeless.)

Initiatives aimed at this population simply wait for the chronically homeless to self-identify by remaining homeless past some temporal threshold. And the effectiveness of the more common drug, social, psychiatric, and other similar services thought necessary to address specific problems of the longer-term homeless is uncertain at best, mostly because experimental studies have not been carried out. Some evidence suggests providing housing, as opposed to providing services, does keep the chronically homeless housed.[18] But these studies do not address the impact of services or housing on those likely to be homeless a long time, but rather wait for the passing of time to identify that population. And studies of the effectiveness of services or housing on those simply homeless (i.e., mixing those likely to be homeless a shorter time with those likely to be homeless a longer time) have not shown what would happen absent these initiatives.

All these empirical difficulties make it hard to say, at present, that individual-based primary, secondary, and tertiary approaches prevent particular kinds of people from becoming or remaining homeless. At the least, our current knowledge base is simply not powerful enough to identify the would-be homeless (or the longer-term homeless) with enough precision, nor do we know enough about what services prevent particular kinds of people from becoming or remaining homeless. Many studies identify risk factors for becoming homeless (see Caton et al. 2005 and cites therein), but with the exception of the few studies analyzed previously, we do not know how these factors translate into likelihoods of identifying and excluding the correct people. Also, few of the many prevention efforts that use psychiatric, cash assistance, case management, or other services rather than provide housing to deter or end homelessness have been studied. And when they have, either effects are scant or our research methods may not be sufficiently powerful to pick them up.

To be sure, a few service efforts have shown promise in helping those already homeless avoid continuing homelessness (e.g., Susser et al. 1997; Shern et al. 2000; Lehman et al. 1997), and a few housing efforts have shown promise for the same population (e.g., Tsemberis, Gulcur, and Nakae 2004; Stojanovic et al. 1999; Culhane, Metraux, and Hadley 2002; Dworsky and Piliavin 2000). At best, however, these studies identify some success in getting particular homeless people housed (e.g., those mentally ill). However, if we are attempting to change the "amount" of homelessness our society produces (e.g., the rate of first-time homelessness), we cannot rely on individual-level prevention. As we explain in the next section, such prevention can only address the causes of particular individuals' becoming homeless, not the causes of the amount of homelessness. That is, successful individual-level prevention means helping some individuals avoid or leave homelessness but leaves in place the forces that will replace them with other homeless individuals.

Structural-Level Prevention

The primary, secondary, and tertiary prevention just described are three forms that individual-level prevention can take. Each focuses on different specific *aggregates* of individuals, attributing the same or different causes across the aggregates.[19] All three forms take social, policy and economic structures as given, if not immutable, and so ignore structural causes as sites for prevention.

One example of the difference between individual- and structural-level prevention is a typical public health issue: averting disease caused by drinking polluted water. Individual-level prevention may try to get people to stop drinking from whatever source they usually drink from. Implicitly, this argues the cause(s) of disease generated by polluted water are individual-level phenomena that lead people to be more likely to drink from polluted sources, such as their choice of where to live, their daily habits, and so forth. An initiative may try to get everyone in a population (primary prevention), those at risk of drinking from that source (secondary), or those already drinking from that source (tertiary) to change their water-drinking ways by, say, trying to get everyone, those at risk, or those already drinking from the source to switch to unpolluted water (e.g., bottled water). By contrast, structural-level prevention focuses on the conditions causing the water to be polluted. One such initiative could be changing the economic or legal incentives to pollute. Thus, structural-level prevention does not expect the behavior of individuals to change absent change in the circumstances in which people find themselves. Importantly, then, prevention efforts aimed at an entire population are not thereby necessarily structural.[20]

The difference between how we conceptualize prevention—individually or structurally—is located in whether we focus on the causes of where particular people fall in the distribution of a problem or on the causes of the distribution of the problem itself. Individual prevention focuses on the former, structural prevention on the latter.[21] These causes are not the same. A relationship may exist between them (e.g., in the case of homelessness, other things being equal, scarce housing stock means that those with a mental illness are less desirable tenants), and such relationships may be weaker or stronger depending on the problem. But who becomes homeless and the distribution of homelessness are two separate phenomena and need to be explained separately (Schwartz and Carpenter 1999). Further, the first and major task is explaining where the distribution comes from; explaining which individuals experience a problem is secondary. We suggest this ordering because we are more likely to be able to explain the distribution than the placement of individuals (Lieberson 1997);[22] because explaining the distribution will aid us in explaining the placement of individuals (Rose 1985, 1992); and because addressing the causes of the distribution will address the situation of individuals (but not vice versa) and, arguably, do so more effectively than trying to address directly the individual placements problem (Schwartz and Diez-Roux 2001). We thus argue that it is both analytically and practically more useful to conceptualize such problems in terms of the causes of a distribution than in terms of the causes of individual placement.

These may not seem to be distinct issues. An argument is commonly made that if we know homeless people are more likely to be, say, very poor, with weak social networks, histories of drug abuse, little employment, and mental, criminal and foster care institutionalization, then we have explained why we have homeless people (see Caton et al. 2005 for a brief overview of the many factors thought to be associated with becoming homeless). This is not correct. Rather, we have explained why we have *these* homeless people. We have homeless people because we have a set of conditions—scarce housing, low subsidies—that make it harder for people to obtain housing who are very poor, with weak social networks and histories of drug abuse, little employment, and mental, criminal, and foster care institutionalization. Knowing whose lives are characterized by these traits tells us who in a population is more likely to fall where in some distribution of homelessness but not why we have that distribution. The answer to that question lies in factors independent of particular individuals—in the distributions of income and wealth, the structure of the local housing market, the availability and amount of government subsidies, and so forth. That is, the distribution is generated by the social, economic, and policy rules of the game; how individuals fare given these rules is determined by their biographies.

We previously pointed out, for example, that studies trying to determine which families were likely to become homeless found a woman's being pregnant or having a newborn child to be a major determinant (Knickman and Weitzman 1989; Shinn et al. 1998). These studies took this finding to be an individual-level cause by definition of the prediction models constructed, implicitly suggesting that pregnancy/a newborn overburdened a household or something similar. However, it was shelter policy at this time to give priority to women pregnant or with a newborn and, thus, such women were more drawn to seeking shelter.[23] The analytic and prevention differences in these two interpretations are great. The study identified pregnancy/ a newborn as a marker for those likely to have a homeless spell and so implies prevention services to help the household stay together. But the rate of sheltered homelessness is unlikely to be thereby changed. By contrast, our analysis argues that a higher rate of homelessness resulted from a policy providing pregnant women an alternative to their current housing and so suggests changing that policy as a way to reduce shelter homelessness.

Note that we are not arguing that encouraging women pregnant or with a newborn to seek shelter is a "good" thing. It may be, and the people who made the policy probably thought so. The point is that a feature of the biographies of certain women (i.e., being pregnant/having an infant) coincided with a shelter policy existing at a particular moment to produce the study's findings. Absent the policy, the study might not have found pregnancy/newborn to be influential. Since the study wasn't done under that condition, we cannot know either way. When the policy was ended, however, the number of women pregnant or with a newborn seeking shelter dropped. As this example also shows, knowing the rules of the game is useful for telling us something about where in a distribution different kinds of individuals will be placed, but, as we have explained, not enough to make identification of these individuals viable for preventing their becoming homeless. And, conversely, knowing particular traits of individuals is not going to tell us much about relevant features of the distribution of homelessness.[24] Such individual-level data may help us gain insight into what causal forces are operating to produce a distribution, but this should not be confused with thinking these individual traits *are* the causal force producing a distribution. Thus, to eliminate homelessness, this analysis suggests focusing on understanding and eliminating the causes of its distribution rather than on the causes of individual placement in that distribution.

Comparing the Two Approaches

We can deepen the distinction between the individual and the structural foci in preventing homelessness. First, consider a common analytic approach that seeks to explain individual homelessness by drawing on both sets of causes. Taking a subset of causes often cited for why people become homeless and creating a causal argument from them, we might construct the following oversimplified model:

Childhood poverty → Poor education → Unemployment → Drug use →
Familial exhaustion → Homelessness

The diagram includes causes commonly thought to be individual (family exhaustion) and structural (childhood poverty). And it displays a particular understanding of how these two sets of causes are ordered: More structural causes are found further away (more upstream or distal) from the actual occurrence of the problem in the life of the individual, and more individual causes are closer (more downstream or proximal) to the occurrence of the problem. Such causal ordering often leads to the argument that we should affect causes more proximal to the problem because those causes are arguably more easily affected (we can convince families to stay together, but we cannot stop their having been raised in poverty) and we have better science concerning them (correlations are higher between the existence of the problem and more proximal causes [Petraitis, Flay, and Miller 1995]).[25]

More generally, the prevention discussion in this argument focuses on where initiatives should enter this causal chain to prevent some outcome, and it argues this decision should be based on expected effectiveness as evidenced, in large part, on the relative certainty of scientific knowledge concerning risks, if not causes. But this approach does not help reduce the size of the problem, we suggest, because it is explaining who becomes homeless rather than the amount of homelessness in a population. The causal diagram is an individual-level diagram that does not explicitly incorporate structural factors but only the expression of structural conditions in the lives of individuals. It provides individual-level hints of structural conditions generating the distribution of homelessness, but these hints do not generate the distribution. The structural factors do.

Further, these models give empirical meaning to distal factors by putting such causes furthest away from the dependent variable in the ordering of all causes. But this ordering is usually temporally based—distal causes are those furthest away from the event in time. Since structural factors are often conceptualized as distal (although not all distal factors need be structural), they are thus thought to have occurred much earlier in the life of the individual than individual-level factors. But this misapprehends how structures work to affect individual-level factors.

Structural conditions are obviously always present in our lives. In the analytical model presented here, they occur at the same time and in the same causal location that unemployment and illegal drug use occur. While being unemployed and using illegal drugs is occurring, we also have a job market with few unskilled positions that may not be easy to access and a certain volume of illegal drugs at a particular cost and degree of accessibility. Obviously, this will be true for various individual-level factors incorporated into such a model. The argument, then, that structural conditions are upstream—in either some temporal or causal modeling sense—is problematic. Also problematic, then, is the claim that because structural conditions are distal, their effects are too causally weak to be an intervention site. Thus the conclusion commonly drawn that we should focus on more immediate causes (in both a temporal and modeling sense)—read individual-level causes—to prevent homelessness becomes problematic.

We recognize that not all individual-level models of homelessness suggest that structural factors operate only in a temporally prior way. Research often discusses such factors as "underlying" conditions, which in this sense can mean either temporally distal or temporally proximal and may not explicitly incorporate these factors into the causal chain. In this context, perhaps a more useful way to understand structural conditions is that they identify the scope conditions of the individual-level theory. That is, they specify invariant circumstances under which the more variable individual factors operate to produce who becomes homeless. Assigning this theoretic role to structural conditions means they cannot be part of the model's causal chain that determines who becomes homeless, since these conditions do not vary (e.g., the price of illegal drugs is the same for everyone). Thus, since they do not enter the individual-level model of the causes of homelessness, structural conditions cannot be—in the logic of the model—objects of intervention to prevent homelessness and, moreover, cannot be changed by intervening at the individual level. (For a similar argument concerning homelessness in particular and more generally, see Schwartz and Carpenter 1999.)

Another distinction between individual-level and structural-level prevention is that, to the extent scientific knowledge is important for prevention, we can more easily gain better knowledge about the causes of a distribution than we can about the causes of the placement of individuals in that distribution. The problems elaborated previously demonstrate how difficult it is to identify causes of placement. Not only are these kinds of studies difficult to carry out correctly (one reason for their rarity), but also evidence from such studies leaves us with specificity and perhaps sensitivity errors that are scientifically and programmatically too high (Shinn et al. 1998). It is relatively easier to carry out studies of how structural conditions cause the distribution of homelessness, as in studies of the relationship between income, the cost of housing, and some rate of homelessness (Burt 1992; O'Flaherty 1996) or how government policies set the parameters for selecting into homelessness (McAllister, Berlin, and Lennon 2004).

This contention may seem at odds with an argument often made that we can gain better knowledge (i.e., stronger associations) of the relationship between more proximal (individual-level) causes than more distal (structural-level) causes (Rothman, Adami, and Trichopoulos 1998). Our contention, however, concerns explaining where a homeless distribution comes from more than explaining why certain people are homeless. The other contention is that we are more able to explain why certain people are homeless by relying on proximal rather than distal individual-level causes. Failure to appreciate this distinction can lead to an error in thinking about homeless prevention. If we think individual-level causes generate effects like the amount of homelessness rather than who becomes homeless, and if we think structural-level causes are more distal and, therefore, either weaker or less causally knowable than individual-level causes, we mistakenly think we are in a better position to reduce homelessness by addressing those better-understood, individual-level, proximal causes.[26]

A third distinction between the two levels of prevention is that we know less about how to treat individual-level causes of homelessness than we do about how to treat structural-level causes. An important structural problem in New York City, for example, has been the sheer lack of low-income housing. Initiatives such as the New York/New York Program—which created about nine thousand apartments for homeless people who are mentally ill—suggest that expanding the supply of housing is more likely to reduce rates of homelessness than treating individual-level problems (for more on NY/NY, see Culhane, Metraux, and Hadley 2002; Metraux, Marcus, and Culhane 2003).

It is, however, likely that the political capacity and, perhaps, fiscal resources needed to address homelessness structurally are less available than the capacity and resources for addressing who becomes homeless. We suspect this is an important reason why prevention tends to focus on individual-level initiatives and why we convince ourselves that it is possible to do something structurally about the problem by focusing resources on the individual level. Such a focus, however, leads us to think of the often cited metaphor of homelessness as a game of musical chairs, where homeless people are the players, a fixed or reduced amount of low-cost housing are the chairs, and the music is the criteria for access to such housing (Sclar 1990). That is, individual-level efforts take structural conditions as more or less fixed (e.g., the amount of low-cost housing) and so lead certain individuals favored by access criteria to gain housing when the music stops, for example, when programmatic eligibility selects certain people to be housed but ignores others equally likely to become homeless who do not fit that eligibility.[27] In this homeless game of musical chairs, we do not reduce or resolve the problem, we simply decide who among those we think likely to become or to remain homeless should be housed.

Logic of Relationship

Critical to the argument we are making is the logic of the relationship between structural-level causes of the distribution of homelessness and individual-level causes of who becomes homeless. It seems pretty straightforward that causes of the distribution can affect who becomes homeless. These causes establish a set of conditions that make it more or less likely for people with particular individual traits to become homeless. So, for instance, if housing is costly, people without the job skills or social network or other capacity to earn a level of income commensurate with the housing market are more vulnerable to becoming homeless than those with these capacities. The degree of impact depends on the strength of the causal relationship between a specified structural condition and a particular characteristic of individuals. But what about the effect of individual-level causes on characteristics of the distribution? It might be suggested that problematic individual traits can affect the distribution, so that treating those traits affects distributional characteristics such as a measure of central tendency or the variance.

Consider the following mental experiment (utilizing our previous hypothetical modeling example): Suppose we know that all illegal drug users become homeless *because* they are illegal drug users and that *only* illegal drug users are homeless. And further imagine that we have an individual-level treatment that completely and totally stops illegal drug use and that we successfully administer this treatment to the entire population of illegal drug users with the result that, because these individuals stop using illegal drugs, they stop becoming homeless. This would seem to be a secondary (individual-level) prevention effort that is successfully affecting the distribution of homelessness, for example, rates of becoming homeless go to zero. However, while illegal drug users might no longer become homeless, the distribution will not change. Different kinds of people will become homeless, such as people who are mentally ill, because the underlying structural conditions that make housing more or less accessible have not been changed. [28] To oversimplify, perhaps the former illegal drug users can now afford the housing previously purchased by people who are mentally ill. Structural conditions are part of what cause individual-level traits—for example, a personal situation plus the availability of drugs causes drug use. But individual traits do not cause structural conditions. [29]

Policy Making and Prevention

We have explained problems with individual-level prevention and distinguished between individual- and structural-level prevention to conclude that, in addressing homelessness, public health should emphasize the latter rather than the former. (More specifically, if public health seeks to end homelessness, then structural-level prevention is required; if it seeks to ameliorate homelessness, then individual-level prevention is sufficient.) Since public health is about practice as well as about analysis, we here consider what this analysis means for public policy making.

Prevention and Forms of Policy Making

We first evaluate the relationship between universalist/particularist policy making and individual-/structural-level prevention. In a commonly made distinction, particularist policy making references initiatives expressly directed at particular subpopulations, for example, income transfers to low-income people through means-tested Medicaid, food stamps, and other similar policies. Universalist policy making references initiatives directed expressly and equally at the entire population—equally in the sense that all get the same level of benefit—for example, income transfers to nearly everyone in the United States through its Social Security program.[30]

On the face of it, our emphasizing structural rather than individual prevention suggests pursuing universalist rather than particularist policies. But our distinction between types of prevention does not track to this policy distinction: Each kind of prevention can be either universalist or particularist, as we show in table 6.1.[31]

Table 6.1 shows that individual-level prevention can be expressed in universalist policy-making strategies that encompass an entire population (educating all students regardless of likelihood for homelessness) or particularist policies that target would-be or currently homeless people (providing services based on specific expectation as to why particular individuals are or will be homeless).

Table 6.1.   **Relationship between Individual-/Structural-Level Prevention and Universalist/Particularist Policy Making**

| | | Prevention Level | |
		Individual	Structural
	Universalist	Primary prevention *Ex:* Educate all high school students in money management	Change structural conditions generally *Ex:* Generate housing production societywide
Kind of Policy Making	*Particularist*	Secondary prevention *Ex:* Provide rent arrears to would-be homeless Tertiary prevention *Ex:* Provide mental health services to current homeless	Change structural conditions for targeted individuals *Ex:* Generate housing production for homeless mentally ill

Structural-level prevention also can be expressed through universalist action (increasing the supply of housing in general) or through action targeted at a particular class of would-be or currently homeless people (increasing the supply of housing for people who are mentally ill). More particular to the argument we have been making, "universalist/structural" policy making has advantages relative to "particularist/structural" policy making that parallel those of structural- to individual-level prevention: figuring out how to identify people with problematic situations and understanding the complex pathways to problems that individuals take are not both required. And Hopper and Barrow (2003) make clear how supported housing for homeless people can be particularist (e.g., homeless mentally ill) and yet have either individualist or structuralist consequences of the kind we describe (e.g., resolving individual problems versus expanding housing supply for those mentally ill).

As the particularist/structuralist cell in table 6.1 suggests, however, initiatives aimed at specific populations of homeless people can affect structural causes in the process. In New York City, for instance, people who are mentally ill and poor may be less likely to become homeless now than in the past because of additions to the supply of income and housing that they can access. Relative to other would-be homeless people, they are more likely to qualify for Supplemental Security Income and are the priority for the NY/NY housing program, which has added about nine thousand units to the supply of low-income housing in that city. One result may be that the rate of homeless shelter use by those leaving mental hospitals declined from 8.5 percent in 1991, before the housing was available, to 4.2 percent in 1994, after the housing was fully available.[32] (Importantly, we do not know whether the rate of shelter use or of homelessness in general showed any displacement effects, nor whether other changes besides NY/NY housing also operated to lower this rate.) Absent policy changes that improve the relationship between income and housing for lower-income individuals, individual-level measures such as taking prescribed drugs, learning household management, or even obtaining housing will not change rates of homelessness, though such policies certainly help the particular people taking the drugs, getting housing, or learning household management.

Prevention and Policy Claims

The distinction between individual- and structural-level prevention addresses the oft-made policy assumption that individual-level prevention will affect structural features of homelessness, such as its rate in a population (e.g., New York City Family Homelessness Special Master Panel 2003). The argument is made that providing services to particular individuals not yet homeless, such as job training or drug abuse treatment, will reduce or "end" homelessness by preventing their becoming homeless.[33] But preventing homelessness among these individuals does not translate into an impact on the structural character of homelessness. These initiatives identify particular types of the would-be homeless in order to provide services that treat the identifying characteristics (the individual-level problems) that make these particular people homeless; they do not treat the reason homelessness exists. Additionally, the argument is made that housing longer-term homeless will "end" chronic homelessness (e.g., U.S. Department of Health and Human Services 2003). But, to the extent efforts to achieve this goal only house people who have already spent a long time in shelters or on streets and do not reduce the cost or increase the availability of low-income housing in general, our argument applies also to this population.

An implication of this discussion is that we need to be clear about the prevention level of proposed or existing policies and initiatives, both to understand better the kinds of impacts we can expect and to analyze better the relative effectiveness on different outcomes.[34] More pointedly, assuming we want to reduce the size of the homeless problem, being clear about the prevention level of our policies means we should focus on structural-level prevention efforts. We acknowledge, as do others making arguments for structurally focused efforts (e.g., Shinn et al. 2001), that individual-level prevention may help particular persons and may be worth doing on those grounds alone. We share this argument to a point. One limit is that individual-level prevention efforts more easily attract funds and carry a lower political and fiscal charge than do structural-level efforts, and acceding the potential individual utility of individual-level prevention contributes to this environment, making support for structural-level prevention more difficult to attain.

A second limit is that individual-level prevention efforts become incorporated in how people become homeless by formalizing how people are selected into or out of homelessness from the population of the would-be homeless (or, actually, from the broader population of poorer people). Individual-level prevention represents a judgment about what kinds of would-be or currently homeless people to help and not to help (Hopper and Baumohl 1994; Rosenheck, Bassuk, and Salomon 1999). In this sense, individual-level prevention is not an unproblematic good provided to people in need. To take one example, a current politically popular interest is "ending" chronic homelessness (Gladwell 2006). An important part of the argument for focusing on longer-term homeless people is that they most need help, as demonstrated by the longevity of their homelessness and by their disproportionate resource use (Gladwell 2006). Evidence shows, however, that other parts of the homeless population are in worse physical and mental health (to take two measures of need) than those chronically homeless (Culhane and Metraux 2006). Thus, insofar as individual-level prevention for the chronically homeless is justified in this way, we may be diverting resources from those physically and mentally worst off, and thus making it more difficult to address their homelessness and related problems.

Prevention and Policy Demands

Paradoxically, individual-level prevention initiatives create additional risk factors—if not individual-level causes—for becoming or remaining homeless. Individual-level prevention efforts favor those more easily identified as likely to become homeless and more easily helped to avoid homelessness. Thus, those with less severe mental illness may be more likely to receive help than those more seriously ill; and those with arguably more tractable problems, such as rent arrears, may be more likely to receive help than those with more difficult problems, such as needing job training to earn income. That is, prevention initiatives are part of the rules of the game—the structural conditions that determine distributions of the problem—and individual-level prevention initiatives select particular winners from the pool of those most susceptible to losing the game. This is not an insignificant outcome for those individuals prevention does help to win. But focusing on these winners causes us to ignore individual prevention's contribution to making it likely that others will lose. Thus, being ineligible for or unable to access individual-level prevention initiatives becomes another set of risk factors for homelessness.

Concomitantly, individual-level prevention places the burden for change on people who have or are at risk for a problem. It avoids analyzing or addressing the social, political, or economic interests generating the conditions to which precariously situated individuals are exposed. Rather, for example, shelter prevention (or deterrent) efforts expect homeless people to figure out how to stay in substandard housing or how to resolve the intrahousehold conflicts that arise from being doubled and tripled up, and so forth (see, e.g., New York City Family Homelessness Special Master Panel 2003). The structural prevention approach, on the other hand, removes causes that generate behaviors that are arguably problematic for maintaining stable housing, such as intrahousehold conflicts.

By contrast, focusing prevention at a structural level politically shifts our focus from housing as a problem of individuals, or of a relatively small subset of individuals, to housing as a societywide problem. More generally, individual-level prevention does not call into question the social, economic, or political conditions that generate or contribute to the problem. By design, such policy making takes these conditions as given, that is, it accepts the distribution of effects caused by these conditions, and, as previously noted, favors certain individuals from among those who fall into the more problematic end of the distribution. If we focus on preventing homelessness by focusing on the problems of individuals we expect to become homeless, we miss deeper developments that are causing housing to become a problem for the population more generally, not just for those most susceptible to dramatic increases in the cost of housing. That is, by focusing on preventing certain individuals from becoming homeless, we distinguish a very small subset of the population as having a unique set of difficulties arising from relatively idiosyncratic causes, rather than recognize their situation as arising from the same set of causes that creates housing problems for much larger segments of the population—the working poor, the working class, and even parts of the middle class. In this way, policy making aimed at individual-level prevention both misses a more widespread problem and, as has often been argued, contributes to the further social exclusion of homeless people (see Titmuss 1987).

It is also often observed that targeting can be politically problematic, especially when those targeted are among those more socially and politically excluded (Skocpol 1991; Wilson 1987; but see Greenstein 1991). Targeted policies allocate resources to socially and economically distinct subpopulations and thus diminish support for these policies precisely because they benefit (or are perceived generally to benefit) only a portion of the population (Rothstein 2000). Also often noted is that targeted policies tend to stigmatize individuals by identifying them as a subpopulation that is, in some important way, different from a perceived mainstream. That is, targeted policies foster social exclusion, something we might think antipodal to public policy making and, more pertinent, to public health.

Caveats

We are not suggesting that understanding who becomes homeless and why they do so cannot be useful for policy making. Nor, more importantly, are we suggesting that it is not important to better understand the relationship between causes of the homeless distribution and causes of who becomes homeless. If we deem it important to alleviate the homelessness of certain kinds of people rather than others, we will need to be able to both identify those people and devise strategies for helping them efficiently and effectively, for example, people who are (or are likely to become) homeless who are also mentally ill or have other problems perhaps thought more worth addressing. And, as we previously noted, understanding individual-level causes of who becomes homeless may give us clues to structural causes. (For instance, we previously cited a study that found being pregnant/having a newborn was associated with families entering shelters. This individual-level finding suggested that a shelter policy existed that prioritized families with pregnant mothers—which turned out to be the case. For a possibly differing argument, see Schwartz and Carpenter 1999.) Further, in the end, it is not sufficient to generally observe that structural-level causes need to be addressed to reduce rates of homelessness (see the critique of the "social determinants" perspective in Blankenship et al. 2006). We also need to evaluate what structural causes affect what rates and how they do so. Paying attention to clues from studies of individual-level causes may help us in this task and may help us better identify policies that have the desired effect.

Finally, structural-level prevention can be problematic on its own terms. Three issues have been well noted, and so we state but do not develop the arguments here. To the extent structural-level policies are universalist, they may face greater political and fiscal hurdles than do structural- or individual-level policies that are targeted (see, e.g., Greenstein 1991).[35] And structural prevention has a built-in prevention paradox: It affects a wide part of the population, but, when it is universalist, its benefits likely accrue to a small proportion of that population (Rose 1985, 1992). Last, as with individual-level prevention, structural-level prevention may create incentives for individuals to act in ways contrary to ostensible policy aims (McAllister, Berlin, and Lennon 2004). For instance, a particularist/ structural policy may create incentives for individuals to meet the criteria defining the targeted population in order to gain the benefits of the policy. These issues may arise with any structural policy, but particularly particularist/structural policies. The question is not whether a structural-level policy creates these kinds of problems, but rather how the particulars of these kinds of problems stack up across the different possible policies generating them. Thus, while ending homelessness requires structural-level policies, not any such policies will do.

Homelessness as a Public Health Issue

We conclude by considering the utility of our analysis for thinking about whether homelessness should be considered a problem to be analytically and practically addressed by the field of public health. The basic argument for why social conditions like homelessness should concern this field is that either they are health problems in and of themselves or they generate or are associated with ill health. To analogize: We think a condition of the body such as, say, diabetes, is a concern of public health because it is itself unhealthy and because it is a component cause of other diseases, such as stroke.

One argument concerning homelessness is that living on the street, in abandoned buildings, or even in certain kinds of shelters is analogous to having a disease. Thus we have findings that, compared to the general population, homeless people have increased rates of infectious and cardiovascular disease, among other health problems (Hwang 2001; Diez-Roux et al. 1999; Zolopa et al. 1994; more broadly, see cites in Caton, Wilkins, and Anderson 2007). A complementary perspective argues that homelessness plays an important role in generating disease. Longitudinal studies have suggested, for example, that homelessness helps produce increased rates of mortality, alcoholism, and mental illness, among other health problems (Hwang 2002; Roy et al. 2004; Fichter and Quadflieg 2003; Kertesz et al. 2005). Evidence of this sort leads researchers to argue that public health should be engaged—analytically and practically—in understanding and changing social and economic conditions to improve health. And Rose (1985, 1992) makes the more intense argument that changing these general conditions has priority over treating individuals, since changing the former has a greater potential for lowering the incidence of health problems (see also Schwartz and Diez-Roux 2001).

An alternative argument is that even if general social and economic conditions like poverty and more particular conditions like homelessness are unhealthy or help generate disease, dealing with this relationship should not be the primary concern of public health. Rather, the field should first be concerned with understanding and addressing the particular causal mechanisms of specific diseases.[36] Analytically, this seems to mean understanding the biological mechanisms of specific diseases, since, it is argued, we are likely to have greater empirical knowledge of the causal relationship between these more proximate mechanisms and the disease. This approach theoretically prefers individuals as the unit of analysis and methodologically prefers experimental designs that randomly sort individuals to control for individual-level factors. As a consequence, this approach to public health means, in practice, prioritizing treating the health problems of individuals as expressions of the individuals rather than as expressions of social, political, and economic conditions. In some versions of this position, the argument is not necessarily opposed to understanding or changing these conditions in order to improve health but sees them as too problematic (e.g., too causally uncertain or too slow to change) to expect much impact from addressing them.

Relative to this debate, the analyses in this chapter support including social and economic conditions like homelessness as a concern of public heath. That is, if homelessness causes ill health, if structural-level prevention is the way to end this source of ill health, and if public health is concerned with understanding and addressing the causes of ill health, then homelessness is a fit concern for that field. As we have shown, prevention that addresses individual-level causes can, at best, palliate the problem by helping particular people. Some who emphasize an individual-level approach seem to recognize this shortcoming, that is, they place greater value on helping just those who can be reached by demonstrated medical interventions, even as the structural causes of the problem affecting a larger part of a population remain unaddressed. Rothman, Adami, and Trichopoulos (1998), for example, emphasize the effective utility of providing vitamin A supplements to prevent the morbidity resulting from malnutrition rather than the utility of addressing the poverty that generates malnutrition. And we note that successfully addressing individual-level causes for the situation of particular kinds of people is not simply palliative but curative for those individuals: It ends their homelessness and so ends the health problems homelessness generates. This is obviously vital for them.

Another concern with incorporating social problems like homelessness within public health is that doing so subjects these problems to clinical conceptualizations, that is, analyses that focus on risk factors and on explaining variation among individuals, and treatments that focus on intervening in the lives of individuals (Meyer and Schwartz 2000). The result is that, at best, certain individuals' problems are resolved even as the societal problem of homelessness remains. This critique is consistent with our analysis, but we draw the conclusion that public health must emphasize structural-level prevention rather than abandon it. In doing so, we suggest a field of public health that is closer to its origins of changing the health-problematic conditions in which people live rather than changing the people themselves. For some, emphasizing social determinants of health suggests (unacceptably) that public health would become a branch of economics or of some other social science (Rothman, Adami, and Trichopoulos 1998). In this context, however, using the tools and reasoning of the social sciences seems no more or less problematic than using the tools and reasoning of the biological and medical sciences, as much of public health currently does.

Acknowledgments

Research support for this chapter was provided by a Robert Wood Johnson Foundation Investigator Award in Health Policy Research and by NIMH grant number R34 MH073651–01. The views expressed imply no endorsement by the Robert Wood Johnson Foundation. We thank Sharon Schwartz for her insightful thoughts on an earlier draft, the editors of and our collaborators in this volume for their useful and encouraging comments on our initial ideas, and Susan Barrow, George Gavrilis, Serban Iorga, and Li Kuang for pointing out lacunae and problems in later drafts. We also thank Li Kuang and Lauren Passalacqua for their thorough research assistance.

Notes

1. Certain living conditions in previous times we might now include under the rubric of homelessness, such as the flophouses of the early twentieth century and the hobo sites of the Great Depression. See Hoch and Slayton 1989.

2. We applied estimates of adults self-reporting homelessness in Link et al. 1994 to the estimate of the number of adults in the United States according to the 2005 American Community Survey (U.S. Census Bureau 2006). Estimates of the size of the homeless population have always varied greatly, depending on the definition of homelessness used, the aspect being counted (incidence or prevalence), the timing of the count, and the methodology used. See Burt, Aron, and Lee 2001 for a relatively recent report on different estimates.

3. We refer to the Center for Homeless Prevention Studies at the Mailman School of Public Health, Columbia University. Two of the authors are participants in this center.

4. These relationships may be thought to be causal in generating the disease (e.g., the effects of class in generating tuberculosis; see Lewontin 1993) or in helping the disease persist or spread (e.g., the role of social networks in spreading sexually transmitted disease; see Morris et al. 2006).

5. The role of being sedentary is qualified in Ewing et al. 2003.

6. "Problems like homelessness" refers to social or economic problems with health implications whose improvement involves allocating scarce resources, that is, the resource cannot be allocated to some without affecting others. Arguably, problems exist that can be resolved without such a consequence, as when we reduce illness through vaccination under certain conditions.

7. In its most extreme form, reducing the size of the problem means "ending" homelessness. Exactly what this can mean is a deep and difficult question. Working through an answer would take us beyond the point of this chapter. For current purposes, we mean ensuring people can obtain housing that meets generally accepted standards of cost and physical and social quality.

8. By "persons" we mean families, couples without children, or any other relational combination of people who are jointly homeless as well as individuals. The emphasis on individuals can be seen in descriptions of prevention programs (Shinn and Baumohl 1999; Shinn, Baumohl, and Hopper 2001; Lindblom 1996; U.S. General Accounting Office 1990) or in the execution of particular programs (Schwartz, Devance-Manzini, and Fagan 1991; O'Connell 2003; New York City Family Homelessness Special Master Panel 2003; White et al. 2005).

9. Estimates of the number of homeless people vary, for reasons observed earlier. For overviews of methods and estimates, see Link et al. 1994; Phelan and Link 1999; and Burt, Aron, and Lee 2001. We focus in this discussion mainly on preventing people or households from becoming newly homeless, since this is a prevention ideal (versus preventing further homelessness among those already homeless), and useful studies have focused on this kind of prevention.

10. To our knowledge (and that of Shinn and Baumohl 1999 and Shinn, Baumohl, and Hopper 2001), these are the only identification studies concerning those becoming homeless (vs. those already homeless) carried out in a way that allows estimating specificity, sensitivity, and "hit" rates, that is, how well risk factors identified would-be homeless families. Without such studies, we cannot construct efficient and effective initiatives to identify would-be homeless people.

11. Knickman and Weitzman also developed other models that identified from 3 to 13 percent of the AFDC population to find different percentages of families requesting

shelter, up to 50 percent of requesting families. The model reported here is arguably the best given the kind and ease of data the model is based on and the percentage of families targeted for the percentage of families correctly identified.

However, this model is less useful than it initially appears. The variable "current pregnancy/child under one" had the largest coefficient, and the authors include it among the risk factors on which the public assistance population could be sorted for vulnerability to homelessness. Its statistical importance, however, is more likely an artifact of New York City shelter policy than of the effect of pregnancy/infant on current living conditions. At the time of the study, city policy gave shelter priority to women pregnant or with an infant, increasing the likelihood of their entering a shelter, other things being equal. This is very different from the implication of the model that pregnant women tended to request shelter because pregnancy or the presence of an infant strained their housing situation to the breaking point, e.g., the mother's having to leave the household because her live-in boyfriend refuses now to support her and the child or because the additional strain on the household is too much for the relatives or friends with whom the mother lives. Absent New York City policy, we suggest, the model would have predicted much less well.

12. Sensitivity is the probability of correctly identifying all those who become homeless from a particular population, and specificity is the probability of correctly identifying all those who will not become homeless from that population.

13. Also, three of these studies defined homelessness as the formal act of entering a shelter. Nonformal acts, such as staying with friends or relatives and sleeping on streets or in abandoned buildings, are much harder to study, making identification even more difficult. Finally, there are a variety of more technical issues, perhaps the most important being the ability to specify a meaningful control (or even comparison) group. We cited the studies here because they did so.

14. Shinn and Baumohl 1999 or Shinn, Baumohl, and Hopper 2001 provides a detailed explication of these programs and of problems with their effectiveness claims. Evidence for the effectiveness of certain kinds of initiatives for those already homeless, especially for longer-term homeless, is stronger; see Susser et al. 1997; Tsemberis, Gulcur, and Nakae 2004. See Shinn and Baumohl 1999 for an overview of some of these efforts.

15. Under a very broad conceptualization of homelessness, being evicted could in and of itself constitute becoming homeless. We agree with some arguments for construing homelessness beyond living in a shelter or on the street, though public policies tend not to.

16. The identification estimate for families is the highest given by the New York City models reported in the text. The estimate for single adults is three-fourths the family estimate: The social amorphousness of this population combined with its mobility suggest that at-risk individuals are harder to identify and to find than families. We think this estimate is conservative. The estimate for the proportion effectively assisted arbitrarily assumes that program services addressing all reasons for homelessness would be half the estimated effectiveness of services that address landlord eviction (New York State Department of Social Services 1990). Because eviction usually has to do with rent or other landlord/tenant disputes, it can be resolved with a grant or with legal representation, both relatively quickly and easily provided. For people with mental or addiction disabilities or social problems, prevention services are much more difficult to provide and take longer to administer, suggesting they will not be as effective as eviction prevention. Again, we think this estimate conservative, in the sense that it will yield an optimistic estimate of program effectiveness.

17. This estimate results from an overly simplified calculation: The proportion of would-be homeless single adults and families identified multiplied by the proportion of those identified avoiding shelters due to prevention program services yields the proportion of the would-be homeless who avoid homelessness because of these programs. Using numbers in the text yields .14, i.e., .14 = ((.15*.4) + (.85*.3)) *.45. The estimates in Burt, Aron, and Lee 2001 are point prevalence rather than incidence. The relationship between these two is unknown, but an implication of Phelan and Link 1999 is that homeless adult households dominate incidence as well.

18. Research suggests that leaving a homeless shelter for one's own housing relative to any other kind of situation (including living with others) decreases the chances of shelter reentry, at least in the short run (see Shinn et al. 1998; Stojanovic 1999; Dworsky and Piliavin 2000). Other studies have analyzed the relative chances of staying housed for those receiving housing first versus receiving psychiatric and social services first and have found the former to be more useful for people remaining housed (Tsemberis 1999; Tsemberis, Gulcur, and Nakae 2004). All these studies, however, mix shorter-term and longer-term shelter users, so the effect for the longer-term homeless is not clear. Finally, some studies have found certain kinds of services at particular points of homelessness to be effective relative to general or no services (Susser et al. 1997) but did not vary postshelter conditions.

19. It may be thought the same cause is operating regardless of the aggregation, for example, poor money management. Or it may be thought, for example, that for the population as a whole the cause of homelessness is poor money management, for those at-risk of homelessness it's poor social networks, and for those already homeless it's poor social or health services.

20. This is partly why we use "structural" rather than "population" to label this kind of prevention. The latter seems generally thought to equate to structural prevention, even when the initiatives it describes are addressing individual-level causes. However, some research does mean structural prevention when using the term population prevention (Rose 1985, 1992). Our meaning also appears largely consistent with that of the "primordial prevention" approach (Strasser 1978; Kaplan and Lynch 1999; Lynch 2001), though we don't share the temporal placement of structural causes that argument seems to have. Other research seems more ambiguous. The term "structural intervention," for example, describes an approach focusing on structural-level and not individual-level policies or programs to, say, reduce HIV transmission (Blankenship et al. 2006; Des Jarlais 2000). But it is not clear whether this approach is trying to address who falls ill, why we have anyone falling ill, or both. This ambiguity also seems to appear in the "social determinants" approach (Link and Phelan 1995).

21. For this discussion, we draw mostly on Lieberson 1997, but the discussion is consistent with Rose 1985, 1992. In our analysis, we refer of course to the distribution of homelessness or to the rate of homelessness. For our purposes, these are conceptually equivalent, and the particular distribution or rate, for example, the distribution or rate of new homelessness or of long-term homelessness, is logically immaterial for our argument.

22. Our earlier discussion on identification also speaks to this point.

23. It's also possible, though less likely, that shelter policy also meant women pregnant or with a newborn were somehow overtly selected for entering a shelter. We think this is less likely to have occurred for three reasons. First, legally, shelters had to accept all requesting shelter. Thus, in theory, shelter capacity was elastic and did not require rejecting applicants. In fact, however, the shelter system was always looking

to reduce demand. Second, the study looked at women applying for shelter, not those actually entering. Third, women would probably have been subjected to whatever shelter-deterrent efforts were then in place after they sought entrance, not before, such as efforts to deter women not pregnant or with a newborn. But since we cannot rule out that such efforts did not occur at this earlier stage, we note here the possibility of shelter prioritization.

24. This may be seen more easily by considering a lottery game (see Lieberson 1997). Assuming the game is not crooked, the distribution of outcomes is determined by the rules of probability, the kinds and amounts of payouts, other rules of the game, and perhaps the number of people playing. It would be absurd to think that knowing the biographies of those winning particular payouts would help us understand the distribution of winners and losers.

25. We are not saying it is easy to convince relatives and friends to continue supporting a potentially homeless person, just that such support is more malleable than childhood poverty and that it has been tried. See, for example, New York City Homelessness Special Master Panel 2003 and similar efforts over the years to deter homeless families from entering shelters.

26. The reasoning why distal factors are thought to be more weakly associated with the outcome follows from path analytic logic. See, for example, Davis 1985. For the reasoning as to why we are likely to have less knowledge about distal factors in individual-level models, see Schwartz and Diez-Roux 2001.

27. The "music" can be things other than program eligibility criteria, such as physical health, psychological well-being, quality of social network, and so forth (see Sclar 1990; Shinn and Baumohl 1999). Note that these are all individual-level traits and that they could, to some extent, be treated programmatically. Thus, the logical status of all these as music is the same. Further, program criteria might be usefully understood as formalizing these traits relative to obtaining housing and so are in practice the same thing. As a result, to the extent access to housing for would-be homeless people goes through programs, programmatic criteria—and not the mere fact of individuals having particular traits—become the crucial music that is playing.

28. This is akin to the argument in the "fundamental causes of health" perspective (see, e.g., Link and Phelan 1995). On the logic of this argument, see Lieberson 1985.

29. Our argument does not distinguish between whether the macro, or social, condition (e.g., rate of homelessness) is caused by other macro conditions (e.g., availability of housing stock) or results from some chain, causal or otherwise, from macro conditions through micro, or individual, behavior back to the macro condition of homelessness rate (see Coleman 1990; Abell 2003). Either is consistent with our argument so long as it is understood that structural conditions constrain individual behavior to generate homelessness rates. We do not here develop a theory of exactly how homelessness rates are generated in either scenario.

30. Skocpol 1991 provides a brief overview of the particularist/universalist distinction. These definitions are based in very practical policy making and, as a result, oversimplify the differences and relationship between particularism and universalism, even in a policy context. For more nuanced analyses, see Titmuss 1987 and Rothstein 2000.

31. The example in our introduction also reflects these distinctions. In addressing sedentariness resulting from the built environment using the format in table 6.1, policies that promote exercise to everyone belong in the upper right cell and to those in the problematic areas or to those in areas with high rates of heart disease in the lower right cell. Policies that design or redesign the built environment fall in the top

left cell, and those that change certain features of the environment only for those either with heart disease or more likely to contract it fall in the bottom left cell.

32. The data and the suggested relationship were presented by Culhane and Metraux (2006). The statistics are based on discharges from a mental hospital within ninety days of entering a homeless shelter.

33. We previously showed that empirical issues with identification and services make it difficult to have great hope, at present, that these kinds of prevention initiatives can work for even the more modest goal of keeping the would-be homeless from the streets or shelters. The argument is also made that housing long-term homeless people will have the same effect. This is the impetus behind ending chronic homelessness (U.S. Department of Health and Human Services 2003). To the extent efforts to achieve this end have only to do with moving longer-term homeless out of shelters without improving conditions like the cost and availability of low-income housing in general, our argument applies also to this population.

34. Hopper and Barrow's (2003) discussion of two kinds of housing initiatives makes clear how efforts can be programmatically similar yet radically different in aiming at structural- or individual-level effects.

35. This contrasts with the more common argument that universalist policies are politically more feasible. As Greenstein points out, the nature, structure, and perceived benefits of policies also affect how politically feasible they are. We can easily imagine particularist homeless policies, even when structural, that would be far less demanding politically and fiscally than universalist policies. See, for example, the NY/NY mental health housing effort (Culhane, Metraux, and Hadley 2002; Metraux et al. 2003).

36. The discussion in this paragraph is based on Rothman, Adami, and Trichopoulos 1998. Other analysts on this side of the debate see utility only in biological, individual-level analysis and treatment (e.g., Zielhuis and Kiemeney 2001).

References

Abell, P. 2003. On the Prospects for a Unified Social Science: Economics and Sociology. *Socio-Economic Review* 1, 1:1–26.

Blankenship, K. M., S. R. Friedman, S. Dworkin, and J. E. Mantell. 2006. Structural Interventions: Concepts, Challenges, and Opportunities for Research. *Journal of Urban Health: Bulletin of the New York Academy of Medicine* 83, 1 (January):59–72.

Breslow, L. 1998. Musings on Sixty Years in Public Health. *Annual Review of Public Health* 19:1–15.

Burt, M. R. 1992. *Over the Edge: The Growth of Homelessness in the 1980s.* New York: Russell Sage.

Burt, M. R., L. Y. Aron, and E. Lee, with J. Valente. 2001. *Helping America's Homeless: Emergency Shelter or Affordable Housing?* Washington, D.C.: Urban Institute Press.

Caton, C. L., D. Boanerges, B. Schanzwer, D. S. Hasin, P. E. Shrout, A. Felix, H. McQuistion, L. A. Opler, and E. Hsu. 2005. Risk Factors for Long-Term Homelessness: Findings from a Longitudinal Study of First-Time Homeless Single Adults. *American Journal of Public Health* 95:1753–1759.

Caton, C. L., C. Wilkins, and J. Anderson. 2007. Characteristics and Interventions for People Who Experience Long-Term Homelessness. Paper presented at the National Symposium on Homelessness Research. Washington, D.C. March.

Caton, C. L., R. J. Wyatt, A. Felix, J. Grunberg, and B. Dominguez. 1993. Follow-up of Chronically Mentally Ill Men. *American Journal of Psychiatry* 150:1639–1642.

Cervero, R., and R. Duncan. 2003. Walking, Bicycling, and Urban Landscapes: Evidence from the San Francisco Bay Area. *American Journal of Public Health* 93:1478–1483.

Coleman, J. S. 1990. *Foundations of Social Theory*. Cambridge, Mass.: Harvard University Press.

Culhane, D. P., and R. Kuhn. 1998. Patterns and Determinants of Public Shelter Utilization among Homeless Adults in New York City and Philadelphia. *Journal of Policy Analysis and Management* 17, 1:23–43.

Culhane, D. P., and S. Metraux. 2006. Institutional Discharges and Homelessness: The Impact of the Child Welfare, Inpatient Mental Health, and Criminal Justice Systems on Public Shelter Admissions. Talk presented at the Columbia Center for Homeless Prevention Studies.

Culhane, D. P., S. Metraux, and T. R. Hadley. 2002. Public Service Reductions Associated with the Placement of Homeless People with Severe Mental Illness in Supportive Housing. *Housing Policy Debate* 13, 1:107–163.

Davis, J. A. 1985. *The Logic of Causal Order*. Beverly Hills, Calif.: Sage Publications.

Des Jarlais, D. C. 2000. Structural Interventions to Reduce HIV Transmission among Injecting Drug Users. *AIDS* 14 (supplement 1): S41–S46.

Diez-Roux, A., M. E. Northridge, A. Morabia, M. T. Bassett, and S. Shea. 1999. Prevalence and Social Correlates of Cardiovascular Disease Risk Factors in Harlem. *American Journal of Public Health* 89:302–307.

Dworsky, A. L., and I. Piliavin. 2000. Homeless Spell Exits and Returns: Substantive and Methodological Elaborations on Recent Studies. *Social Service Review* 74, 2:193–213.

Ewing, R., T. Schmid, R. Killingsworth, A. Zlot, and S. Raudenbush. 2003. Relationship between Urban Sprawl and Physical Activity, Obesity, and Morbidity. *American Journal of Health Promotion* 18:47–57.

Feins, J., L. C. Fosburg, and G. Locke. 1994. *Evaluation of the Emergency Shelter Grants Program*. Vols. 1–3. HUD-PDR-1489. Washington, D.C.: U.S. Department of Housing and Urban Development, Office of Policy Development and Research.

Fichter, M. M., and N. Quadflieg. 2003. Course of Alcoholism in Homeless Men in Munich, Germany: Results from a Prospective Longitudinal Study Based on a Representative Sample. *Substance Use and Misuse* 38, 6:395–427.

Gladwell, M. 2006. Million Dollar Murray: Why Problems Like Homelessness Might Be Easier to Solve Than to Manage. *New Yorker*, February 13, 96–105.

Greenstein, R. 1991. Universal and Targeted Approaches to Relieving Poverty: An Alternative View. In *The Urban Underclass*, ed. C. Jencks and P. E. Peterson. Washington, D.C.: Brookings Institution.

Hoch, C., and R. A. Slayton. 1989. *New Homeless and Old: Community and the Skid Row Hotel*. Philadelphia: Temple University Press.

Hopper, K., and S. Barrow. 2003. Two Genealogies of Supported Housing and Their Implications for Outcomes Assessment. *Psychiatric Services* 54, 1:50–54.

Hopper, K., and J. Baumohl. 1994. Held in Abeyance: Rethinking Homelessness and Advocacy. *American Behavioral Scientist* 37, 8:522–552.

Hwang, S. W. 2001. Homelessness and Health. *Canadian Medical Association Journal* 164, 2:229–233.

———. 2002. Is Homelessness Hazardous to Your Health? *Canadian Journal of Public Health* 93, 6:407–410.

Jencks, C. 1994. *The Homeless*. Cambridge, Mass.: Harvard University Press.

Kaplan, G. A., and J. Lynch. 1999. Socioeconomic Considerations in the Primordial Prevention of Cardiovascular Disease. *Preventive Medicine* 29, 6: S30–S35.

Kertesz, S. G., M. J. Larson, N. J. Horton, M. Winter, R. Saitz, and J. H. Samet. 2005. Homeless Chronicity and Health-Related Quality of Life Trajectories among Adults with Addictions. *Medical Care* 43, 6:574–585.

Knickman, J. R., and B. A. Weitzman. 1989. *Forecasting Models to Target Families at High Risk of Homelessness, Final Report*. Vols. 3–4. New York: Health Research Program, New York University.

Krieger, J., and D. L. Higgins. 2002. Housing and Health: Time Again for Public Health Action. *American Journal of Public Health* 92, 5:758–768.

Kuhn, R, and D. P. Culhane. 1998. Applying Cluster Analysis to Test a Typology of Homelessness by Pattern of Shelter Utilization: Results from the Analysis of Administrative Data. *American Journal of Community Psychology* 26, 2:207–232.

Last, J. M. 1988. *A Dictionary of Epidemiology*. New York: Oxford University Press.

Lehman, A. F., L. B. Dixon, E. Kernan, B. R. DeForge, and L. T. Postrado. 1997. A Randomized Trial of Assertive Community Treatment for Homeless Persons with Severe Mental Illness. *Archives of General Psychiatry* 54, 11:1038–1043.

Lewontin, R. C. 1993. *Biology as Ideology*. New York: HarperCollins.

Lieberson, S. 1985. *Making It Count: The Improvement of Social Research and Theory*. Berkeley: University of California Press.

———. 1997. Modeling Social Process: Some Lessons from Sports. *Sociological Forum* 12, 1:11–35.

Lindblom, E. 1996. Preventing Homelessness. In *Homelessness in America*, ed. J. Baumohl, 187–200. Phoenix, Ariz.: Oryx Press.

Link, B. G., and J. Phelan. 1995. Social Conditions as Fundamental Causes of Disease. *Journal of Health and Social Behavior* (extra issue): 80–94.

Link, B. G., E. Susser, A. Stueve, J. Phelan, R. E. Moore, and E. Struening. 1994. Lifetime and Five-year Prevalence of Homelessness in the United States. *American Journal of Public Health* 84, 12:1907–1912.

Lynch, J. 2001. Socioeconomic Factors in the Behavioral and Psychosocial Epidemiology of Cardiovascular Disease. In *Integrating Behavioral and Social Sciences of Health*, ed. N. Schneiderman, M. A. Speers, J. M. Silva, H. Tomes, and J. H. Gientry, 51–71. Washington, D.C.: American Psychological Association.

McAllister, W., and G. Berlin. 1994. Homeless Policymaking: Prevention and Shelter Population Dynamics. Typescript. Author files.

McAllister, W., G. Berlin, and M. C. Lennon. 2004. *Policymaking and Caseload Dynamics: Homeless Shelters*. ISERP Working Paper No. 04–04. New York: Institute for Social and Economic Research and Policy, Columbia University.

Metraux, S., and D. P. Culhane. 1999. Family Dynamics, Housing, and Recurring Homelessness among Women in New York City Homeless Shelters. *Journal of Family Issues* 20, 3:371–396.

Metraux, S., S. C. Marcus, and D. P. Culhane. 2003. The New York–New York Housing Initiative and Use of Public Shelters by Persons with Severe Mental Illness. *Psychiatric Services* 54, 1:67–71.

Meyer, I. H., and S. Schwartz. 2000. Social Issues as Public Health: Promise and Peril. *American Journal of Public Health* 90, 8:1189–1191.

Mobley, L. R., E. D. Root, E. A. Finkelstein, O. Khavjou, R. P. Farris, and J. C. Will. 2006. Environment, Obesity, and Cardiovascular Disease Risk in Low-Income Women. *American Journal of Preventive Medicine* 30, 4:327–331.

Morris, M., M. S. Handcock, W. C. Miller, C. A. Ford, J. L. Schmitz, M. M. Hobbs, M. S. Cohen, K. M. Harris, and J. R. Udry. 2006. Prevalence of HIV Infection among Young Adults in the United States: Results from the Add Health Study. *American Journal of Public Health* 96, 6:1091–1097.

New York City Department of Homeless Services. 2006. Historic Data, www.nyc.gov/html/dhs/html/statistics/statistics.shtml.

New York City Family Homelessness Special Master Panel. 2003. *Family Homelessness Prevention Report*. New York: City Government of New York.

New York State Department of Social Services. 1990. *The Homelessness Prevention Program: Outcomes and Effectiveness*. Albany: Office of Program Planning, Analysis and Development and Office of Shelter and Supported Housing Programs.

O'Connell, M. E. 2003. Responding to Homelessness: An Overview of US and UK Policy Interventions. *Journal of Community and Applied Social Psychology* 13:158–170.

O'Flaherty, B. 1996. *Making Room: The Economics of Homelessness*. Cambridge, Mass.: Harvard University Press.

Petraitis, J., B. R. Flay, and T. Q. Miller. 1995. Reviewing Theories of Adolescent Substance Use: Organizing Pieces in the Puzzle. *Psychological Bulletin* 117:67–86.

Phelan, J. C., and B. G. Link. 1999. Who Are the Homeless: Reconsidering the Stability and Composition of the Homeless Population. *American Journal of Public Health* 89, 9:1334–1338.

Phinney, R., S. Danziger, H. A. Pollack, and K. Seefeldt. 2007. Housing Instability among Current and Former Welfare Recipients. *American Journal of Public Health* 97, 5: 832–837.

Redburn, S. F., and T. F. Buss. 1986. *Responding to Homelessness: Public Policy Alternatives*. New York: Praeger.

Robertson, M. J., R. A. Clark, E. D. Charlebois, J. Tulsky, H. L. Long, D. R. Bangsberg, and A. R. Moss. 2004. HIV Seroprevalence among Homeless and Marginally Housed Adults in San Francisco. *American Journal of Public Health* 94, 7:1207–1217.

Rose, G. 1985. Sick Individuals and Sick Populations. *International Journal of Epidemiology* 14, 1:32–38.

———. 1992. *The Strategy of Preventive Medicine*. New York: Oxford University Press.

Rosen, G. 1958. *A History of Public Health*. New York: MD Publications.

Rosenheck, R., B. Bassuk, and A. Salomon. 1999. Special Populations of Homeless Americans. In *Practical Lessons: The 1998 Symposium on Homelessness Research*, ed. L. Fosburg and D. Dennis. Washington, D.C.: U.S. Department of Housing and Urban Development and U.S. Department of Health and Human Services.

Rossi, P. H. 1989. *Down and Out in America: The Origins of Homelessness*. Chicago: University of Chicago Press.

Rothman, K. J., and S. Greenland. 2005. Causation and Causal Inference in Epidemiology. *American Journal of Public Health* 95: S1:S144–S150.

Rothman, K. J., H.-O. Adami, and D. Trichopoulos. 1998. Should the Mission of Epidemiology Include the Eradication of Poverty? *Lancet* 352:810–813.

Rothstein, B. 2000. The Future of the Universal Welfare State. In *Survival of the European Welfare State*, ed. S. Kuhnle. London: Routledge.

Roy, E., N. Haley, P. Leclerc, B. Sochanski, J. F. Boudreau, and J. F. Boivin. 2004. Mortality in a Cohort of Street Youth in Montreal. *JAMA* 292:569–574.

Saegert, S. C., S. Klitzman, N. Freudenberg, J. Cooperman-Mroczek, and S. Nassar. 2003. Health Housing: A Structured Review of Published Evaluations of US Interventions to Improve Health by Modifying Housing in the United States, 1990–2001. *American Journal of Public Health* 93, 9:1471–1477.

Schwartz, D.C., D. Devance-Manzini, and T. Fagan. 1991. *Preventing Homelessness: A Study of State and Local Homelessness Programs.* East Orange and New Brunswick: National Housing Institute and American Affordable Housing Institute, Rutgers, the State University of New Jersey.

Schwartz, S., and K. M. Carpenter. 1999. The Right Answer for the Wrong Question: Consequences of Type III Error for Public Health Research. *American Journal of Public Health* 89, 8:1175–1180.

Schwartz, S., and A. Diez-Roux. 2001. Commentary: Causes of Incidence and Causes of Cases: A Durkheimian Perspective on Rose. *International Journal of Epidemiology* 30:435–439.

Sclar, E. D. 1990. Homelessness and Housing Policy: A Game of Musical Chairs. *American Journal of Public Health* 80, 9:1039–1040.

Shern, D. L., S. Tsemberis, W. Anthony, A. M. Lovell, L. Richamond, C. J. Felton, J. Winarski, and M. Cohen. 2000. Serving Street-Dwelling Individuals with Psychiatric Disabilities: Outcomes of a Psychiatric Rehabilitation Clinical Trial. *American Journal of Public Health* 90:1873–1878.

Shinn, M., and J. Baumohl. 1999. Rethinking the Prevention of Homelessness. In *Practical Lessons: The 1998 National Symposium on Homelessness Research*, ed. L. B. Fosburg and D. L. Dennis, 13–1–13–36. Washington, D.C.: U.S. Department of Housing and Urban Development and U.S. Department of Health and Human Services.

Shinn, M., J. Baumohl, and K. Hopper. 2001. The Prevention of Homelessness Revisited. *Analyses of Social Issues and Public Policy* 1, 1:95–127.

Shinn, M., B. C. Weitzman, D. Stojanovic, J. R. Knickman, L. Jiminez, L. Duchon, D. James, and D. H. Krantz. 1998. Predictors of Homelessness among Families in New York City: From Shelter Request to Housing Stability. *American Journal of Public Health* 88, 11:1651–1657.

Skocpol, T. 1991. Targeting within Universalism: Politically Viable Policies to Combat Poverty in the United States. In *The Urban Underclass*, ed. C. Jencks and P. E. Peterson. Washington, D.C.: Brookings Institution.

Sosin, M., and S. Grossman. 1991. The Mental Health System and the Etiology of Homelessness: A Comparison Study. *Journal of Community Psychology* 19, 3:337–350.

Stojanovic, D., B. C. Weitzman, M. Shinn, L. E. Labay, and N. P. Williams. 1999. Tracing the Path out of Homelessness: The Housing Patterns of Families after Exiting Shelter. *Journal of Community Psychology* 27:199–208.

Stoner, M. R. 1989. *Inventing a Non-Homeless Future.* New York: Peter Lang.

Strasser, T. 1978. Reflections on Cardiovascular Disease. *Interdisciplinary Science Review* 3:225–230.

Susser E. S., E. Valencia, S. Conover, A. Felix, W-Y. Tsai, and R. J. Wyatt. 1997. Preventing Recurrent Homelessness among Mentally Ill Men: A "Critical Time" Intervention after Discharge from a Shelter. *American Journal of Public Health* 87, 2:256–262.

Titmuss, R. M. 1987. Universal and Selective Social Services. In *The Philosophy of Welfare: Selected Writings of Richard M. Titmuss.* London: Allen and Unwin.

Torrey, E. F. 1988. *Nowhere to Go: The Tragic Odyssey of the Homeless Mentally Ill.* New York: HarperCollins.

Towber, R., and C. Flemming. 1989. *The Housing Alert Program: A One Year Evaluation.* New York: City of New York, Human Resources Administration.

Tsemberis, S. 1999. From Streets to Homeless: An Innovative Approach to Supported Housing for Homeless Adults with Psychiatric Disabilities. *Journal of Community Psychology* 27, 2:225–241.

Tsemberis, S., and R. F. Eichenberg. 2000. Pathways to Housing: Supported Housing for Street-Dwelling Homeless Individuals with Psychiatric Disabilities. *Psychiatric Services* 51, 4:487–493.

Tsemberis, S., L. Gulcur, and M. Nakae. 2004. Housing First, Consumer Choice, and Harm Reduction for Individuals Who Are Homeless with Dual Diagnoses: A 24-Month Clinical Trial. *American Journal of Public Health* 94:651–656.

U.S. Census Bureau. 2006. American Community Survey. Washington D.C.: U.S. Government Printing Office.

U.S. Department of Health and Human Services. 2003. *Ending Chronic Homelessness: Strategies for Action: Report from the Secretary's Working Group on Ending Chronic Homelessness.* Washington, D.C.: Department of Health and Human Services.

U.S. General Accounting Office. 1990. *Homelessness: Too Early to Tell What Kinds of Prevention Assistance Work Best.* Washington, D.C.: U.S. Government Printing Office.

Weitzman, B., and C. Berry. 1994. *Formerly Homeless Families and the Transition to Permanent Housing: High-Risk Families and the Role of Intensive Case Management Services.* New York: New York University.

White, S., K. Nauer, S. Lerner, and B. Glenn. 2005. *Spanning the Neighborhood: The Bridge between Housing and Supports for Families.* New York: Center for New York City Affairs, New School University.

Wilson, W. J. 1987. *The Truly Disadvantaged: The Inner City, the Underclass, and Public Policy,* Chicago: University of Chicago Press.

Wong, I., D. P. Culhane, and R. Kuhn. 1997. Predictors of Exit and Re-Entry among Family Shelter Users in New York City. *Social Service Review* 71, 3:441–462.

Zielhuis, G. A., and L. Kiemeney. 2001. Social Epidemiology? No Way. *International Journal of Epidemiology* 30, 1:43–44.

Zlotnick, C., M. J. Robertson, and M. Lahiff. 1999. Getting off the Streets: Economic Resources and Residential Exits from Homelessness. *Journal of Community Psychology* 27, 2:209–224.

Zolopa, A. R., J. A. Hahn, R. Gorter, J. Miranda, D. Wlocdarczyk, J. Peterson, L. Pilote, and A. R. Moss. 1994. HIV and Tuberculosis Infection in San Francisco's Homeless Adults: Prevalence and Risk Factors in a Representative Sample. *JAMA* 272, 6:455–461.

Dealing with Humpty Dumpty

Research, Practice, and the Ethics of Public Health Surveillance

Alice considered [the idea of un-birthday presents] a little. "I like birthday presents best," she said at last.

"You don't know what you're talking about!" cried Humpty Dumpty. . . . "There are three hundred and sixty-four days when you might get un-birthday presents. . . . And only one for birthday presents, you know. There's a 'glory' for you!"

"I don't know what you mean by 'glory,'" Alice said.

Humpty Dumpty smiled contemptuously. "Of course you don't—till I tell you. I meant 'there's a nice knock-down argument for you!'"

"But 'glory' doesn't mean 'a nice knock-down argument,'" Alice objected.

"When I use a word," Humpty Dumpty said in a rather scornful tone, "it means just what I choose it to mean—neither more nor less."

—Lewis Carroll, *Through the Looking Glass*

The last third of the twentieth century witnessed the articulation of the ethics governing human subjects research. The federal research legislation and guidelines passed and promulgated in the 1970s built on the Nuremberg Code of 1947 and the 1964 Declaration of Helsinki. All drew upon a common set of principles that stressed the absolute need to prioritize the rights of the individual over those of society: There could be no exceptions to voluntary participation and informed consent of competent adults in any research protocol (Ackerman 1996). But while affirming the principle that no one could be conscripted into research projects, the guidelines, as Robert Levine (1996, 250) has noted, "were not addressed to the entire field of research involving human subjects as that field is currently understood."

In response to the new federal research protections, epidemiologists and ethicists began to discuss whether the principle of informed consent extended to the use of records, and whether the insistence on individual consent would render epidemiological research virtually impossible (Gordis, Gold, and Seltzer 1977; Gordis and Gold 1980; Gostin 1991; Capron 1991; Cann and Rothman 1984; Hershey 1985; Rothman 1981). In 1981, U.S. Department of Health and Human Services regulations for the protection of human subjects explicitly exempted from informed consent requirements epidemiological research that involved already existing data, provided that the risk to subjects was minimal, the research did not record data in a way that was individually identifiable, and the research could not otherwise be conducted (U.S. Department of Health and Human Services 1991).[1] In short, federal regulations balanced the rights of subjects against the general welfare, specifying clear conditions under which informed consent and voluntary participation might be waived.

But the discussion regarding research ethics and restrictions to records-based research did not extend to public health surveillance. Surveillance is a practice that often involves epidemiological research mandated by state and local law. It is thus based on a principle fundamentally different from that animating biomedical research ethics; individuals may be compelled to do or not do things to protect the common good.

In the context of the AIDS epidemic, however, as the Belmont principles were increasingly used to define the limits of public health practice in light of patients' civil rights, the nature of surveillance itself was called into question. The 1991 *International Guidelines for Ethical Review of Epidemiological Studies*, issued by the Council for International Organizations of Medical Sciences (CIOMS), epitomize the efforts of those concerned with the ethics of human subjects research to consider the questions posed not only by epidemiological investigations but also by public health surveillance. The guidelines employed a relatively narrow

definition of public health surveillance to justify exemptions from the requirement of ethical review: "An exception is justified when epidemiologists must
investigate outbreaks of acute communicable diseases. Then they must proceed
without delay to identify and control health risks. They cannot be expected to
await the formal approval of an ethical review committee." By focusing on the
urgency of some surveillance efforts, though, the committee excluded the vast
majority of surveillance, which is routine and ongoing. While the CIOMS guidelines stressed that investigators "as far as possible" were still obliged to respect
individual rights, freedom, privacy, and confidentiality, they left open the question of what rules should govern surveillance more broadly understood. The
guidelines stated: "Practice and research may overlap, as for example, when both
routine surveillance of cancer and original research on cancer are conducted by
professional staff of a population-based cancer registry" (Council for International
Organizations of Medical Sciences 1991, 255, 249). When it was difficult to distinguish research from practice, CIOMS called for the guidance of ethical review
committees.

Shortly after CIOMS issued its epidemiological guidelines, the question of
how to view surveillance—as research or as public health practice—would
become a pressing issue in the United States. Some AIDS advocates would
come to argue that the rules of research should be applied not only to HIV name
reporting but to all forms of disease surveillance.[2] Nonetheless, it was not HIV
name reporting that would give rise to the first critical challenge to surveillance; it was the Centers for Disease Control and Prevention's (CDC) blinded
HIV seroprevalence studies among childbearing women—a personally unintru-
sive but nonetheless highly controversial form of surveillance—that would
cause critics to charge that the CDC was engaged in research and that the rules
of human subjects protections should apply.

As a result of this complaint, the CDC developed guidelines to help distinguish between research and practice. But in reviewing the history of this
political controversy it becomes clear that the issue remains unsatisfactorily
unresolved and, indeed, that it will not be resolved by further attempts at defi-
nitional clarification of the distinction between research and practice. This history serves as a call to master not vocabulary but ethics.

Blinded HIV Serosurveillance and the Challenge to Surveillance

In 1993, National Institute of Health's (NIH) Office for the Protection from
Research Risks (OPRR) received written complaints regarding two CDC studies:
a measles vaccine trial intended to compare two vaccination schedules that the

CDC had contracted out to the Kaiser Foundation Research Institute and its own blinded HIV seroprevalence surveillance of childbearing women. In each case, the complaints alleged noncompliance with human subjects research regulations, but it was the serosurvey that raised questions about the bounds between research and practice within the context of federal human research regulations.

The CDC had begun to explore the feasibility of tracking the HIV epidemic through blinded testing at sentinel hospitals in 1986. When subject to ethical review in the 1980s, experts deemed such screening unproblematic (Bayer, Levine, and Wolf 1986; Office for the Protection from Research Risks 1988; Government of Canada Federal AIDS Centre 1988; World Health Organization Global Programme on AIDS 1989). It involved samples of blood, not identifiable individuals. The privacy of no one could be violated. Informed consent was hence unnecessary (Bayer 1993). But what made the studies—based on testing without subjects' consent—ethically acceptable also precluded notification of infected individuals. Since there was little that could be done for people with asymptomatic HIV infection in the late 1980s, there was widespread consensus that the blinded surveys were ethically permissible and served a critical public health need (Fairchild and Bayer 1999).

Because of the controversial nature of the studies and the negative press attention that the agency had received when it first became known that it was contemplating blinded surveillance, however, CDC officials decided to consult with their own Institutional Review Board (IRB), which reviewed and approved the protocol in 1987.[3] The CDC then requested further review from Office for Protection from Research Risks (OPRR), which had ultimate oversight authority over human subjects research.

A twelve-member OPRR ad hoc advisory group determined that serosurveillance did not fall within the regulatory definition of human subjects research because it met both of two key criteria: first, it "caused no interaction or intervention with living individuals (i.e., the activity resulted in no collection of information or specimens that would not otherwise be obtained)," and, second, it "utilized no information or specimens that could be linked, directly or indirectly, to identifiable living individuals" (OPRDHSP 1995, 7). The CDC proceeded as it would in normal surveillance activities with the exception that its own IRB continued to review the survey annually.

It was after this series of reviews and the initiation of the blinded studies that OPRR received a written complaint that the blinded survey violated human subjects regulations. The letter charged that the studies failed to obtain the informed consent of the childbearing women whose babies were anonymously tested.[4] The OPPR subsequently conducted a three-day onsite investigation.

While OPRR ultimately maintained its position that serosurveillance did not represent human subjects research and therefore did not require informed consent, the office came to the sweeping conclusion that "discussions with CDC personnel indicated that the distinction between human subjects research and routine, non-research public health practice was poorly understood and inconsistently applied" (OPRDHSP 1995, 11).[5]

In its report, OPRR reflected a larger NIH predisposition to view all data collection as research. It noted that because "a variety of otherwise routine public health practices" could evolve into human subjects research—the sometimes urgent need to investigate disease outbreaks notwithstanding—"it may be advantageous to invoke the provision in HHS regulations" and develop "IRB review arrangements that are suited to the particular challenges faced . . . in meeting unique public health responsibilities" (OPRDHSP 1995, 14). But while OPRR raised the prospect of formal IRB review for almost all surveillance activities, they required only that CDC develop a program for educating personnel about the regulatory requirements of human subjects research, as well as written guidelines for distinguishing research from practice.

The CDC received the final OPRR report in the summer of 1995 and began to deal with it in terms of three areas where public health practice was particularly difficult to distinguish from research: surveillance, emergency responses (for example, emergency responses to infectious or food-borne disease outbreaks), and program evaluation. Dixie Snider, the CDC's associate director for science in the Office of the Director, assigned Marjorie Speers, his deputy director, the task of addressing the OPRR report. Speers came to the CDC from academia, where all studies are considered research, unaware that surveillance "was such a sacred cow," as she told me in a 2002 interview.[6]

Prior to its internal examination of what constituted research, Speers explained, the CDC had traditionally employed a procedure-based approach to determining whether an activity required IRB review: "If they did a blood draw," for example, "they were defining it as research."[7] Scientists at the CDC were profoundly resistant to labeling an activity research, she said, in part because of a concern that such a designation would invoke a lengthy IRB review and require informed consent.

It was precisely these concerns that had so worried epidemiologists and other social science researchers following passage of the Privacy Act and National Research Act in 1974. (The National Research Act mandated evaluation of all federally funded human subjects research by IRBs.) Regulations requiring the protection of privacy and informed consent, they feared, would effectively put an end to their research efforts (Brody 1998). At the CDC, the concerns of epidemiologists were compounded by the way in which health officials tended to see the relationship between surveillance efforts and the central mission of public health. Speers recalled numerous occasions on which CDC scientists—on hearing that she had determined a protocol to be human subjects research requiring IRB review—told her, "You are killing people because you are making me go to the IRB." This stance reflected the legacy of the CIOMS and, indeed, OPRR formulation of "urgency" as representing grounds to exempt an activity from oversight. In short, the new application of the research regulations "wreaked havoc" on the way things had been done for a century (Centers for Disease Control and Prevention 1996, 5).

Viewing herself as an outsider who was "not a product of the system," Speers began to tackle this problem by considering the meaning of research in the law. While the Declaration of Helsinki had, in 1964, distinguished between therapeutic and nontherapeutic research, it was not until the formation of the National Commission for the Protection of Research Subjects of Biomedical and Behavioral Research in the United States that a body was given the task of " 'consider[ing] the boundaries between biomedical or behavioral research and the routine and accepted practice of medicine'" (Levine 2002).[8] It was the National Commission's 1979 *Belmont Report* that formally distinguished research from practice.

The *Belmont Report* observed that "the distinction between research and practice is blurred partly because both often occur together" (National Commission for the Protection of Research Subjects of Biomedical and Behavior Research 1979). Jay Katz—a central figure in the development of contemporary medical ethics—described differentiating between these two endeavors as "the most difficult and complex problem facing the Commission." The need to make the distinction was rooted in the ways that Americans came to see a tension between clinician and researcher. Thomas Chalmers, who sat with Katz on the National Commission, explained that drawing the distinction was so difficult because "every physician is carrying out a small research project when he diagnoses and treats a patient" for "episodes of illness and individual people are so variable" (Levine 1988, 3).

The *Belmont Report* defined practice as "interventions that are designed solely to enhance the well-being of an individual patient or client and that have a reasonable expectation of success." Research, in contrast, "designates an activity designed to test a hypothesis, permit conclusions to be drawn, and thereby to develop or contribute to generalizable knowledge (expressed, for example, in theories, principles, and statements of relationships). Research is usually described in a formal protocol that sets forth an objective and a set of procedures designed to reach that objective" (National Commission for the Protection

of Research Subjects of Biomedical and Behavior Research 1979). The NIH subsequently used the *Belmont Report* as the basis for the definition of research in
its 1981 regulations governing human subjects research: "research is a systematic investigation, including research development, testing and evaluation,
designed to contribute to generalizable knowledge" (U.S. Department of Health
and Human Services 1991).

Speers was convinced that underlying these definitions was the question
of intent.[9] After all, Robert Levine, who drafted the first definition of research
for the National Commission, defined research as an activity "done with the
intent" of generating new knowledge. But while Levine maintained and has
continued to maintain that intent must be the basis for distinguishing research
from practice, as he said in our interview on December 2, 2002, in New Haven,
Connecticut, the National Commission's Joseph Brady took issue with the idea
of linking the definition of research to intent. A Skinnerian from Johns Hopkins,
Brady argued that it was impossible to measure intent. The Belmont compro-
mise used the language of design.

Although the National Commission formally rejected the notion of intent,
the first set of CDC guidelines drafted in 1996 made the case that intent differentiates public health surveillance from pure research: Public health practice is
undertaken with "the primary goal . . . to monitor the health of a given population for the purpose of taking public health action." Whereas "the *intent* of
research is to contribute to or generate generalizable knowledge; the *intent* of
public health practice is to conduct programs to prevent disease and injury and
improve the health of communities" (Snider and Stroup 1997, 30, 32).

While OPRR approved this CDC draft, they simultaneously but paradoxically advanced the notion with their own draft document that all surveillance
was research. This formulation alarmed the CDC as well as the Council of State
and Territorial Epidemiologists (CSTE), which protested the position. According
to the CDC (1996): "The implications of calling public health surveillance
research are broad and far reaching. There are 2,088 health departments and
over 100 surveillance systems. If all surveillance activities were research, it
might mean each local health department would have to form institutional
review boards (IRBs) and secure [special CDC assurances that human subjects
were being protected] for each system. Whether the surveillance system is mandated by state law is irrelevant. If the research activity is federally funded, it
requires assurance of human subjects protection." To the CDC, this was more than
a bureaucratic consideration: If surveillance activities were designated research,
the CDC feared that "people with TB could prevent their names from being
reported to the health department or refuse to provide information about their

contacts" (Snider and Stroup 1997, 30). OPRR, however, did not press the alternative position that all data collection represented research: "The bottom line is that OPRR is prepared to live with a certain amount of ambiguity as long as we are convinced that CDC is making a genuine effort to define these distinctions in a reasonable manner, that the definitions are not being abused, and that CDC has an effective gatekeeper . . . to ensure consistency in its decision-making."[10]

The Effort to Distinguish Research from Practice

By 1997, the CDC had begun working with CSTE on refining its guidelines for distinguishing between research and practice. Although the state health officials expressed from the outset their concerns that a range of state-level activities, including surveillance, outbreak investigation, and program evaluation, "be considered public health practice, not public health research," it was not until 1999 that the profoundly different ways in which the states and the federal government drew the boundary between research and practice began to become clear.

The CDC, which notably relies on the voluntary reporting of surveillance data by the states, is rarely involved in the use of surveillance for public health interventions like contact tracing. It is thus open to considering many of its activities as directed toward generating "new" knowledge based on the collective experience of the states. To be sure, CDC considers their "human subjects research" as "intricately associated with other public health activities, such as public health surveillance," and consequently as "strongly public health- and prevention-oriented and carried out with a clear public health purpose" (Snider 2000). But however practical their research might be, it remains research that requires IRB review, in the minds of many CDC officials.

States, typically operating under statutes mandating departments of health to collect and act on individual-level disease data for the explicit purpose of controlling disease, tended to view most public health surveillance activities as practice (CDCP/CSTE 1999, 22).[11] New York State, for example, described the range of activities it undertook to control a typhoid outbreak in 1989, which included not only case reporting and testing but also one cohort and two case control studies conducted by phone on the sixth day of the outbreak (8–9). In the case of the two phone studies, participation was not mandatory, but outbreak investigators were not required to inform individuals about what cooperation was required.[12] Again, the example that New York called upon to make the point that surveillance must not be captured by the IRB system relied on the urgency of these endeavors.

While the CDC and the states generally agreed that activities such as outbreak investigation should not be defined as research, the federal government and the states defined research and practice differently when it came to routine surveillance (CDCP/CSTE 1999, 15). These differences were not merely semantic but carried broad consequences. John Middaugh, Alaska's state epidemiologist, described an instance in which his state was given legislative authority to conduct birth defects surveillance using federal funds. The funding agency viewed the project as research and demanded a state-level IRB review: "Alaska eventually returned the grant funds because the Attorney General did not want to delegate the decision-making process to an IRB" (11).[13] The same scenario was repeated when the state attempted to use federal funds to conduct surveillance for fetal alcohol syndrome (FAS), though in this instance OPRR concluded that the surveillance effort was not research and therefore did not require IRB review. But in states where FAS surveillance was not mandated by law, the OPRR could and did demand IRB review (12).

In response to the comments from a meeting with CSTE, the CDC in its June 1999 draft "Guidelines for Defining Public Health Research and Public Health Non-Research" sought to describe more specifically the activities that constituted research. These efforts at clarification provoked more pointed objections on the part of state and local health officials. The guidelines stated that "if the primary intent is to prevent or control disease or injury and no research is intended at the present time, the project is non-research. If the primary intent changes to generating generalizable knowledge, then the project becomes research." That is, "if subsequent analysis of identifiable private information is undertaken in order to generate or contribute to generalizable knowledge, the analysis constitutes human subjects research that requires IRB review." Thus, a hallmark of public health practice that was not research was that the "intended benefits of the project are primarily or exclusively for the study participants; data collected are needed to assess and/or improve the health of the participants" (Centers for Disease Control and Prevention 1999a, 3, 4).

The New York City Department of Health responded that "the very essence" of its mission was "to prevent or control disease and injury." In doing so, the department argued: "We derive knowledge that may protect the particular 'victims' before us. However, it may also be that it is too late to help the particular victims, but that the activity, or the information derived from it, becomes generalizable so as to protect the general population."[14] CSTE concurred, arguing that "we are rarely able to conduct an investigation that provides any medical benefit to those already infected." For example, in the case of food-borne outbreak investigations, the "major benefit has been to others than those we identified and obtained data and specimens from."[15]

New York City gave the example of an outbreak of hepatitis A among young gay men that investigation determined was associated with sexual practices rather than consumption of contaminated food or water; vaccination "was then directed not to the original victims but to the general population of young men who have sex with men. At what stage of this investigation did the Department shift from its 'primary intent' of preventing disease or injury to 'generating generalizable knowledge'?" The department thus adamantly insisted that "generalizable knowledge can be derived from public health epidemiological investigations, and such investigations can still be deemed not to be human subjects research where there is sufficient statutory authority to conduct the investigation."[16] And, indeed, New York State public health law specifically noted that "human research shall not . . . be construed . . . to include epidemiological investigations" (New York State Public Health Law Section 2441[2]). For New York City, because surveillance carried the potential for public health impact, broadly construed, this made it practice rather than research, regardless of any research implications it might also carry: "If an inquiry may result in a public health intervention, such as contact notification, Commissioner's Orders or perhaps even rulemaking, then such should be viewed as an epidemiologic investigation" that does not constitute research.[17]

Just as surveillance may not always benefit directly the populations from which it was drawn, health officials also drew a distinction between immediate intent and primary intent. CSTE thus explained that it consistently collected data with an eye not only to the present but also to the future: "Ongoing analysis" of previously collected data sets was "routinely conducted for most, if not all, of the diseases for which data are collected under state law." By review of previous investigations of trichinosis outbreaks, for example, the state health department in Alaska not only developed an early diagnostic test for the disease but also identified an animal species not previously known to harbor trichinella, as well as a new subspecies of the disease-causing organism. "We do not view these activities as research" when conducted by the state; yet "if conducted by an entity other than the state public health agency, we would define it as research and require an outside researcher to obtain IRB approval."[18] Thus it was the provenance of the undertaking that determined whether an activity was research or practice. By definition, then, what public health departments did was not research.

Most alarming to state and local officials was the very narrow conception of when surveillance clearly represented pure practice. The CDC described as practice only disease reporting "conducted to monitor the frequency of occurrence and distribution of disease or a health condition in the population" and surveillance regimes "in which no analytic (etiological) analyses can be conducted." "Longitudinal data collection systems (e.g. follow up surveys and registries)" in which "the scope of the data is broad" and includes "more information than occurrence of a health-related problem," in which "analytic analyses can be conducted," and in which "cases may be identified for subsequent studies" were, according to the CDC guidelines, "likely to be research" (Centers for Disease Control and Prevention 1999a). The CSTE described this as a contradiction in terms: After all, "by its very nature, mandatory disease reporting is intended to be longitudinal data collection" and "to detect the causal agent to prevent future disease or injury."[19]

But it also represented a catch-22 for states: New York City and some states found the narrow definition of nonresearch surveillance "very troubling" because it conflicted with their legal mandate to collect data.[20] For example, the New York State Sanitary Code (10 N.Y.C.R.R.24–1.1), in creating the AIDS registry, authorized the health commissioner, after receiving an initial case report, to collect all information "as may be required for the epidemiologic analysis and study of Acquired Immune Deficiency Syndrome." Thus, for many public health officials, "if an intervention or action is delegated to the health officer by statute or regulation, such intervention is per se ethical and is not human subjects research."[21] CSTE broadly concurred that "what distinguishes the activities as non-research at the state level is that the public health authority undertakes them and the data are collected under the authority of explicit state law."[22]

In the end, the CDC addressed the states' concerns not by altering its guidelines to meet any of the specific challenges raised by the states (Centers for Disease Control and Prevention 1999b), but by holding that "intent is different under the authority of a state/local health department versus a university" and that legal authority or mandate to protect the public health also shaped intent: States acted with such power, the CDC did not (CDCP/CSTE 1999, 19, 26; Council of State and Territorial Epidemiologists 1996; Patrick 2001). In short, as the former associate director for science at the CDC's National Center for HIV, STD, and TB Prevention Jim Buehler said, "activities can be viewed differently at federal and state levels."[23]

Putting Humpty Dumpty Together Again?

It is clear that public health surveillance is simultaneously both research and practice, in some instances more heavily favoring one component than the other. Key stakeholders, moreover, can draw the boundary differently at different moments or recognize it not at all. In 1998 and 1999, for instance, the CDC commissioned the drafting of a Model Public Health Privacy Act to help ensure that states keep all surveillance data secure without impeding surveillance efforts. Some AIDS advocates challenged not only the model act but also the very legitimacy of public health surveillance. Advocates did not explicitly frame the debate in terms of whether surveillance should be considered research or practice, but they worried about how easy it was for health officials to conduct research with surveillance data under the model law and thus attempted to require informed consent for all surveillance for all diseases in a way that would have brought even state-mandated data collection under strict human subjects regulation. But not all disease advocates agree that informed consent is desirable. In the context of cancer surveillance, breast cancer advocates led the fight against efforts to make inclusion in state tumor registries voluntary (National Committee on Vital and Health Statistics 1998, 17).

It may be that there are few practical consequences for individuals if an activity is defined as practice rather than research, for health officials may protect the rights of citizens as vigilantly as IRBs protect the rights of those same people when they are defined as research subjects. But using the intent of surveillance to determine whether it is research or practice is a sleight of hand that in the end is conceptually unsatisfying, even if it represents a politically necessary response to the historical legacy of how research was originally defined and what was initially conceived as research. Some health officials have found that they do not distinguish between research and practice consistently and that they sometimes face political pressure to define an activity as practice rather than research.

Thus, the time has come, first, to articulate ethical principles for public health practice that both justify and limit data collection and use and, second, to envision a mechanism for oversight. To be sure, ethical guidelines governing public health practice would not eliminate the thorny problem of determining when surveillance should be governed by the ethics of medical research and when it should be governed by the ethics of public health practice. Nor would such an ethics provide a practical mechanism for challenging legal mandates for states to acquire, use, and disclose surveillance data. But it would provide a systematic means for evaluating legal mandates to conduct surveillance: A practice is not automatically ethical simply because it is mandatory. As important, a framework for ethical review of practice would render what has been an ongoing and tortured effort to distinguish such activities from research less momentous. No one should underestimate the resistance that such a proposal will confront: As Humpty Dumpty might say, there will be a "glory" for you.

Acknowledgments

I thank Ronald Bayer, Alison, James Colgrove, Alison Bateman-House, and the participants in the seminar series at the Program in the History of Science, Medicine, and Technology, Johns Hopkins University. This research was funded by grants from the National Institutes of Health and the Robert Wood Johnson Foundation.

Notes

1. National and international guidelines typically share a common set of ethical principles that guide the discussions of research ethics. They were first formally articulated in the United States in the 1979 *Belmont Report* by the United States National Commission for the Protection of Research Subjects of Biomedical and Behavior Research. Respect for persons necessitates respect for the choices of competent individuals and protection of vulnerable persons. The right of informed consent derives from this principle. Beneficence (the charge to do good) and its counterpart, nonmaleficence (the admonition to do no harm), necessitate maximizing benefits and minimizing research harms. Justice demands equal treatment and, in the research context, refers to fairly distributing benefits and burdens.

2. And, indeed, that this might happen was a concern early in the epidemic, as ethicists began to develop guidelines for AIDS research in a fashion that the CDC feared did not adequately set surveillance apart. Memo from J. R. Allen, MD, Chief, Surveillance Section, AIDS Activity, Centers for Disease Control, regarding Meeting on Confidentiality and Research into AIDS, Hastings Center, New York, November 7, 1983, copy in author files.

3. Tim Dondero, interview by R. Bayer and the author, Atlanta, June 11, 2002.

4. In addition, the letter alleged that the study violated Public Health Service policy on informing individuals who were tested for HIV about their serostatus and that the IRB review was improper due to conflicts of interest (OPRDHSP 1995, 8).

5. Further, it determined that policy on informing individuals of their test results did not apply to blinded tests. It did, however, question the diversity of the CDC's IRB and recommended changes on the grounds that "it is especially critical that no real or apparent conflict of interest undermine respect for [federal agency] IRBs' advice and counsel in safeguarding the rights and welfare of human subjects" (ibid., 10–11).

6. Margery Speers, interview by the author, Washington, D. C., March 13, 2002.

7. Speers interview. See also R. Bernier, Centers for Disease Control and Prevention, e-mail to M. Speers, Centers for Disease Control and Prevention, September 20, 1999, copy in author files. When the controversy over research and practice between the CDC and the states began to unfold, Speers said, an idea was put forth regarding the use of "telltale signs" as a means to distinguish research from practice based not on intent but on "what is actually done."

8. For the Declaration of Helsinki, see World Medical Association 1989. The distinction between therapeutic and nontherapeutic research—the subject of substantial criticism—would persist virtually unchanged until the 2000 revision of the code, when it was substantially modified (Levine 1988). In 2000, the Declaration of Helsinki provided principles governing all of medical research with special principles for research combined with care. It is also in this year that references to "investigators" or "researchers" replace all references to "physicians."

9. Robert Levine, who had been an instrumental informant and consultant to the National Commission in formulating the *Belmont Report*, had indicated to Speers that, indeed, intent had at one time been included in the definition.

10. Tom Puglisi, Office for Protection from Research Risks, e-mail to Marjorie Speers, CDCP, October 4, 1999, copy in author files.

11. Patricia Fleming, interview by R. Bayer and the author, Atlanta, June 11, 2002.
12. In Minnesota, in contrast, state law required that public health investigators inform the public that participation is voluntary in addition to why data are being collected and how they will be used. CDCP/CSTE 1999, 13.
13. Minnesota law, in contrast, prohibits legally mandated public health activities from undergoing IRB review. CDCP/CSTE 1999, 12.
14. Benjamin Mojica, MD, MPH, Deputy Commissioner of Health, City of New York Department of Health, to Donna Knutson, Executive Director, Council for State and Territorial Epidemiologists, August 25, 1999, 3, copy in author files.
15. John Middaugh, memo to Marjorie Speers, CDCP, regarding Comments on "Draft of Revised Document for Defining Research," June 7, 1999, copy in author files.
16. Mojica to Knutson.
17. Ibid.
18. Middaugh to Speers; see also Mojica to Knutson, 4.
19. Middaugh to Speers.
20. Guthric Birkhead, New York State Department of Health AIDS Institute, e-mail to Marjorie Speers, CDCP, June 1, 1999; Kristine Moore, CSTE and Minnesota State Department of Health, e-mail to Marjorie Speers, CDCP, June 9, 1999; Diane Simpson, Texas State Department of Health, e-mail to Donna B. Knutson, CSTE, July 20, 1999, copies in author files. For general objections to the distinctions between research and practice, see Memo from the Director, NIOSH, Department of Health and Human Services, to Marjorie Speers, CDCP, May 28, 1999, copy in author files.
21. Mojica to Knutson, 2.
22. Middaugh to Speers. See also Birkhead to Speers; Moore to Speers; Simpson to Knutson; Stephen Waterman, California Department of Health Services, e-mail to Fran Reid-Sanden, CDCP, March 3, 1999, copy in author files. Colorado, in contrast to all the other states commenting on the CDC draft guidelines, did not object to any of the distinctions drawn between research and practice but rather to the fact that research protocols had to undergo IRB review at both the state and federal levels. Richard Hoffman, Colorado State Department of Public Health and Environment, e-mail to Guthric Birkhead, New York State Department of Health AIDS Institute, August 26, 1999, and Richard Hoffman, Colorado State Department of Public Health and Environment, e-mail to Dixie Snider, CDCP, March 3, 1999, copies in author files.
23. James Buehler interview by author, Atlanta, July 8, 2002.

References

Ackerman, T. H. 1996. Choosing between Nuremberg and the National Commission: Balancing of Moral Principles in Clinical Research. In *The Ethics of Research Involving Human Subjects: Facing the 21st Century,* ed. H. Y. Vanderpool. Frederick, Md.: University Publishing Group.

Bayer, R. 1993. The Ethics of Blinded HIV Surveillance Testing. *American Journal of Public Health* 83:496–497.

Bayer, R., C. Levine, and S. M. Wolf. 1986. HIV Antibody Screening: An Ethical Framework for Evaluating Proposed Programs. *JAMA* 256:1768–1774.

Brody, B. A. 1998. *The Ethics of Biomedical Research: An International Perspective.* New York: Oxford University Press.

Cann, C. I., and K. J. Rothman. 1984. IRBs and Epidemiologic Research: How Inappropriate Restrictions Hamper Studies. *IRB: A Review of Human Subjects Research,* July/ August, 5–7.

Capron, A. M. 1991. Protection of Research Subjects: Do Special Rules Apply in Epidemiology? *Law, Medicine, and Health Care* 19:184–190.

CDCP/CSTE. See Centers for Disease Control and Prevention and Council of State and Territorial Epidemiologists.

Centers for Disease Control and Prevention. 1996. Minutes, Protection of Human Research Subjects in Public Health, Centers for Disease Control and Prevention, Atlanta, March 18–19.

———. 1999a. *Draft Guidelines for Defining Public Health Research and Public Health Non-Research.* Revised June 1999. Atlanta: Centers for Disease Control and Prevention.

———. 1999b. *Guidelines for Defining Public Health Research and Public Health Non-Research.* October 4. www.cdc.gov/od/ads/opsp0111.htm (accessed November 14, 2003).

Centers for Disease Control and Prevention and Council of State and Territorial Epidemiologists [CDCP/CSTE]. 1999. Minutes, Meeting on Research, Atlanta, March 4–5.

Council for International Organizations of Medical Sciences. 1991. *International Guidelines for Ethical Review of Epidemiological Studies.* Geneva: CIOMS. Reprinted in *Law, Medicine, and Health Care* 19:247–258.

Council of State and Territorial Epidemiologists. 1996. CSTE Position Statement 1996–8, "Definition of Public Health Research." www.cste.org/ps/1996/1996–08.htm (accessed November 14, 2003).

Fairchild, A., and R. Bayer. 1999. The Uses and Abuses of Tuskegee. *Science* 284:919–921.

Gordis, L., and E. Gold. 1980. Privacy, Confidentiality, and the Use of Medical Records in Research. *Science* 207:153–156.

Gordis, L., E. Gold, and R. Seltzer. 1977. Privacy Protection in Epidemiologic and Medical Research: A Challenge and a Responsibility. *American Journal of Epidemiology* 105: 163–168.

Gostin, L. 1991. Ethical Principles for the Conduct of Human Subject Research: Population Based Research and Ethics. *Law, Medicine, and Health Care* 19:191–201.

Government of Canada Federal AIDS Centre. 1988. *Guidelines on Ethical and Legal Conditions in Anonymous Unlinked HIV Seroprevalence Research.* Ottawa, Ont.: Government of Canada Federal AIDS Centre.

Hershey, N. 1985. IRB Jurisdiction and Limits on IRB Actions. *IRB: A Review of Human Subjects Research,* March/April, 7–9.

Levine, R. J. 1988. *Ethics and Regulation of Clinical Research.* New Haven: Yale University Press.

———. 1996. International Codes and Guidelines for Research Ethics: A Critical Appraisal. In *The Ethics of Research Involving Human Subjects: Facing the 21st Century,* ed. Harold Y. Vanderpool. Frederick, Md.: University Publishing Group.

———. 2002. "Should All Disciplines Be Subject to the Common Rule?" Presentation to the National Human Research Protections Advisory Committee. July 31, 2002.

National Commission for the Protection of Research Subjects of Biomedical and Behavioral Research. 1979. *The Belmont Report.* Reprinted in *The Ethics of Research Involving Human Subjects: Facing the 21st Century,* ed. Harold Y. Vanderpool. Frederick, Md.: University Publishing Group.

National Committee on Vital and Health Statistics. 1998. Transcript of the Roundtable on Privacy and Confidentiality, January 29. Copy in author files.

Office for the Protection from Research Risks. 1988. *HIV Seroprevalence Survey of Childbearing Women: Testing Neonatal Dried Blood Specimens on Filter Paper for HIV Antibody.* Atlanta: Centers for Disease Control.

Office for Protection from Research Risks, Division of Human Subject Protections [OPRDHSP]. 1995. *Evaluation of Human Subject Protections in Research Conducted by the Centers for Disease Control and Prevention and the Agency for Toxic Substances and Disease Registry.* Rockville, Md.: Office for Protection from Research Risks, National Institutes of Health.

OPRDHSP. See Office for Protection from Research Risks, Division of Human Subject Protections.

Patrick, S. L. 2001. CDC Efforts to Ensure Human Subjects Protection in Applied Epidemiologic Activities. *American Public Health Association Epidemiology Section Newsletter,* Fall, 6–7. www.apha.org/private/newsletters/epifa112001.htm.

Rothman, K. J. 1981. The Rise and Fall of Epidemiology, 1950–2000 A.D. *New England Journal of Medicine* 304:600–602.

Snider, D. E. 2000. Comments for the External Review Panel: Characteristics of CDC-Supported Research. Presented at Human Subjects Review Processes at CDC: Summary of External Consultants Meeting, Atlanta, March 24.

Snider, D. E., and D. F. Stroup. 1997. Defining Research When It Comes to Public Health. *Public Health Reports* 112:29–32.

U.S. Department of Health and Human Services. National Institutes of Health. 1991. Office for Protection from Research Risks. Code of Federal Regulations, Title 45, Public Welfare, Part 46, Protection of Human Subjects (45 CFR 46).

World Health Organization Global Programme on AIDS. 1989. *Unlinked Anonymous Screening for the Public Health Surveillance of HIV Infections Proposed International Guidelines.* Geneva, Switz.: World Health Organization.

World Medical Association. 1989. *Declaration of Helsinki.* Reprinted in *Law, Medicine, and Health Care* 19:264–265.

Health Production

A Common Framework to Unify Public Health and Medicine

Examining commonalities between public health and medicine might be more fruitful for advancing the public's health and well-being than would another effort to delineate their differences.

While stark differences between public health and medicine are apparent in every category of comparison (see table 8.1), the ultimate social purpose of both is to protect and improve the health and well-being of individuals and populations while reducing health inequalities. This purpose has compelling empiric bases.

The United States ranks in the bottom third in comparisons of population health among the economically developed member nations of the Organization for Economic Cooperation and Development (OECD). Further, when the distribution of health status across the population of each nation is plotted against social, economic, or educational status, the distribution of health in the United States is among the most unequal in OECD.

Before proceeding further to develop the concept of health production, we pause here to identify an impediment to joining public health and medicine within a common framework.

Avedis Donabedian, professor of epidemiology at the University of Michigan, envisioned the health care system as consisting of three intersecting parts: structure, process, and outcomes. Structure consists of fixed components such as health plans; hospitals and clinics; the health care workforce; the organization, financing, and regulation of medical services; and the people and populations served. Process refers to the activity of providing health services, including diagnostic procedures and therapies—what actually transpires in the doctor, nurse, pharmacist, or allied health professional interaction with

Table 8.1. **Public Health and Medicine Compared**

	Public Health	Medicine
Focus	Populations as a whole	Individual persons (one by one)
	Strategies based on population health sciences	Strategies based on human biology, medical technology, and engineering
	Interventions begin with public policies	Interventions begin in doctors'/nurses' offices
Purpose	Monitor and enforce government regulations regarding food and water supplies, sanitation	Provide individualized medical services (diagnose, treat, relieve suffering, restore function, counsel, refer)
	Defend population against epidemics of infection, chronic disease, humanmade and natural disasters, contaminant toxins	
Organized Structure	Financing: public, tax supported health agencies within federal, state, county, and municipal governments	Financing: public and private combo, employer contributions, individual self-pay, public insurance (Medicare, Medicaid, VAH)
	Agenda-setting: principally public sector: federal leadership, U.S. Public Health Service, surgeon general, assistant secretary for health, U.S. Department of Health and Human Services; and by state and local boards of health and health departments	Delivery systems: principally private sector: health plans and hospital systems on a fee-for-service basis
		Leadership: Largely private sector and professional self-regulation
Outcomes Assessment	Air-water-soil-food hygiene, industrial effluent monitoring, sanitation systems oversight	Structure and process measures: insured rates, access
	Responsiveness to health crises (humanmade and natural) and infectious epidemics	Outcomes measures: Patient satisfaction, patient functional capacity, morbidity and mortality rates over time, patient safety, cost-effectiveness ratios
	Epidemiologic data monitoring systems	
Accountability	Governments: federal, state, county	Mandatory accreditation, certification, and licensure
	Local health agencies and boards	Professional self-regulation
	Minimal credentialing	High individual provider autonomy
		Accountable to health plans
		Regulation and monitoring by Medicare, Medicaid, Social Security, veteran's health care, insurance companies

(Continued)

Table 8.1. **(Continued)**

	Public Health	**Medicine**
Workforce Training	Locations: schools of public health, nursing, business and administration, and community colleges	Locations: schools of medicine, osteopathy, nursing, allied health professions, and teaching hospitals
Research	Funding: federal (NIH, CDC, NCHS), local (tax revenues) Locations: universities, CDC, local jurisdictions Annually appropriated research expenditures	Funding: federal (NIH, AHCQR, CMM, FDA, NCHS), private (pharmaceutical industry, medical device manufacturers) Locations: universities, teaching hospitals, pharmaceutical laboratories Mostly multiyear research appropriations

patients in the doctor's office, hospital, home, or long-term care facility. Outcomes are the end results, the consequences of interventions. In individual patients, outcomes include changes in physical health, mental health, sense of well-being, functional capability in everyday activities, and relief of pain, suffering, and other symptoms. Outcomes in a whole population include changes in morbidity or mortality rates for specific disease categories; regional differences in disease rates, treatments, and health outcomes; aggregated rates of work absenteeism and disability; and cost effectiveness of health gains.

Assessments of medical care are most often related to access to care, the number of uninsured people, patient satisfaction with health services, annual increases in health care expenditures, and shifting of costs from employers to employees and to governments. These assessments are not direct indicators of health but primarily relate to structural and process performance. The outcomes assessed in public health are diverse and reflect the wide variations of functions a noncentralized public health system undertakes. Although public health does provide a wide array of services that respond to the public's health needs, trends in the incidence and prevalence (epidemiology) of disease is its major focus. Monitoring public health effects in terms of direct measures of health and well-being is, by and large, underemphasized.

If health improvement becomes an operational objective, public health and medicine in the United States will be shown to have been not cost effective. Approval to introduce expensive new diagnostic and therapeutic technology does not require solid evidence that these technologies will improve health outcomes. That U.S. expenditures on health exceed by 30 percent or more those of other developed countries whose health is superior to ours does not support a conclusion that health care has been a cost-effective instrument for improving population health in the United States.

In the past fifty years advancements in measurement of health status and outcomes have been made at the level of both the individual and the population. For measuring individual health at a single moment, as well as for monitoring an individual's health over time, assessing physical and mental functional capacity by means of patient-completed brief questionnaires has proven sensitive, reliable, and valid. These brief individual survey measures of health can be aggregated for a whole population to also assess population health status. Other simple and inexpensive measures that integrate health assessment with social circumstances, such as Quality Adjusted Life Years (QUALYs) or Disability Adjusted Life Years (DALYs) have been developed and tested. These permit comparison of trends in population health among diverse populations and settings. It is technically feasible now to adopt a health outcomes measurement system for use by both public health and medicine that would capture their effectiveness in health production. Such a unified health assessment system could become an important facilitative asset for establishing common ground and synergistic interventions by public health and medicine for health production purposes.

Moreover, the distinction between a focus on population health or on individual health has become blurred. Increasingly, research has illuminated more clearly the causes of ill health, especially social contextual factors that have been identified as fundamental to the production of health and health inequalities.

The era in which disease production is considered primarily a biological aberration is giving way to a more sophisticated understanding of the complex interactions among genetic makeup, social context, social policy, physical environment, health behaviors, the ecology of all living things, the brain, psychological and biological adaptation, and medical care. These complex interactions can be usefully thought of as constituting an integrated system of health production (Tarlov, forthcoming).

Health production could become an underlying framework that joins public health and medical care in a common purpose to protect and improve the health of individuals and populations while reducing health inequalities. Although a crossover of interest between public health and medicine is evident in some works (Aday 2005), effectiveness in pursuing common purposes could be enhanced by adoption of an integrated social-ecologic-biologic conceptualization of health production. Among the consequences, social policy could become a primary intervention in health.

A comprehensive model of health production is needed to provide guidance for efforts to improve health and reduce disparities. Such a model might have three sections: (1) circumstances of living that include factors external to the body such as social context and experiences that affect us every minute of every day; (2) biological adjustments within the body that are in response to, and adaptive to, the external circumstances of living. These adjustments to circumstances, beginning in utero and continuing over the life course, are physiological adjustments of many biological regulatory processes. The adjustments seem to be upregulatory reactions to external threats, and quantitatively are in inverse proportion to levels of education, job class, and income (Tarlov, forthcoming). These adaptations appear to become permanently imprinted or embedded in the biology of each individual in response to social status in a process referred to in this chapter as socio-psycho-biological-health translation; (3) consequences, or outcomes, which refer to the wide variations in health that are observable across every population. The health variations are highly correlated with social position; that is, in almost a straight-line relationship, higher levels of health accompany increased levels of education, job classification, and income. This relationship is referred to as the social-health gradient and is the basic concept behind health disparities.

In the next sections, six conceptual frameworks help integrate circumstances of living, biologic adjustments, and health outcomes into an understanding of health production. That understanding will help broaden the formulation of policies and interventions to improve health and reduce health inequalities.

Integration of Multiple Conceptual Frameworks into an Explanation of Health Production

The production of health is complex and affected by a large number of factors embedded in a viscous matrix of social, economic, and political organization that initially resists change but ultimately adapts to consensus public expectations. The conceptual frameworks relevant to health production include: (1) influences (determinants) of health; (2) social context; (3) the health gradient; (4) life course; (5) parallel production of brain development, child development, human development, and health; and (6) socio-psycho-biological-health translation. A more inclusive, integrated, and coherent framework can provide a broader range of interventional possibilities for research and public policy formulations for the production of improved health and common ground to unify public health and medicine.

Conceptual Framework #1. Health Influences (Determinants)

This conceptual framework includes five general categories of factors that directly influence health.[1] They are genomic, behavioral, medical care, physical environmental, and social context. By common custom these factors have been labeled "determinants." But that is a misnomer. Each of these factors interacts with all the others. The interactions comprise a complex system of positive and negative feedbacks, cancellation effects, enhancements, synergies, and so forth. None of the categories of influence are autonomous or solely determinant. They are highly interdependent. For example: Gene activity is highly dependent on environments, both the physical and social environments; medical care produces variable results, partly because of genetic variations in a population, differences in health behaviors (diet or tobacco smoking), and variations in the physical environment (particulate matter and noxious chemicals in patients having asthma), and partly because lower socioeconomic groups respond less favorably to medical care. In this chapter the term "determinants" will be avoided in favor of "influences." The following sections briefly elaborate on each category of influence.

Genomic Influences

There are substantial data about the role of genetic inheritance in explaining variations in child development and in health status. (This section addresses the role of genetic inheritance in health production; later, I address the role of genetic inheritance with respect to the health gradient.)

Weatherall, at Oxford University, has for thirty years analyzed data on the frequency of genetic diseases, the health burden on populations, and the clinical load on medical practitioners and hospitals. When he began his work, only single mutant gene disorders were known. Currently, single mutant genes are found in 4.5 to 14.0 per 1000 population (0.4 to 1.4 percent of the population). Another type of inherited disorder, chromosomal abnormalities (0.7 percent of the world population) occurs when an extra chromosome is inherited, such as XXY in Down Syndrome, or when a piece of one chromosome breaks off and becomes attached to another. Common disorders such as diabetes mellitus and some other chronic conditions have been discovered to be associated with the genetic transmission of a distinctive combination of six to twelve normal genes on normal chromosomes, referred to as polygenic inheritance, that predispose to a specific disease when they interact with environmental factors. Congenital malformations that include cleft lip and congenital heart disease might affect 2 percent of the population, and some proportion has a genetic basis (Weatherall 1991). Mitochondrial DNA inheritance, somatic mutations in cancer, and others have revealed a fuller range of possibilities for genetic inheritance.

Health Behaviors

Rose and Marmot (1981), using British male data, and Lantz, House, and colleagues (1998), using U.S. male and female data, reported that about 12–20 percent of the differences in mortality (the gradient) across their samples were attributable to differences in health behaviors. The health behaviors referred to included diet, body mass, exercise, tobacco use, alcohol intake, and untreated high blood pressure. Although a lower percentage than researchers thought twenty-five years ago, 12–20 percent is not trivial.

Medical Care

The quantitative effect of medical care on health has been a contentious issue. Thomas McKeown and Ivan Illich, writing throughout the 1960s and 1970s, were among the most prominent of the many commentators who voiced great skepticism about the supposed contribution of medical care to individual and population health (McKeown 1976, 1979; Illich 1976). When the British adopted the National Health Service in 1948, many expected the provision of universal access to medical care to reduce or eliminate inequalities in health. But in 1980, the Black Report noted that "despite more than thirty years of a National Health Service expressly committed to offering equal care for all, there remains a marked class gradient in standards of health. Indeed, that gradient . . . in certain respects has been becoming more marked" (Townsend and Davidson 1982; Berridge and Blume 2003). More recently, Fogel (2004), an economic historian, concluded that technological improvements in agriculture and in other organized productivities were responsible for the doubling of life expectancy and the 50 percent increase in body size since 1700.

Bunker and colleagues undertook a critical review of outcomes data from clinical trials of medical and surgical interventions in diseases that account for most of the mortality in the United States (Bunker, Frazier, and Mosteller 1994). They estimated that 16 percent of the life expectancy gain in the twentieth century was due to beneficial results of medical care. Bunker (1995) reported that the proportion attributed to medical care appeared to be greater than 16 percent in the decades toward the end of the twentieth century. He hypothesized that medical care might be shown to be more effective if change in functional capacity over time is substituted for morbidity and mortality as the major indicator of medical care's effect (Bunker 2001a,b).

The effect on children of lack of access to medical care is more certain. Failure to vaccinate against common infectious diseases, failure to detect hearing, vision, and development defects and lack of attention to remediable mental health problems play a large role on a population basis in delays or failures in learning and development. Children's vulnerability to these health problems is greater in families of low socioeconomic status. The impact of unattended to health problems on early childhood education is largely due to inability to concentrate or fully participate in school, absenteeism, delayed socialization, the potential for permanent functional losses, and so forth (Landry 2005).

Physical Environment

Data do not exist to estimate the population health effects of toxic contamination of air, water, and soil. The direct effects of radioactivity on health and mortality at Hiroshima and Nagasaki were measured, and some estimates have been made at Chernobyl and environs. The threat to human health from radioactive materials will rise as the world's energy needs inevitably become more dependent on nuclear energy, as the proposed agreement on March 2, 2006, between President Bush and President Singh of India confirms (Bumiller and Sengupta 2006). Add to radioactivity the toxic effects of chemicals from mining, manufacturing, and farming, and the continuing growth of the world's population and consumption, and one can easily forecast that the coming threat not only to human health but also to the ecology of all living things will be large. Yet, at this time the effects of contamination on population health, although dramatic on an individual case basis, are not large on a population basis.

Social Context

Social context includes all elements of social organization, that is, governing institutions, public services, politics, policies, business, the economy, law, history, culture, faith, ideology, business practices, education, work, income, income distribution across the population, hierarchical class structures, attitudes toward race and ethnicity, social and material inequality, disparities in social advantage, and so forth. Every minute of every day, social context envelops individuals, friendships, families, schooling, work, and the social order. Variations in social context powerfully influence the unequal distribution of social advantage and health. Social context is such a critical element of health production that, in addition to its place as one of the categories of determinants, it will be presented as a conceptual framework in its own right.

Conceptual Framework #2. Social Context

The representation of social context in figure 8.1 is a simplification in which a series of concentric spheres envelop the population (families, i.e., mothers, fathers, children). The proximal sphere refers to the immediate surroundings of the family: neighborhood features (such as average family income), other

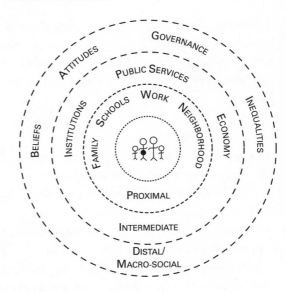

Figure 8.1   Social Context

families, interpersonal relationships, schools, work, and so on. The intermediate sphere comprises regional characteristics such as governance, provision of public services, public health measures, medical care access and quality, the regional economy, jobs, inequalities, and the like. The distal sphere includes the overall characteristics of the society as a whole, such as its history, culture, governance, and laws; its business practices, tax codes, and redistributive policies; its attitudes toward race, ethnicity, and gender, and so forth.

The dashed lines around each sphere convey porosity and interaction among components within and among the spheres. As an example, national tax codes set in the distal sphere influence the intermediate-level economy, the availability of public services, the accessibility and quality of public health and medical services, and the profile of social inequalities in the region, and at the proximal level the availability and quality of work, the neighborhood characteristics, the socioeconomic norms, and the material well-being of the family, including income, assets, homeownership, and security. The social context is a complex, pervasive, highly interactive system that confers specificity and identity on each population group, even at the neighborhood or block level.

In some ways the social context is fluid, but in others it is viscous and resistant to change. Initiatives to improve opportunities for strong family development and health, for example, will require understanding the dynamics of social context and adopting strategies to overcome the large resistances to social change. Investments in early childhood education and development, education K through 12, job training, and good paying jobs are important to health over the life course. Other large forces that might not be obviously relevant to health include literacy training, wage levels, family support services, housing, transport, and medical and nutrition services. Opportunities for community connectedness and social capital building will be important through neighborhood or community organizations, churches, and other institutions such as schools. Multiple targets for coordinated intervention must be selected at different levels (spheres) within a well-financed and sustained strategy. Families and their health do not stand alone in their own context. Underestimating the resistance power of social context is a common reason social policy fails.

The social context is perhaps among the most powerful of the influences and has been a principal focus for research on health and development during the last twenty-five years. The social context is a critical component of health production, but not yet fully addressed by public health, medicine, public policies, education, and the media. Its mechanism for influencing health appears to be through effects on equality-inequality and advantage-disadvantage dynamics in society.

Conceptual Framework #3. The Gradient: Inequalities in Health Generated by the Social Context

Wide disparities (inequalities) in health have been noted since ancient times. The modern era of advanced research on health disparities began with the Whitehall study in the United Kingdom in the 1970s. In 1978, Marmot, Rose, and colleagues reported on the ten-year longitudinal study of a cohort of seventeen thousand civil servants, stratified by job classification (for example, manual workers, clerical workers, professionals, administrators). All the civil servants were fully employed and had unrestricted access to insured medical care under the National Health Service. They reported their health status and health behaviors at each visit to their physician.

Coronary heart disease relative risk (probability of having a heart attack, for example) varied fourfold with job classification in the Whitehall study. The least skilled workers (groundskeepers, messengers) were at greatest risk, while the top ministers and executives (administrators) were at least risk. The fourfold gradient did not simply define the top compared to the bottom; there was a continuous gradient of risk across the four job classes. Another important finding was that health behaviors explained only a fraction of the risk in each job class (recall the prior discussion of health behaviors in the conceptual framework of health influences).

Case, Lubotsky, and Paxson (2002) at Princeton University have studied health in children. Using data from the National Health Interview Survey and the Panel Study of Income Dynamics, they discovered a gradient relationship that ranged from excellent to poor between family income and child's health status as assessed by the parent. They also studied the presence of fourteen medical conditions that afflict children. Progressively higher family income was associated with progressively better health status and lower rates of disease in the children. In poor families the health of children worsened with age, and on average those children entered adulthood with lower socioeconomic status, poorer health, and fewer years of education relative to children of higher-income families.

Case, Fertig, and Paxson in a 2005 publication show that the income-health gradient seen in adult populations has antecedents in childhood. Their work demonstrates that the socioeconomic-health relationship is observable from birth and continues to be observable and have a lasting impact over the entire life course.

Work by dozens of scientists from many of the industrialized nations on all continents confirms and expands the gradient work using alternative indicators of social position and health. Similar gradients were discovered using other measures of inequality such as job class, income, assets, education, and social class. Further, the gradient was reproduced using almost all health status indicators, including death, prevalence rates for almost all diseases, disability rates, school or work absenteeism, functional status measures, and infant mortality.

The unequal distribution of development and health in a population is the result not of bad luck but to a major extent of the systematic unequal distribution of social advantage-disadvantage associated with hierarchical social arrangements. Link and Phelan (1995) and Phelan and Link (2005) have effectively advanced the concept of social conditions as fundamental causes of disease. The social-health gradient is a universal feature of all industrialized economies, although the steepness of the gradient varies. Nations with steeper gradients (e.g., the United States) signifying greater inequalities in health are almost uniformly associated with poorer average health when compared to nations with gentler gradients (e.g., Japan, Sweden).

Variations in health are partly owing to genetic inheritance, as discussed earlier in this chapter. It can be said justifiably that every individual human trait is influenced to some extent by the individual's genome. But genetic inheritance does not adequately explain the health variations illustrated in the gradient. What about genetic inheritance of the other component of the gradient, social status?

Most genetics scholars would agree with the arguments of Holtzman (2002), who concluded that the roots of social status differences do not lie in our genes. Although it is probably correct that genetic inheritance does affect development and health to some extent, and that disordered development and health can influence social position to some extent, the influence of genetic inheritance on the gradient is not large and cannot come close to explaining the large inequalities in social advantage that exist in all economically developed nations.[2]

Conceptual Framework #4. Life Course: Variations and Continuities in the Production of Health

From the left side of figure 8.2 to the right, the life course progresses from conception to old age. Through adolescence the manifestations of disordered development are predominantly related to developmental lags, educational underachievement, aberrant behaviors, and social deviance. Health effects may be manifested at birth (premature birth, low birth weight, birth defects), during infancy (nutritional deficiencies, failure to thrive), and in childhood or young adulthood (sinusitis, bronchitis, hay fever, asthma, hearing and vision disorders) (Case, Lubotsky, and Paxson 2002). Developmental, learning, behavioral and social effects are more visible in infancy, childhood, and adolescence. Later, during work life, retirement, and elderly stages, the more conventionally recognized dimensions of declining health become obvious, including chronic disease, multiple prescription drug taking, functional disabilities, work absenteeism, the need for hospitalization, frailty, dependence, and so on. Mustard (2000) in Canada and van der Gaag (2000) in the Netherlands were among the earliest to point out the obligate interdependence over the life course among brain development, child development, human development, learning, behavior, and health.

Using a cascade metaphor, figure 8.3 illustrates positive life-course effects of advantaged development and health. The graphic depicts a progression of positive developmental outcomes throughout life, assuming a successful early childhood education and development experience prior to kindergarten and high-quality subsequent schooling through primary and secondary education.

The headwaters at the top form at birth, when visible human dissimilarity is perhaps the least. The downstream flow traverses successive phases of child and adolescent development, when variations in the social context and of life's experiences and relationships produce the infinite diversity of human beings that is a cardinal feature of the species. As diversity defines greater and greater individual characteristics, the cascade widens until it becomes the open archipelago of adulthood, with the cascade's greatest expanse of differences in human development and health. Success at each level in this flow depends on each individual's prior experiences and successes in development, education, and life.

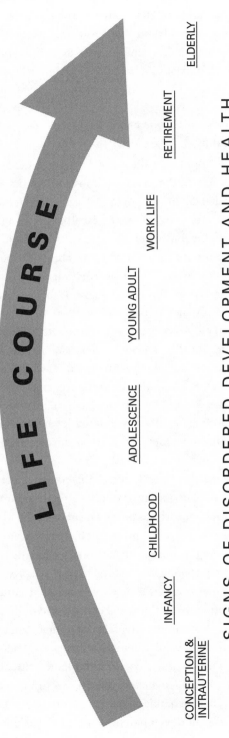

Figure 8.2 Social-Societal Context

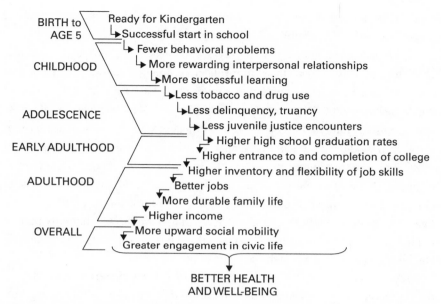

Figure 8.3 Cascading Effects of Enhanced Early Childhood Education and Development: A Lifecourse Perspective

A disturbance in one part of the flow can limit an individual's downstream potential in another part.

Differences between groups in level of preparedness for kindergarten provide an instructive illustration. Consider two populations that as adults have lost their jobs in an economic downturn. An opportunity is presented to both to acquire a new set of job skills. Group A individuals entered kindergarten years ago with a foundation of past experiences and relationships that helped them become successful and confident learners. On average they progress through the challenges in subsequent education and development, are able to acquire new skills better suited to the new economy, and are the first to be rehired. Thus, Group A on average copes successfully with job layoffs, resumes earned income, contributes to the economy, pays taxes, retains family stability, resumes active life as community members, and is more likely to enjoy good health and a positive sense of well-being throughout the life course.

Group B individuals, however, begin school not ready for kindergarten, experience lack of success as learners, become disinclined to embrace the learning environment as a mechanism to avoid failure and humiliation, evince behavioral problems, make fewer friends, move into delinquency, suffer poor health, and so forth down the cascade. Job retraining doesn't "take" in Group B, family income and assets disappear, family breakup may follow, and Group B on average may be committed to a lifetime of underemployment, minimum wages, dependence on public funds, and poor health.

Another fact of the cascade deserves emphasis: Interventions to promote child development and health are more effective, and more cost effective, the earlier in the cascade they are applied (Reynolds et al. 2002; Carneiro and Heckman 2003; Heckman 2006; Reynolds, Ou, and Topitzes 2004). The most cost effective and successful interventions are in the 0–5 age group, the preschool phase of early childhood development that prepares children to be successful upon entry to kindergarten, producing a return to the individual and to society of seven to eight dollars for each one dollar invested (Heckman 2006). Investments later in childhood and adolescence still yield a positive return but at a reduced rate. Even job retraining yields a return, but at a still lower rate. Part, but only part, of the decline in return on investment when the intervention starts later in the life course is owing to fewer remaining years of life for earnings.

Incorporating a life-course framework into a development and health production model produces a more informative and practically useful understanding of the coproduction of development and health, and the design of more effective and economically efficient public policies and interventions. Good schools for three- and four-year-olds is an example of social synergy through the life-course cascade that can yield gains in education and development, improved population health, a more skilled and flexible labor force, productivity enhancement, and improved economic development. It is easy to imagine that public health and medicine working collaboratively can play complementary, even synergistic, benevolent roles in health production over the life course.

Conceptual Framework #5. The Parallel Production of Brain Development, Child Development, Human Development, and Health

The levels of human development and of health achieved over the life course are highly correlated and vary systematically with social class. Progressively higher levels of social class, from lower class up through the middle classes to the upper class, are accompanied by higher levels of both development (skills, knowledge) and health. This is exemplified in children by the association of lower cognitive test scores with higher rates of school absenteeism due to illness; in adolescence by the association of lower rates of encounters with the criminal justice system with low rates of asthma; and in mid and later years by the association of higher cognitive and linguistic capacities on average with lower rates of cardiovascular and other diseases (Keating and Hertzman 1999; Power and Hertzman 1999; Mustard 2000; Case, Lubotsky, and Paxson 2002; and Case, Fertig, and Paxson 2005; McCain, Mustard, and Shanker 2007).

Recently, the linkage in time and function between brain development and early childhood development has been demonstrated (Levitt, forthcoming; McCain, Mustard, and Shanker 2007). It also appears that the levels of brain development, early childhood development, human development, and health production follow parallel courses in any one individual over the life course and may be cogenerated by the same set of influences. Sometime in the future we might use the omnibus concept of "brain development, early childhood development, human development, human capital formation, and health" to connote their related production. An etiological relationship among these factors would substantially broaden the choices of public policies to improve health. A public policy and intervention platform might be adopted that would be complementary and mutually reinforcing for both public health and medicine.

The association of human development and health might be coincidental. Or the association could be owing to superior development's providing the resourcefulness or accessibility to education, information and services that are instrumentally related to health improvement through either self-help or access to expert services. Or the fundamental influences of poor or delayed development in children may be the same influences that render those individuals more susceptible to almost all diseases. Whatever the case, observational data allow a tentative assumption that development and health have common origins. This area of knowledge has important relevance to the conceptual foundation and roles of public health and medicine.

Conceptual Framework #6. Socio-Psycho-Biological-Health Translation

Social equality-inequality and advantage-disadvantage are social states, whereas brain development, child development, human development, and health have major biological components. If the relationships between social advantage-disadvantage to disease are causal, biological adjustments to social circumstances might at least in part mediate the translation of social status. Variations along the continuum of social disadvantage-advantage might be systematically proportional to variations in the level of biological adjustment, that is, might represent a social-biological gradient. Socio-psycho-biological-health translation might be the connecting link between social inequality and the health gradient.

There is much evidence in humans as well as in apes and monkeys for adjustments according to social status in the resting state of several physiological regulatory processes.[3] For example, McEwen has postulated (McEwen 2002; McEwen with Lasley 2002) that the damaging effects of long-term stress are mediated through a mechanism he has termed allostatic load. Allostasis is the normal adaptive mechanism for maintaining physiological stability under circumstances that are stressful. The body's allostatic systems include the autonomic nervous system, hypothalamic-pituitary-adrenal system, immune system, and so forth. If the body encounters stressful circumstances repeatedly, or chronically, McEwen argues, the appropriate adaptive system and the organs it serves ultimately suffer fatigue or wear and tear (allostatic load). Ultimately, illnesses such as cardiovascular disease, heart failure, and asthma may ensue.

The evidence is highly suggestive, but not yet definitive, that elevated resting cortisol levels in disadvantaged baboons (Sapolsky 1993) and disadvantaged human beings (Lupien et al. 2000; Gunnar et al. 2001; Gunnar and Vasquez 2001) are causally related to poorer health outcomes in individuals of lower social rank. Allostatic physiologic processes are facts of primate physiology. Geronimus (1996) applies the term "weathering" (wear and tear) to help explain the lower health status in African Americans compared to non-Hispanic whites. Weathering and allostatic load might refer to the same pathophysiologic mechanism. Lu and Halfon (2003) apply the weathering idea to explain the higher incidence of low birth-weight infants born to African American mothers. McEwan's allostatic load concept is biologically plausible (Seeman et al. 1997, 2004).

These findings seem to be regulatory adaptations in reaction to adverse or threatening circumstances related to social position, that is, the lower the social position, the greater the adaptive response. As more studies are reported, and especially as life-course perspectives have been applied, many of these adaptations appear to have begun in childhood, or even in infancy when maternal-child attachment bonds can fail for one reason or another. Moreover, these adaptations appear to become permanently embedded in the biology of the individual, or at least to remain stable over time.

These research findings are remarkable for their relevance to child development, adult capability, health, and public policy. The physiological departures from normative levels in numerous reactive regulatory systems (summarized in Tarlov, forthcoming) have been discovered in infants, children, and adults alike, and in both men and women, although with some quantitative differences. The adaptations occur in many if not all the major regulatory pathways, as a generalized regulatory alert in each individual. There is extraordinary similarity in physiological responses to social position in humans, apes, and New World monkeys, suggesting a homologous beginning in our common ancestral past in distant evolutionary history. The evidence suggests that the physiologic reactivity is a general up-regulatory response to social circumstances that the individual does not welcome. Let's probe further.

For decades an inference has been advanced in genetics that gene action is affected by environmental circumstances (Lewontin 2000). The inference of gene-environment interaction can be accepted as a biological principle, as demonstrated by Suomi (2004, 2005). Suomi showed that the inheritance of a variant of the serotonin transport gene resulted in highly inheritable, inappropriate, impulsive aggression and low levels of central nervous system serotonin in monkeys that had experienced insecure attachment bonds to their mother. In contrast, in experiments in which the rearing histories of newborns were manipulated so that strong and secure attachment bonds were formed with their mother, despite inheriting the same aberrant gene, both the lower serotonin levels and the impulsive aggressive behavior were averted. The Suomi experiments demonstrate that gene-environment interactions, in this case where "environment" refers to the social context within the family and troop, can substantially modify gene expression, developmental trajectories throughout the life span, behaviors, biological pathways, and health outcomes.

In a study of two- to four-year-old children in childcare settings, and monkeys in a primate research center, Boyce (2004) discovered: (1) both young children and monkeys form dominant and subordinate social hierarchies; (2) subordinates, both children and monkeys, demonstrate exaggerated cortisol and autonomic nervous system reactivity to challenge together with higher rates of chronic medical conditions in children and higher rates of violent injury in monkeys; and (3) in both children and monkeys the combination of reactivity to stress, naturally occurring stressors, and social position (dominance or subordinate position within their group) are predictive of health status. The appearance of dominate-subordinate positional arrangements among two-, three- and four-year-old children in preschools with measurable cortisol stress reactivity that are predictive of health outcomes is striking for its similarity in both primate species (monkey and human), and for its resemblance to the social position: biological reactivity:health relationship in adults. Is it possible that adult development and health have their trajectoral origins in the social organization, development, and health of early childhood?

Boyce and Ellis (2005) have pushed forward the frontier of biologic reactivity to stress by incorporating into their models the social context in which the stress is experienced. This yields a sharply different concept of stress reactivity than previously held. They title their model "biological sensitivity to context" (BSC). Although gene inheritance does play a role, they posit that early developmental experiences (context) interact with the genome to establish plasticity of the stress response system. Each individual calibrates his system to match the environment experienced in childhood. Early childhood exposure to either an extremely protective environment or to an extremely stressful environment results in heightened reactivity, with most children not at the extremes having adopted lower (normative) levels of stress reactivity. High reactivity in children can have either positive or damaging health consequences depending on their social context, supportive or stressful, respectively.

Figure 8.4 sketches an outline of a hypothesized mechanism by which social context, social status, and advantage-disadvantage influence development and health. Briefly, one's experiences in a social context of inequality are received by sensory systems (visual, auditory, smell, touch) and transmitted to the mind. In this depiction the major routes to development and health pass through the mind, the body's command and control center. In the mind the information is processed into emotional states, coping and adaptation responses, stress, and so forth. The state of mind is then converted to signals that modulate or activate the body's physiological regulatory systems. Once activated, these systems send messages chemically, or through the nervous system, to responsive organs (the heart, lungs, pancreas, adrenal glands, lymph nodes, and so forth), where the organ activates its response. Over time, if the signaling is maintained, even if at a low amplitude, adaptations in the organs, perhaps calibrated to gene-social circumstance interaction, might set the circumstances for either protection from or vulnerability to disease or for successful or delayed development (Tarlov 1996; forthcoming).

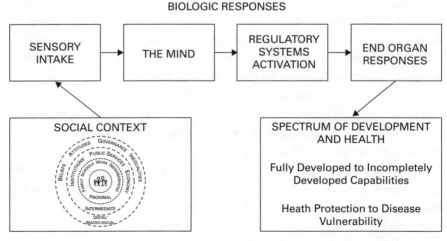

Figure 8.4 Conversion of Social Context into Biologic Processes That Affect Development and Health

Health Production: A Unifying Conceptualization

A large literature has assigned population health to the dominion of public health and individual health care to the realm of medicine.[4] Past arguments seem to be too heavily weighted toward finding distinctions that confer independent legitimacy on each profession, as if one or the other's professional status, vitality, or even survival is at risk. From where does this quest for distinctiveness come? Are its roots in competition for funds or for postcollege applications for professional training? Is there a hierarchical priority setting within the universities that creates a kind of academic class structure? There must be good reasons for pursuing distinctiveness, but is professional vanity a factor?

There is much value to the distinction between population health and individual health, promoted decades ago by the eminent epidemiologist Sir Geoffrey Rose (1992). Using the two definitions to distinguish the roles and identities of public health and medicine in the contemporary era might be carrying the distinction too far. True, the underlying factors affecting population health are more deeply rooted in social organization and are more likely to be affected by social policy. The causes of individual health variations are more likely to have origins in genetics, biology, health behaviors, and medical care and are more likely to be affected by individual treatment modalities. But clearly there is significant overlap between the two. From an epidemiologic viewpoint, population health often is simply an average of aggregated health indicators based on the sum of individual person measurements. But in the reality of health production, causal pathways by which a patient has suffered an acute myocardial infarction are likely to be a blend of factors from the concepts of both population health and individual health. These factors include position in the stratified social advantage-disadvantage structure as well as individual factors such as genomically mediated risk, health behaviors such as tobacco use, overeating, and physical inactivity, and failures and successes of medical care.

Whether oriented toward population health or individual health, the interplay of determinant influences, social context, interpersonal supportive relationships, and experiences over the life course evokes biological adjustments that affect brain development, child development, human development, vulnerability or resistance to disease, and the incidence and aggressiveness of disease, whether within a population or in a single individual. The end product regardless is health, whether measured by morbidity, mortality, functional capacity, disability, or health capability. The challenge to both public health and medicine is to protect and improve health and well-being, and to reduce health inequalities. The structures and processes adopted by public health and medicine are merely the means to common ends: to improve, promote, and enhance the production of health. The focus on structure and process and the lack of emphasis on health outcomes are distracting. There is something real in the aphorism that you become what you measure. Seeking to highlight boundaries in terms of structure and process, including population health versus individual health, obfuscates commonality of purpose and dilutes effectiveness. A jointly evolved conceptual foundation in health production could generate a recharged sense of public purpose and enhance the effectiveness of both public health and medicine.

Notes

1. Child, indeed human, development and health are influenced by hundreds of factors on multiple levels of daily living that comprise a complex interconnected web of interactions. I pursue summarization and brevity in this chapter to favor understandability of the overall concepts. The references I cite provide more detailed information.
2. For more information on social context and the gradients in development and health, I recommend Bunker, Gomby, and Kehrer 1989; Evans, Barer, and Marmor 1994; Amick et al. 1995; Blane, Brunner, and Wilkinson 1996; Marmot and Wilkinson 1999; Adler et al. 1999; Kawachi, Kennedy, and Wilkinson 1999; Tarlov and St. Peter 2000; Berkman and Kawachi 2000; Davey Smith 2003; Marmot 2004; Wilkinson 1996, 2005.
3. See Blum 2002; Boyce 2004; Boyce and Ellis 2005; Brunner 2000; Cacioppo et al. 2002; Cohen et al. 2004; Gunnar et al. 2001; Gunnar and Vasquez 2001; Lupien et al. 2000; McEwen 2002; Suomi 2000, 2004, 2005; Sapolsky 1993, 1995; Sapolsky, Romero, and Munck 2000; Shively 2000.
4. See Kilbourne and Smillie 1969; Burton and Smith 1970; Institute of Medicine 1988, 2003; White 1991; White and Connelly 1992; Lasker and the Committee on Medicine and Public Health 1997; Marmot 2004.

References

Aday, L. A., ed. 2005. *Reinventing Public Health: Policies and Practices for a Healthy Nation.* San Francisco: John Wiley (Jossey-Bass).

Adler, N. E., M. Marmot, B. S. McEwen, and J. Stewart, eds. 1999. *Socioeconomic Status and Health in Industrial Nations: Social, Psychological, and Biological Pathways.* Vol. 896 of the *Annals of the New York Academy of Sciences.* New York: New York Academy of Sciences.

Amick, B. C., III, S. Levine, A. R. Tarlov, and D. C. Walsh, eds. 1995. *Society and Health.* New York: Oxford University Press.

Berkman, L. F., and I. Kawachi, eds. 2000. *Social Epidemiology.* New York: Oxford University Press.

Berridge, V., and S. Blume, eds. 2003. *Poor Health: Social Inequality before and after the Black Report.* London: Frank Cass.

Blane, D., E. Brunner, and R. Wilkinson, eds. 1996. Health and Social Organization: Towards a Health Policy for the Twenty-First Century. London: Routledge.

Blum, D. 2002. Love at Goon Park: Harry Harlow and the Science of Affection. Cambridge, Mass.: Perseus.

Boyce, W. T. 2004. Social Stratification, Health, and Violence in the Very Young. *Annals of the New York Academy of Sciences* 1036:47–68.

Boyce, W. T., and B. J. Ellis. 2005. Biological Sensitivity to Context: I. An Evolutionary-Developmental Theory of the Origins and Functions of Stress Reactivity. *Development and Psychopathology* 17:271–301.

Brunner, E. 2000. Toward a New Social Biology. In *Social Epidemiology*, ed. L. F. Berkman and I. Kawachi, 306–331. New York: Oxford University Press.

Bumiller, E., and S. Sengupta. 2006. Bush and India Reach Pact That Allows Nuclear Sales. *New York Times*, March 3.

Bunker, J. P. 1995. Medicine Matters After All. *Journal of the Royal College of Physicians* 29:105–112.

———. 2001a. The Role of Medical Care in Contributing to Health Improvements within Societies. *International Journal of Epidemiology* 30: 1260–1263.

———. 2001b. *Medicine Matters After All: Measuring the Benefits of Medical Care, a Healthy Lifestyle, and a Just Social Environment.* Nuffield Trust Series 15. London: Nuffield Trust for Research and Policy Studies in Health Services.

Bunker, J. P., H. S. Frazier, and F. Mosteller. 1994. Improving Health: Measuring Effects of Medical Care. *Milbank Quarterly* 72:225–258.

Bunker, J. P., D. S. Gomby, and B. H. Kehrer, eds. 1989. *Pathways to Health: The Role of Social Factors.* Menlo Park, Calif.: Henry J. Kaiser Family Foundation.

Burton, L. E., and H. H. Smith. 1970. *Public Health and Community Medicine: For the Allied Medical Professions.* Baltimore. Williams and Wilkins.

Cacioppo, J. T., G. G. Berntson, R. Adolphs, C. S. Carter, R. J. Davidson, M. K. McClintock, B. S. McEwen, et al., eds. 2002. *Foundations in Social Neuroscience.* Cambridge: MIT Press.

Carneiro, P., and J. Heckman. 2003. *Human Capital Policy.* Working Paper 9495, National Bureau of Economic Research, Cambridge, Mass. www.nber.org/papers/w9495 (accessed April 2005).

Case, A., A. Fertig, and C. Paxson. 2005. The Lasting Impact of Childhood Health and Circumstance. *Journal of Health Economics* 24:365–389.

Case, A., D. Lubotsky, and C. Paxson. 2002. Economic Status and Health in Childhood: The Origins of the Gradient. *American Economic Review* 12: 1308–1334.

Cohen, S., W. J. Doyle, R. B. Turner, C. M. Alper, and D. P. Skoner. 2004. Childhood Socioeconomic Status and Host Resistance to Infectious Illness in Adulthood. *Psychosomatic Medicine* 66:553–558.

Davey Smith, G., ed. 2003. *Health Inequalities: Lifecourse Approaches.* Bristol, Eng.: Policy Press.

Evans, R. G., M. L. Barer, and T. R. Marmor, eds. 1994. Why Are Some People Healthy and Others Not? The Determinants of Health of Populations. New York: Aldine de Gruyter.

Fogel, R. W. 2004. *The Escape from Hunger and Premature Death, 1700–2100: Europe, America, and the Third World.* Cambridge: Cambridge University Press.

Geronimus, A. T. 1996. Black/White Differences in the Relationship of Maternal Age to Birth Weight: A Population-Based Test of the Weathering Hypothesis. *Social Science and Medicine* 42:589–597.

Gunnar, M. R., S. J. Morison, K. Chisholm, and M. Schuder. 2001. Salivary Cortisol Levels in Children Adopted from Romanian Orphanages. *Development and Psychopathology* 13:611–628.

Gunnar, M. R., and D. M. Vasquez. 2001. Low Cortisol and a Flattening of Expected Daytime Rhythm: Potential Indices of Risk in Human Development. *Development and Psychopathology* 13:515–538.

Heckman, J. J. 2006. Skill Formation and the Economics of Investing in Disadvantaged Children. *Science* 312:1900–1902.

Holtzman, N. A. 2002. Genetics and Social Class. *Journal of Epidemiology and Community Health* 56:529–535.

Illich, I. 1976. *Medical Nemesis: The Expropriation of Health.* New York: Pantheon Books.

Institute of Medicine. 1988. *The Future of Public Health.* Washington, D.C.: National Academies Press.

———. 2003. *The Future of the Public's Health in the Twenty-First Century.* Washington, D.C.: National Academies Press.

Kawachi, I., B. P. Kennedy, and R. G. Wilkinson, eds. 1999. *Income Inequality and Health.* Vol. 1 of *The Society and Population Health Reader.* New York: New Press.

Keating, D. P., and C. Hertzman, eds. 1999. *Developmental Health and the Wealth of Nations.* New York: Guilford Press.

Kilbourne, E. D., and W. G. Smillie, eds. 1969. *Human Ecology and Public Health.* Fourth ed. London: Collier-Macmillan.

Landry, S. H. 2005. *Effective Early Childhood Programs: Turning Knowledge into Action.* University of Texas-Houston and Rice University. www.uth.tmc.edu/circle/publications.htm and www.tecec.org.

Lantz, P. M., J. S. House, J. M. Lepkowski, D. R. Williams, R. P. Mero, and J. Chen. 1998. Socioeconomic Factors, Health Behaviors, and Mortality: Results from a Nationally Representative Prospective Study of U.S. Adults. *JAMA* 279:1703–1708.

Lasker, R. D., and the Committee on Medicine and Public Health. 1997. Medicine and Public Health: The Power of Collaboration. New York: New York Academy of Medicine.

Levitt, P. Forthcoming. Building Brain Architecture and Chemistry: A Primer for Policy Makers. In *Nurturing Early Childhood Development: Evidence to Support a Movement for Educational Change,* ed. A. R. Tarlov and M. P. Debbink. New York: Palgrave Macmillan.

Lewontin, R. 2000. *The Triple Helix.* Cambridge, Mass.: Harvard University Press.

Link, B. G., and J. C. Phelan. 1995. Social Conditions as Fundamental Causes of Disease. *Journal of Health and Social Behavior* (Extra issue): 80–94.

Lu, M. C., and N. Halfon. 2003. Racial and Ethnic Disparities in Birth Outcomes: A Life-Course Perspective. *Maternal and Child Health Journal* 7: 13–30.

Lupien, S. J., S. King, M. J. Meaney, and B. S. McEwen. 2000. Child's Stress Hormone Levels Correlate with Mother's Socioeconomic Status and Depressive State. *Biological Psychiatry* 48:976–980.

Marmot, M. 2004. *The Status Syndrome: How Social Standing Affects Our Health and Longevity.* New York: Times Books, Henry Holt.

Marmot, M., G. Rose, M. Shipley, and P.J.S. Hamilton . 1978. Employment Grade and Coronary Heart Disease in British Civil Servants. *Journal of Epidemiology and Community Health* 32:244–249.

Marmot, M., and R. G. Wilkinson, eds. 1999. *Social Determinants of Health.* Oxford: Oxford University Press.

McCain, M. N., J. F. Mustard, and S. Shanker. 2007. *Early Years Study 2: Putting Science into Action.* Toronto, Ont.: Council for Early Childhood Development.

McEwen, B. S. 2002. Protective and Damaging Effects of Stress Mediators. In *Foundations in Social Neuroscience,* ed. J. T. Cacioppo, G. G. Berntson, R. Adolphs C. S. Carter, R. J. Davidson, M. K. McClintock, B. S. McEwen, et al., 1127–1140. Cambridge: MIT Press.

McEwen, B. S., with E. N. Lasley. 2002. *The End of Stress As We Know It.* Washington, D.C.: Joseph Henry.

McKeown, T. 1976. *The Modern Rise of Population*. London: Edward Arnold.

———. 1979. *The Role of Medicine: Dream, Mirage, or Nemesis?* Second ed. Princeton: Princeton University Press.

Mustard, J. F. 2000. *Early Child Development and the Brain: The Base for Health, Learning, and Behavior throughout Life*. Presentation to the World Bank Conference, Investing in our Children's Future, Washington, D.C., April 10–11.

Phelan, J. C., and B. G. Link. 2005. Controlling Disease and Creating Disparities: A Fundamental Cause Perspective. *Journals of Gerontology* Series B, 60B (Special issue): 27–33.

Power, C., and C. Hertzman. 1999. Health, Well-being, and Coping Skills. In *Developmental Health and the Wealth of Nations*, ed. D. P. Keating and C. Hertzman, 41–54. New York: Guilford Press.

Reynolds, A., S. Ou, and J. Topitzes. 2004. Paths of Effects of Early Childhood Intervention on Educational Attainment and Delinquency: A Confirmatory Analysis of the Chicago Child-Parent Centers. *Child Development* 75:1299–1328.

Reynolds, A., J. A. Temple, D. L. Robertson, and E. A. Mann. 2002. Age 21 Cost-Benefit Analysis of the Title I Chicago Child-Parent Centers. *Educational Evaluation and Policy Analysis* 24:267–303.

Rose, G. 1992. *The Strategy of Preventive Medicine*. New York: Oxford University Press.

Rose, G., and M. G. Marmot. 1981. Social Class and Coronary Heart Disease. *British Heart Journal* 45:13–19.

Sapolsky, R. M. 1993. Endocrinology Al Fresco: Psychoendocrine Studies of Wild Baboons. *Recent Progress in Hormone Research* 48:437–468.

———. 1995. Social Subordinance As a Marker of Hypercortisolism: Some Unexpected Subtleties. In *Stress: Basic Mechanisms and Clinical Implications*, ed. G. P. Chrousas, R. McCarty, K. Pace, G. Cizza, E. Sternberg, P. W. Gold, and R. Kvetnansky. Vol. 771 of *Annals of the New York Academy of Sciences*. New York: New York Academy of Sciences.

Sapolsky, R. M., M. Romero, and A. Munck. 2000. How Do Glucocorticoids Influence Stress Responses? Integrating Permissive, Suppressive, Stimulatory and Preparative Actions. *Endocrine Reviews* 21:55–89.

Seeman, T. E., E. Cummins, M. H. Huang, B. Singer, A. Bucur, T. Gruenwald et al. 2004. Cumulative Biological Risk and Socio-economic Differences in Mortality: MacArthur Studies of Successful Aging. *Social Science and Medicine* 58:1985–1997.

Seeman, T. E., B. H. Singer, J. W. Rowe, R. I. Horwitz, and B. S. McEwan. 1997. Price of Adaptation—Allostatic Load and Its Health Consequences: MacArthur Studies of Successful Aging. *Archives of Internal Medicine* 157:2259–2268.

Shively, C. A. 2000. Social Status, Stress, and Health in Female Monkeys. In *The Society and Population Health Reader*. Vol. 2. *A State and Community Perspective*, ed. A. R. Tarlov and R. E. St. Peter, 278–289. New York: New Press.

Suomi, S. J. 2000. Early Development in Monkeys. In *The Society and Population Health Reader*. Vol. 2. *A State and Community Perspective*, ed. A. R. Tarlov and R. E. St. Peter. 131–142. New York: New Press.

———. 2004. How Gene-Environment Interactions Shape Biobehavioral Development: Lessons from Studies with Rhesus Monkeys. *Research in Human Development* 1:205–222.

———. 2005. How Gene-Environment Interactions Shape the Development of Impulsive Aggression in Rhesus Monkeys. In *Developmental Psychobiology of Aggression*, ed. D. M. Stoff and E. J. Susman, 252–268. Cambridge: Cambridge University Press.

Tarlov, A. R. 1996. Social Determinants of Health: The Sociobiological Translation. In *Health and Social Organization*, ed. D. Blane, E. J. Brunner, and R. G. Wilkinson, 71–93. London: Routledge.

———. Forthcoming. The Co-Production of Human Development and Health. In *Nurturing Early Childhood Development: Evidence to Support a Movement for Educational Change*, ed. A. R. Tarlov and M. P. Debbink. New York: Palgrave Macmillan.

Tarlov, A. R., and R. F. St. Peter, eds. 2000. *A State and Community Perspective*. Vol 2. of *The Society and Population Health Reader*. New York: New Press.

Townsend, P., and N. Davidson, eds. 1982. *Inequalities in Health: The Black Report*. Harmondsworth, Middlesex, Eng.: Penguin Books.

van der Gaag, J. 2000. *From Child Development to Human Development*. Presentation to The World Bank Conference, Investing in Our Children's Future, Washington, D.C., April 10–11.

Weatherall, D. J. 1991. *The New Genetics and Clinical Practice*. Third ed. Oxford: Oxford University Press.

White, K. L. 1991. *Healing the Schism: Epidemiology, Medicine, and the Public's Health*. New York. Springer-Verlag.

White, K. L., and J. E. Connelly, eds. 1992. *The Medical School's Mission and the Population's Health: Medical Education in Canada, the United Kingdom, the United States, and Australia*. New York. Springer-Verlag.

Wilkinson, R. G. 1996. *Unhealthy Societies: The Afflictions of Inequality*. London: Routledge.

———. 2005. *The Impact of Inequality: How to Make Sick Societies Healthier*. New York: New Press.

Part III

Public Health in the Post-9/11 World

The three chapters in this section address the critical question of how public health is changing in the context of disasters both natural and human made, and find that consensus on the appropriate boundaries remains distant. David Rosner and Gerald Markowitz analyze the ways that the attacks of September 11, the subsequent mailing of anthrax spores, and the plan to forestall a bioterrorist attack with smallpox through mass vaccination altered the expectations among politicians, policy makers, and the public about the roles of public health. They conclude that, in spite of the ongoing threats such as SARS and avian flu, the momentum to reinvigorate, strengthen, and expand the nation's public health infrastructure has been lost. Nicole Lurie, Jeffrey Wasserman, and Christopher Nelson, drawing on a series of desktop preparedness exercises, describe the capacity of local and state health departments to respond to health emergencies. In spite of the enormous attention given to the weaknesses of public health, these authors, like Rosner and Markowitz, conclude that the nation's health agencies still have a long way to go before reaching an acceptable level of capacity or consistency in the services they offer. Beatrix Hoffman analyzes the response to the flooding in the wake of Hurricane Katrina in August and September of 2005. Contrasting the governmental response to Katrina with the aftermath of September 11, Hoffman notes that Congress refused to pass legislation extending health coverage for Katrina victims, a step it had taken in the earlier national emergency. Hoffman shows that the two disasters forced a recognition that providing health coverage is an essential component of both disaster preparedness and response—an idea that remains controversial in the current political climate.

The Challenge of 9/11 to the Ideologies of Population and Public Health

September 11, 2001, affected virtually all aspects of American life, from foreign policy and domestic security to philanthropy, social services, and health policy. We now increasingly understand social welfare, public health, health care, and environmental issues, generally seen as separate spheres, as interrelated components of a traumatized nation's and city's mental and social well-being and emergency preparedness, and the opportunities to integrate these concerns are immense. The experience of September 11 has highlighted the interrelationships among biological, sanitary, medical, social, and economic factors that together affect the well-being of populations. Perhaps more directly than at any time in the recent past, September 11 has illustrated that a population's health "encompasses a broader array of determinants of health than the field of public health has previously addressed" and has made all the more critical the "emerging theory and practice of population health," one that incorporates "the traditional concerns of public health" with "such issues as the effects on health status of . . . relative income and social status, racial and gender disparities, *and educational achievement*" (Fox 2001, xix). This shifting terrain reminds us of the importance of political and economic realities in shaping our perceptions of what public and population health are and are not. As the director of CDC's National Center for Infectious Diseases, James Hughes, noted in our telephone interview on October 12, 2004: "You of course know Bill Foege [former director of CDC], who said that public health is where politics and science come together. We are at that interface."

The Expanding Boundaries of Public Health

The newspaper headlines in the fall of 2001 were stark and eerie: "Efforts to Calm the Nation's Fears Spin out of Control"; "Local Public Health Officials Seek Help"; "This Is Not a Test"; "State Can't Handle Bioterrorist Attack"; "Scared into Action" (Schwartz 2001; Copeland 2001; Kristof 2001; Burress 2001; Abate 2001). And the pictures that accompanied them were worse: space-suited investigators, smallpox-ridden children, cold, stark laboratories staffed by masked personnel. State and local health departments were now supposed to be on a "war footing," as one headline noted (Connolly 2001). Health officials, knowing that their historical role was as the first line of defense against infectious disease, were at once energized and terrified by the prospect that their actions could be responsible for protecting or damaging the health of an entire state, even nation. How should they react? What were their goals? Their limitations?

Public health is a methodical discipline, historically rooted in the collection of data, the tracking of disease outbreaks, and laboratory and epidemiological investigation, often working in the background, out of the public eye. But the events of September 11 and the October anthrax incidents placed state public health agencies in the spotlight to a degree not experienced since the great epidemics of influenza, polio, whooping cough, and similar illnesses during the first half of the twentieth century. Many officials felt overwhelmed. The limitations of the public health surveillance system, laboratories, and treatment and social services became all too apparent. Almost overnight, state public health services were pulled into a cooperative campaign as part of the nation's defenses. Beleaguered staff and limited laboratory space and supplies, along with the general inexperience with bioterrorism, led to a profound reevaluation—sometimes naïve, sometimes quite sophisticated—of the place of population health services in the country's antiterrorism and emergency preparedness systems.

Fear of terrorism—and of bioterrorism specifically—thrust public health onto center stage in the broader arena of emergency preparedness and national security. Academics and public commentators alike argued that a new conception of traditional emergency responders was now upon us. "Firefighters, police officers, and other first responders will be on the front lines of a terrorist attack. . . . But in a bioterrorist attack, the people on the front lines will be the practicing physicians who will diagnose and treat diseases, and public health epidemiologists and laboratory personnel who will determine who has been exposed" to a host of biological and chemical agents (Evans, Clements, and Shadel 2001). From established academics and public health professionals to conservative think tanks and state officials, everyone agreed that "nowadays protection from disease is nothing short of national defense" (Satel 2001). State government agencies were called upon to play a new and crucial role in emergency preparedness.

In his opening address to the American Public Health Association (APHA) annual meeting just a few weeks after the initial anthrax attacks, the then secretary of the U.S. Department of Health and Human Services, Tommy Thompson, pledged: "We must take this opportunity to do everything we can to strengthen the public health system" (quoted in Terhune 2001). Public health spokespeople and even commentators across the political spectrum seized upon the promise of federal bioterrorism money as a possible salve for the system's inadequacies and as a motivation to rethink its scope and purpose. Further, it was used to buttress ideological and political goals. A fellow of the conservative American Enterprise Institute criticized public health leadership for having a "social justice agenda" that crowded out its true calling: "The upheaval of September 11 poses a momentous opportunity for public health to reclaim its proper focus: to protect the population from disease," a function, she argued—citing the 1988 Institute of Medicine study that described the public health infrastructure as being in "disarray"—that "has suffered for many years" (Satel 2001). Mohammed Akhtar, executive director of the APHA, disagreed that public health should be narrowly construed but agreed that severe weaknesses existed in the public health system that were the "result of neglect of many decades. . . . Since we conquered many infectious diseases, there have been no major outbreaks, so we continued to cut down on the system. It is at a point that it needs to be rebuilt and modernized" (quoted in Christian 2001).

Views differed on what constituted preparedness in general and bioterrorism preparedness in particular. Local health officials, worried about the weaknesses in their agency programs, sometimes came into conflict with general government—state elected government officials and their staffs—whose focus was a broader array of population health needs. Those concerned with public health at the state level hoped that new federal money would allow state and local agencies to rebuild, even expand, their infrastructures. They hoped that the money could be used both to prepare the nation and to bolster general public health programs. But even in the immediate weeks after September 11, some public health agency administrators feared that the new focus on bioterrorism would distort public health priorities. A narrow focus on health as an adjunct to national defense could undermine their broader mission to provide a variety of services not necessarily tied to bioterrorism and emergency preparedness.

Unlike public health officials whose perspectives were framed by their agencies' pressing needs, many legislators, governors, and members of their staffs focused on the glaring weaknesses in the social services system, on hospital care facilities, and on the broader threat of terrorism and bioterrorism alike. In addition, they were dismayed that more had not been done to strengthen intrastate and interstate coordination for emergency response.

National crisis and broad social, economic, and political events framed these early hopes and fears. The near cessation of travel and consumer spending that followed the terrorist attacks greatly exacerbated the economic recession in progress before September 11. Strained state budgets led to the need to reduce spending in numerous sectors of the states' bureaucracies, including health. As legislators moved further and further away from the events of late 2001, population health preparedness became just one of a number of different budget priorities that they needed to consider in tough fiscal times. In early 2002, federal grants through CDC and the Health Resources and Services Administration (HRSA) provided a substantial infusion of funds for specific health-related activities and programs aimed at improving the public health infrastructure as a part of general bioterrorism preparedness. Even though these funds could not be used to supplant existing programs, the federal mandate in late 2002 for a major smallpox inoculation campaign dramatically affected debates within state governments about where resources should be spent and how personnel should be allocated. In the end, the rapidly developed smallpox program planning and inoculation campaign provided an additional challenge to those in general government concerned with bioterrorism preparedness and to state public health officials who saw the new infusions of federal funds as enabling them to buttress the general public health infrastructure.

Fiscal crisis and political agendas were not the only forces reshaping thinking about population health after September 11. The attempt to stimulate new and revised law through the draft Model State Emergency Health Powers Act (which we hereafter refer to as the draft Model Act) and, according to many of the public health officials we interviewed, the poor federal handling of the anthrax episode (as embodied in the confusing messages sent out by Secretary of Health and Human Services Tommy Thompson) and smallpox inoculation campaign highlighted the difficult interface between the public health community and those whose focus was law enforcement and national security. These factors also helped encourage a discussion regarding regional and even national public health response to the threat of biological or chemical attacks.

Even years after the attacks, many public health officials believed that there was still tremendous ambiguity about what emergency preparedness for bioterrorism really means. Some saw it as synonymous with strengthening the existing public health infrastructure. Some saw it as building population health services more broadly. Others saw it as narrowly focused on smallpox, anthrax, emergency care, border protection, and the like. While all these formulations are obviously complementary, they often created competing demands for scarce resources.

The Challenge of Bioterrorism

The initial expectations of public health officials waxed and waned as 9/11 receded. At first, many believed that the federal emphasis on bioterrorism would allow for the revitalization of their field. Indeed, important improvements addressed serious weaknesses in the public health infrastructure. But many public health agency and government officials at the state level were wary that the emphasis on national defense could undermine other key programs necessary for improving the population's health.

The federal promises of money in late 2001 and early 2002 raised expectations that what many considered to be the long neglect of state and local public health agencies had, at long last, come to an end. For those in state public health agencies, the events of late 2001 were seen as potentially empowering, reversing what they perceived to be a century-long decline in status and authority. "Before, they left public health out [at the state level]," said Anne Harnish, assistant director of the Ohio Department of Health, in our telephone interview on April 1, 2003. "But bioterrorism brought us to the table and showed that we do have expertise." Similarly, in our telephone interview April 4, 2003, Ronald Cates, chief operating officer of the Missouri Department of Health and Senior Services, reflected the ideology of many public health officials: "A lot of people who couldn't spell 'public health' now saw public health as the equivalent of the Department of Defense." Even in Massachusetts, a state with well-established public health traditions and the oldest department of health in the country, administrators and politicians believe that "public health was never really an equal partner at the table . . . in the past," that is, in the past half-century, but "became an equal partner as it was called upon to safeguard our water supply," protect the airports, and protect against the importation of biological agents into the state (telephone interview with Harriette Chandler, April 15, 2003).

Some state officials outside public health had a somewhat different perception of its place in history and in emergency preparedness. For Massachusetts state senator Harriette Chandler, the discussion of anthrax fundamentally transformed state officials' perception of public health. "The anthrax scare that we had was more than a public safety scare," Chandler recalled in our interview. "It required public health, it required testing, and it required knowledgeable people. But it also required the two groups [public safety and public health] to work together and to understand where the FBI comes in, local and state police, and if there's a role for municipal authorities. In that paradigm public health was basically the quarterback. We've never had that before." For Chandler, the need for a public health response was part of a broader problem. "It also showed all of the weaknesses that we have in terms of a national disaster or emergency."

Even in states whose government agencies were vigilant in regard to planning for and coping with natural disaster, administrators in departments of health saw the anthrax episode as a watershed. In California, where earthquakes, fires, floods, and drought were a central concern of state emergency planning agencies, Angela Coron, associate director of the California Department of Health Services, remembers that "we took advantage of bioterrorism funds for California and Los Angeles to expand our capacity to respond statewide." California, like many states, has a decentralized system, with sixty-one jurisdictions for public health. Moreover, public health came to be "included in emergency preparedness more and more," Coron said in our April 2, 2003, telephone interview, because anthrax and smallpox are "where bad bugs and bad guys come together."

Across the country, administrators saw bioterrorism as an enormous opportunity to effect a sea change in public attitudes. They hoped that the money could be used both to prepare the nation and to bolster general public health programs. Dennis Perrotta (telephone interview, April 10, 2003), then state epidemiologist for the Texas Department of Health, and now associate professor of epidemiology and biosecurity, Center for Biosecurity and Public Health Preparedness, at the University of Texas School of Public Health, reflects the perception of the public health community that in most disasters public health was "always in the back helping. In bioterrorism, we moved to the driver's seat of the bus. . . . We have been brought to the front table. Sometimes in the past we have been well received, and sometimes not well received, but now the other players are our best friends." In Arizona, Catherine Eden, once a state legislator but then director of the state's Department of Health Services, and David Engelthaler, then chief of the State Office of Bioterrorism and Epidemic Preparedness and Response and now state epidemiologist for the Arizona Department of Health Services (telephone interview, March 23, 2003), thought it was "interesting [that] the military, police, and fire . . . now know they very much need us." But that is "very new for public health to be so far out in the forefront," and it did not occur without a major effort by public health officials. "We had to insert ourselves into the emergency management/response community, and there has been a major culture shift in emergency management, perhaps across the country but definitely in Arizona. . . . We were able to get an understanding of the emergency management/response community and give them an understanding of us."

Catherine Eden (telephone interview, March 21, 2003), perhaps because her background was in politics, not public health, was able to see the profound change in the culture of the department as public health personnel gained "respect with the legislature and the press." State legislators paid closer attention to the role that departments of health could play in antiterrorist planning. Similarly, Mary Kramer (telephone interview, April 11, 2003), then president of the Iowa State Senate and subsequently a U.S. ambassador, recalled that anthrax led to "including public health people for the first time in our emergency planning efforts." In Missouri, Ronald Cates (telephone interview, April 4, 2003), chief operating officer of the state's Department of Health, believed that "public health is the lead agency." Throughout the nation, the events of 2001 led those in public health to reevaluate the accuracy of their fifty-year-old ideology as an underfunded and unappreciated stepchild of government.

For the first time in many years, state and local departments of health were engaging in the kind of long-term planning that could result in the provision of services that would protect against bioterrorist emergencies and also protect population health in their states. Emergency preparedness could result in fundamental reform of public health practice. Rice Leach (telephone interview, March 19, 2003), commissioner of the Kentucky Department for Public Health, believed that public health was recovering its old, lost focus: "This [was] the first time since polio in the 1940s and 1950s that public health has had the opportunity to shine. It's a hell of a situation, but it gives us an opportunity to strut our stuff." Public health has "dealt with these things in the past, . . . but since polio and tuberculosis have declined, we have not had to handle things that affected the entire system" (Leach, quoted in Wolfe 2002).

Whatever loss of prestige the field had suffered was immaterial in light of its now very relevant special skills and methodologies. The growing importance of new federal initiatives to address disease in general and infectious diseases more specifically paralleled the perceived decline of public health's state and local standing in the second half of the twentieth century. Most important was the creation in 1946 of the Communicable Disease Center (renamed the Center for Disease Control in 1970, the Centers for Disease Control in 1980, and the Centers for Disease Control and Prevention in 1992) in the U.S. Public Health Service. This federal agency honed epidemiology, laboratory science, health surveys, and disease surveillance and reporting. Anthony Moulton (telephone interview, April 2, 2003), codirector of the CDC's Public Health Law Program, points out that the CDC built on state and local department strengths. Public health agencies routinely are engaged in "monitoring health of communities, including the surveillance for infectious disease, . . . and monitoring unusual cases and patterns of disease and injury." Also central is close coordination with medical and public health professionals, such as private doctors and emergency room nurses and physicians, who are often the first to notice unusual diseases or disease patterns. "One or more observant people see something amiss and may initiate quarantine [or isolation] and notify state/local public health agencies, which in turn would notify the CDC." Some very traditional public health activities that have been used during natural disasters in various states "applied equally to biological, chemical, and radiological threats."

Once possible disease outbreaks are identified, public health authorities use public health laboratories and a panoply of tools such as inspection, isolation (the segregation of those with symptoms), and quarantine (the segregation of those possibly exposed but not symptomatic) to limit the impact of the disease on the population. Finally, public health authorities ideally do what Moulton described as a "postmortem of the whole operation—seeing what went right and wrong—and planning for training courses" and infrastructural improvements. Rice Leach summarized these traditional mechanisms in our interview: "In any emergency preparedness you have to detect, identify, intercept, neutralize, and recover. In public health we do surveillance for detection, we use labs and epidemiology for identification, we use vaccines, antibiotics, and quarantine to neutralize, and we are the only ones who can certify that we have recovered from a problem, whether it be bioterrorism or meningitis."

The public health and emergency response communities had not been caught completely unaware by the September 11 attacks and the anthrax episodes. Before September 11, the federal government had engaged in a number of exercises aimed at assessing the nation's preparedness for bioterrorist and chemical attacks. Two efforts were especially relevant for public health officials. In May 2000 the federal government organized a mock attack on three cities, "simulat[ing] a chemical weapons event in Portsmouth, New Hampshire, a radiological event in the greater Washington, D.C., area, and a bioweapons event in Denver, Colorado." Called TOPOFF for its involvement of top officials of the U.S. government, the exercise "illuminated problematic areas of leadership and decision making; the difficulties of prioritization and distribution of scarce resources; the crisis that contagious epidemics would cause in health care facilities; and the critical need to formulate sound principles of disease containment." Also, in 1999 the federal government had "made grants available in five focus areas for bioterrorism preparedness" (Inglesby, Grossman, and O'Toole 2001).

In June 2001 the nonprofit Center for Strategic and International Studies, the Johns Hopkins Center for Civilian Biodefense Studies, the ANSER Institute for Homeland Security, and the Oklahoma National Memorial Institute for the Prevention of Terrorism "hosted a senior-level war game examining the national security, intergovernmental, and information challenges of a [smallpox] attack on the American homeland," called Dark Winter. The exercise spanned thirteen days and came to some troubling conclusions about the readiness of the nation to confront a bioterrorist attack, including lack of planning and coordination at state and federal levels (ANSER Institute for Homeland Security 2003). Not insignificantly, national concerns about the possibility of a computer system meltdown at the turn of the new century, commonly referred to as Y2K, had also forced some state agencies to address emergency preparedness planning. Y2K revealed a great deal about the absence of coordination within government and between government and health care organizations.

As a result of these and other efforts, some states had been in the process of planning for the possibility of massive disruptions before September 11. For example, Norma Gyle (telephone interview, April 8, 2003), a former legislator and now deputy commissioner of the Connecticut Department of Public Health, notes that her state was "very fortunate," for it had been preparing studies during the previous two years. Because of the concerns surrounding Y2K, when in 1999 massive computer failures and disruptions were seen as a real possibility, the state had "organized a command center that stood [Connecticut] in good stead." Because there was at least "one general convinced that there would be no milk left on the shelves," officials were "well organized." Also, California was in relatively good shape, despite low morale due to the state's ongoing budget crises. A well-developed emergency response program had been sharpened in the face of recurrent natural disasters, from earthquakes and mudslides to brushfires and chemical spills. Philip Lee, previously assistant secretary in the Department of Health and Human Services in both the Johnson and Clinton administrations and now at the University of California at San Francisco's Institute for Health Policy Studies, said that "overall, California is better off than most states in bioterrorism preparedness. Historically, it has had a strong system of public health laboratories. . . . Chemical spills have honed the skills of hazardous materials containment teams—skills that translate well in the handling of both biological and chemical warfare attacks." Colorado's and Nebraska's labs, among others, were also identified as in relatively good shape in comparison with those of most other states (Lee quoted in Russell 2001). In addition, the *Denver Post* reported, the Colorado "Department of Public Health and Environment has discovered ways to more rapidly test for such things as anthrax and plague" (Seibert 2002).

Such planning did not cease when the predicted disasters did not occur. Before September 11, the Department of Public Health in Connecticut, like those in forty-three other states, had received a Health Alert Network grant from the CDC to improve its electronic communications systems, Deputy Commissioner Gyle said in our interview. The department had "made communications a major early priority . . . [and launched] a Web site that linked health care professionals and public safety officials with the health department." This would, in the words of Warren Wollschlager, chief of staff for the Department of Public Health, "provide nearly instant information on critical resources, such as available medicines and empty hospital beds," so that the "state is much better prepared to deal with a germ attack today than it was a year ago" (quoted in Condon 2002).

But most state departments of health were grossly unprepared for September 11 and its aftermath. Georges Benjamin, then director of the Maryland Department of Health and also president of the Association of State and Territorial Health Officials, noted in October 2001, just weeks after the attacks on the World Trade Center and the Pentagon, that "in a field where communication can save a life, some state health departments" did not have an effective e-mail communication system with their local and county departments (quoted in Thompson 2001). The *Atlanta Journal-Constitution*, citing Benjamin, reported that "public health officials have been warning for years that the [public health] system is antiquated" (Nesmith 2002). The lack of planning was one problem, but equally important was insufficient financial support. "Public health funding has been woefully inadequate and it needs a boost," Benjamin pronounced. The basic infrastructure of public health needed to be "enhanced . . . at local levels to fund disease-surveillance systems, to do basic medical detective work, to coordinate with local officials, hospitals, and labs" (quoted in Thompson 2001). The National Association of County and City Health Officials (NACCHO), in its study "Local Public Health Agency Infrastructure: A Chartbook," and others pointed out that "most public health departments are not accessible 24 hours a day; 10 percent of the 3,000 local health departments don't have e-mail, let alone a computer network that links to hospitals and other health departments that would allow information about suspicious events to be distributed quickly" (Hajat, Brown, and Fraser 2001).

Benjamin, now the executive director of the American Public Health Association (APHA), recalled in our telephone interview March 12, 2003, that "September 11 brought home the fact that we had to do something about public health preparedness. Before, there was a small cadre of people concerned about bioterrorism and a small amount of money from the CDC on bioterrorism that was a specialty program and not well funded." And those people were not listened to but "were seen as doomsayers. The West Nile virus episode put people into a response mode, at least on the East Coast. They became tuned in to inter-agency cooperation to respond to an environmental event. Anthrax rolled out very slowly, insidiously. We knew it was about to come but hoped that it wouldn't . . . and then [were] shocked that it happened, but still there was an avoidance of its implications." After some days of confusion, there was "a quick response and great concern about the impact."

Benjamin's views reflected the growing worries about the public health infrastructure, which preceded the attacks. A CDC report published only months before September 11 detailed the terrible state of most public health departments across the country. Of the three thousand county and city health departments, approximately 78 percent were directed by people with no graduate training. The CDC found that "only one-third of the U.S. population [were] effectively served by public health agencies." Even the most mundane technologies were lacking in many health departments around the country. "In a test of e-mail capacity, only 35 percent of messages to local health departments were delivered successfully" (Centers for Disease Control and Prevention 2002b). The CDC lamented that "the U.S. public health infrastructure, which protects the nation against the spread of disease and environmental and occupational hazards, is still structurally weak in nearly every area," and in summary, found that "our local public health agencies lack basic equipment. . . . Our public health labo-ratories are old and unsafe. . . . Our public health physicians and nurses are untrained in new threats like West Nile virus and weaponized microorgan-isms" (Centers for Disease Control and Prevention 2001).

In the two years following the attack, state departments of health through-out the country sought to determine their own preparedness status and to define exactly what "preparedness" meant. According to Ron Kampeas report-ing in Southern California's *North County Times*, one nationwide survey found "90 percent of county governments were . . . unprepared for biological or chem-ical attacks." Kampeas quoted Tom Milne, former executive director of NAC-CHO, who reported that "a significant number of local health departments have no high-speed access to the Internet, no way of sharing data." In fact, Illinois doctors reporting outbreaks have to phone in or mail a form to the state, "basi-cally 1920s technology for monitoring disease," said John Lumpkin, formerly the state's public health chief. In Illinois the state's three labs—in Chicago, Springfield, and Carbondale—were not linked electronically. "The Springfield and Carbondale labs also need to be upgraded so they can perform more sophis-ticated tests on site . . . and new equipment that can deliver results of biological tests in one hour, as opposed to 48 hours, under conventional testing methods is needed." Iowa was in a similar position. "'Our personnel are very limited,' said [Mary] Gilchrist, who runs the University hygienic laboratory in Iowa City" and who was president of the Association of Public Health Laboratories (Lumpkin and Gilchrist quoted in Graham 2001).

To help remedy the flaws in the public health infrastructure that the anthrax attack had highlighted, President George W. Bush signed into law on January 10, 2002, a bill to send $1.1 billion to the states, territories, and three cities—Chicago, Los Angeles, and New York—to "develop comprehensive bioterrorism prepared-ness plans, upgrade infectious-disease surveillance and investigation, enhance the readiness of hospital systems to deal with large numbers of casualties, expand public health laboratory and communications capacities, and improve connectiv-ity between hospitals, and city, local, and state health departments to enhance dis-ease reporting" (U.S. Department of Health and Human Services 2002).

The moneys were distributed to the states in three components. All the states received 20 percent of their per capita allotment upfront, in most cases several million dollars, to develop plans for how they would use the money and, after review, received the remaining allocation. The moneys were divided into two parts. The first and significantly larger part consisted of grants from the CDC specifically "targeted to supporting bioterrorism, infectious diseases, and public health emergency preparedness activities." The second, provided through the Health Resources and Services Administration (HRSA), provided funding to "be used by states to create regional hospital plans to respond in the event of a bioter-rorism attack" (Centers for Disease Control 2002a). To get the money, the gover-nor's office, often relying on its department of health, submitted bioterror preparedness plans to the U.S. Department of Health and Human Services and was required, among other things, "to provide for at least one epidemiologist . . . for each metropolitan area with a population greater than 500,000, [and to] develop a communications system that provides a 24/7 flow of health information among hospital, state, and local health officials and law enforcement" (Guiden 2002). In addition, the CDC targeted "preparedness planning and readiness assessment, surveillance and epidemiology capacity, laboratory capacity, Health Alert Network/communications, risk communication and health information dissemi-nation, and education and training" (Staiti, Katz, and Hoadley 2003).

In some measure, a disjuncture of expectations developed between federal officials and those at the state level. For state officials, the billions of dollars pledged to the states seemed like a huge bonanza that promised a possibility of saving the public health infrastructure that they saw as having been eviscerated by years, if not decades, of neglect. But to officials responsible for the federal budget—for the hundreds of billions of dollars devoted to the maintenance of the nation's public health, defense, and health care infrastructure—the money made available to the states through the CDC and HRSA augured only modest promise for improving the infrastructure.

Years before anthrax made bioterrorism a household word, some experts were suggesting that there was no contradiction between improving the overall public health infrastructure and meeting the nation's growing need to protect itself from bioterrorist attacks. In 1999, in a prescient article describing the government's growing attention to bioterrorism as a real threat, S. J. Freedberg and M. Serafini quoted Harvard's terrorism expert Richard Falkenrath, then of the Kennedy School of Government, on the benefits of bioterrorism money as a salve for the problems plaguing state departments of health. "Even in the crucial area where existing assets are inadequate—public health—filling the gaps has benefits far beyond biowar. New multipurpose drugs, new vaccines, and above all, a revived public health surveillance system are all independently desirable because they help you get a handle on naturally occurring diseases which are in all respects more common and more damaging to American citizens." James M. Hughes, director of the National Center for Infectious Diseases at CDC, agreed: "This money is going to be well-spent, strengthening national, state and local capacity to deal with infectious agents, even if a biological attack does not occur. . . . To stop both biowar and natural disease outbreaks, the steps you have to take are the same." Surgeon General Satcher saw these bioterrorism funds as a way to counter what he described as "decades of decay and neglect to the public health system." Fortunately or unfortunately, "bioterrorism has really gotten the attention of people, [when] perhaps we've had trouble getting their attention before" (Falkenrath, Hughes, and Satcher quoted in Freedberg and Serafini 1999).

In the immediate aftermath of the anthrax episode, these hopes for the dual benefits of bioterrorism funding were revived. Washington State secretary of health Mary Selecky, among many others, asked: Was this money going to be there for the long term? And would it support the public health infrastructure generally and not just the short-term fashion of bioterrorism? "We have had numerous communicable diseases many times before we had anthrax last fall, and we're using the same systems." But would there "be a sustained, long-term investment, so . . . if headlines subside, we don't drop our attention?" (quoted in Guiden 2002). Others asked a similar question. Officials in Chicago, for example, hoped that federal funds would go "beyond hazardous-materials suits and stockpiles of penicillin to computer networks, personnel training, modern laboratories, and updated equipment that is critical in times of crisis and in routine work." Patrick Lenihan, the deputy commissioner of the Chicago Department of Public Health, was quoted as saying, "The day-to-day stuff that is taken for granted is just what is called upon in a threat of bioterrorism." Epidemiology and surveillance were as essential to the tracking of syphilis and tuberculosis as to that of anthrax and smallpox (Christian 2001). Some state administrators see the efforts around bioterrorism as having had lasting positive effects on the public health infrastructure in their states.

While many state officials saw the federal involvement in bioterrorism and emergency preparedness as generally beneficial or at least a mixed blessing, American Public Health Association executive director Georges Benjamin (then president of the Association of State and Territorial Health Officials) and others developed a fundamental critique of the effect of federal funding for bioterrorism on population health. Within a few months of the World Trade Center disaster, Benjamin was cited in a February 5, 2002, *New York Times* article: "While public health officials view bioterrorism preparedness as important . . . it should not come at the expense of other programs. They note that just five Americans have been killed by bioterrorism over the last year, while thousands die each year of chronic illnesses and infectious diseases. 'We will be very concerned if we are funding one thing at the expense of another,' said Georges C. Benjamin. . . . 'If you really want to push people towards better health, you have got to keep these programs in place'" (Stolberg 2002a).

The concern was prompted by the call in a new federal budget proposal "for a $57 million cut in the CDC's program for chronic disease prevention and health promotion. Infectious disease control, meanwhile, would be cut by $10 million, at a time when public health officials are particularly concerned about the threat of new and emerging infections." The budget for other programs, including "childhood immunization, environmental health, preventing birth defects, and sexually transmitted diseases, including AIDS," would remain flat. Advocates worried that their own public health priorities would be short-changed. The same *New York Times* article quoted Marsha Martin, executive director of AIDS Action, who said that President Bush was sending "a clear message that our nation's public health has fallen off the administration's radar screen." Martin also asked for a broader definition of emergency preparedness: "Homeland security also means investing in prevention and care services for people at risk and living with HIV" (Stolberg 2002a).

Further concern arose over the panicked and erratic reaction of federal officials who were sending out mixed messages about future funding and priorities. "'Yo-yo funding has been the history of public health,' said Georges C. Benjamin. Leslie M. Beitsch, the former health commissioner in Oklahoma, said, 'I think it's a very significant commitment, but the question then becomes, is it a long-term commitment?'" State health officials echoed these fears, saying they "were eager for the money [for bioterrorism preparedness] but were concerned that it would not last" (Stolberg 2002b).

Effects of Budget Crises on Public Health and Emergency Preparedness

Whatever the conflicting views of state officials about federal bioterrorism money in general, there was a broad consensus that the budget problems that most states began to suffer in 2002 have had a deleterious impact on states' abilities to respond to both bioterrorism and population health needs. The economic downturn that devastated most state budgets undermined the positive effects of the federal bioterrorism funding in various states, and the distortions in services and attention created by that infusion of money were amplified as state legislatures attempted to cope with huge deficits and falling tax revenues. The stock market decline and the effects of terrorist attacks on the World Trade Center and the Pentagon had exacerbated the beginnings of an economic recession. As John M. Colmers, Scott D. Pattison, and Sheila Peterson (2005) explain: "The recession itself also stimulated countercyclical spending by states as citizens unemployed as a result of the recession or the jobless recovery that followed it, turned to their state governments for assistances." As a result, "leaders of the executive and legislative branches in the states" had to "make difficult decisions in order to balance their budgets, as 49 states are constitutionally required to do."

Overall, the economic problems of the states were immense. More than half the states saw their budget for public health decline in FY 2003, fifteen states suffered further declines in FY 2004, and fifteen more states had their public health budget increase by 3 percent or less (Trust for America's Health 2004). In a detailed analysis of state health expenditures before and after September 11, Colmers, Pattison, and Peterson (2005), writing on behalf of the National Association of State Budget Officers and the Reforming States Group, found that "under the most difficult budgetary pressures in a generation, escalating health care costs for the poor and frail trumped the repair of a decaying public health infrastructure in state houses around the country." Although "total state health expenditures grew from $271 billion in FY 2000 to $358 billion in 2003" most of this $86 billion increase "is attributable to Medicaid spending ($66 billion), which by itself is the largest share of state health spending." Population health spending represents only 5.4 percent of the total. The authors conclude that the states' fiscal distress and the increased Medicaid expenses "trumped the states' ability to improve the infrastructure of population health. The important but unglamorous categories of infectious disease prevention, chronic disease control and population health infrastructure will have to wait for budget increases until the economy recovers sufficiently to generate substantial increases in tax receipts."

The effects of these budget cuts on public health departments and programs were severe, especially in states that had invested a significant amount of state money in building up population health programs. Ironically, states that had relied entirely on federal grant funding were affected less severely when state budget deficits forced a contraction of state health programs.

If state budget crises were not enough to cause disruptions and potential disasters for the public health departments around the country, the smallpox vaccination campaign initiated in December 2002 added strain to the system. This federal program proposed to inoculate half a million health care workers in the first stage of what was described as a three-stage process. At first, the national attention to public health and its needs that the program created was a great boon to the field. Citizens who had not thought about the source of their pure water, air, or food now came to understand the enormous effort that went into assuring their purity. In the context of the general mobilization around the war in Iraq and the discussion about the danger of biological warfare, the smallpox vaccination campaign and the public health system's role in protecting the country from bioterrorism led to support for a national campaign to prepare for a possible smallpox attack. But as the campaign continued and it became clear that this effort, far from building support for and strengthening population health initiatives in the states, was actually draining resources and energies, support began to wane. While some officials praised the stimulus to plan for possible future bioterrorist events, soon an uncommitted public health community, a resistant public, and health providers who did not volunteer to become vaccinated virtually stopped the campaign in its tracks. Across the country, state administrators referred to the distortions in program and policy that the smallpox campaign caused.

Georges Benjamin takes a long view of the entire recent history of bioterrorist threats. Anthrax helped focus the nation on the dangerous possibility of infectious diseases as a terrorist tool and the ways in which the infusion of federal money to combat that threat could be used: "Lots of money was poured in for all-hazards management to build up the public health infrastructure," he said in our 2003 interview. But the smallpox inoculation campaign is another matter. Even though "smallpox has become the new mandate," it "has been underfunded"; furthermore, the single-minded attention to it has "sacrificed core public health activities," pulling money and people from other public health programs. Not only has it undermined core public health programs, but "we have also sacrificed an all-hazards management (bioterrorism) approach to concentrate on one specific disease."

Benjamin summarizes the general uneasiness of many in the public health community as well as in the broader population:

> Many public health practitioners believe the case for smallpox inoculation has not been effectively made and is taking away resources and personnel from things we know we should be doing. It is pulling people away from screening for HIV and the counseling of AIDS patients, prenatal care clinics, other immunizations, and inspection programs for other diseases. A basic surveillance system is already lacking. And money is being used to deal with a theoretical disease. . . . Already people are being laid off in disease and inspection programs but are being hired in bioterrorism. They are being funded by shifting moneys around. Phase 1 was supposed to inoculate 500,000 people, but only about 12,000 have been inoculated so far. It is well behind schedule; it is stalled.

Regional Coordination

Perhaps the most glaring weakness that was revealed by the events of September 11 and the subsequent anthrax episode was the very fragile, virtually non-existent relationship among the various state health departments throughout the country. Significantly, throughout the twentieth century there has been an enormous expansion in the scope of federal power and authority in numerous aspects of American life. Washington, D.C., has assumed responsibilities and powers that were once the province of the states. Labor legislation, commerce, environmental regulation, food and drug safety, and a host of other policy concerns have moved from the state and local to the national arena. While public health is addressed in national agencies such as the Public Health Service and the National Institutes of Health within the Department of Health and Human Services, many critical powers and decisions that affect the nation's health and well-being still reside at the state and local level (Gostin 2000). Practically, this has meant that preparation for bioterrorism and coordination between states is largely nonexistent. For the most part, administrators of each of the state departments of health acted independently of one another. Administrators in some states, it appears, have simply gone back to business as usual and remain isolated from their colleagues in other states.

Lessons for the Future

September 11 presented the public health community and those involved with population health more generally a great opportunity to revitalize and rethink the health agenda for the nation. Politicians, administrators, and the general public came to appreciate the vital role that public health agencies could play in a national emergency and in the fight against terrorism; public health administrators and advocates hoped that they could capture and perhaps recapture the potential they believed public health had had in a bygone era. Some observers called for a revamping of the nation's health insurance system so that more of the population was covered as a means of improving the surveillance of disease; some called for an expansion of the scope of traditional public health activities so that the growing barriers between prevention and care would be reduced; some called for the extension of the social service system and its integration with the health care and public health systems; others called for the upgrading of the public health infrastructure as a necessary tool in the fight against terrorism. Yet others cautioned that simply increasing budgets and financial resources might do little to address the long-term problems affecting public and population health programs in the various states. While those in general government—elected officials and members of their staffs—and public health agencies agreed on many points, those in general government were not expecting increased funding for public health department activities per se to solve decades of problems.

In examining the public health community's response in the various states, we conclude that the very definition of emergency response must continue to expand the purview of public health so that professionals in the field understand the breadth of social and medical activities that determine a population's health and well-being. For much of the past century, public health officials, administrators, and city agencies in general clung to very traditional notions of what constituted dangers to the public's health: they created discrete functions regarding sanitation, emergency care, scientific data collection, and surveillance to address these dangers. But this narrow definition of public responsibility has broadened considerably over the past few generations. The events of the past five years have spurred this redefinition, forcing government officials—indeed, all of us—to rethink what health is, which agencies are responsible for a population's health, and what the public's role is in defining what is considered a healthful or unhealthful environment.

After September 11, 2001, officials and legislators in state government were buffeted by geopolitical events and federal government decisions that dramatically altered the basic assumptions under which they operated. Rural county officials, often isolated and laboring far from the seats of power at the state or federal levels, could hardly be expected to be fully prepared for their new responsibilities for developing plans for bioterrorist or chemical attack. At the state level, legislators and state officials responsible for population health and well-being focused on a broader array of social service, public health, and health care needs that all demanded scarce state and federal resources. Public health agency heads, both at the county and state level, concentrated on the need to improve traditional public health infrastructural services such as lab capacity, surveillance systems, intra- and interagency communication, border protection, and other specific needs of their agencies. Certainly, the mobilization around public health needs resulted in the allocation of significant resources and in what many of our respondents called "progress."

In the early months after the World Trade Center attack and the anthrax episodes, public health officials and those in general government believed that the new resources of the federal government could be used to address long-standing weaknesses in the public health infrastructure as well as to meet the new federal mandates to protect citizens from bioterrorist or chemical attack. Many officials understood that the cause of the day gets massive funding and that when that cause changes, the money may disappear. But this time, they believed, would be different. Because of the pain of September 11, many state officials hoped that the federal government would finally fund public and population health programs at a level that not only would protect the country from narrowly defined bioterrorist threats but also would protect the population from SARS and other infectious diseases. Some even hoped that essential population health services such as improved health care and health insurance availability would be addressed. There was no intrinsic contradiction between the traditional goals of public health departments to investigate, monitor, and perform laboratory investigations and to provide services for well babies and the uninsured, and the new goal of participating as full members in an emergency response team. Yet while those in general government and those in public health agencies agreed on many of the same goals, those in state legislatures and their staffs were obligated to balance their budgets, with entitlement programs (such as Medicaid) representing about 80 percent of those budgets, whereas those in public health agencies sought to maintain or protect the programs more traditionally associated with preventive services.

It is clear from the interviews and our reading of published and unpublished reports and media coverage that in the years since September 11, much has been accomplished in terms of providing resources, legal reform, improved surveillance, and communication. The focus of the CDC and HRSA programs has expanded beyond smallpox and preparations for war against Iraq. The CDC and HRSA grant programs are a clear indication that the federal government remains committed to addressing bioterrorism and terrorism in general, with the grant awards for fiscal years 2003, 2004, and 2005 matching those of 2002. The strengthening of the public health infrastructure (together with rising employment as a result of the recovery from the recession) has resulted in a modest improvement in access to health care and health insurance, general childhood inoculation programs, well-baby services, and mental health care services. It has also aided agency and interagency coordination for emergency response and improved laboratory capacity in some communities. The CDC identifies a number of significant improvements in public health preparedness at the state level as a result of federal initiatives, grants, and programs. Through its grants, the CDC has fostered the development of surveillance systems, management information systems, interagency cooperative agreements, twenty-four-hour-a-day public health emergency response systems, and identified physicians to serve as consultants in diagnosis and treatment of infectious diseases in an emergency. Among the concrete accomplishments were stronger relationships between law enforcement and health providers, enhanced epidemiological capacity, better training for possible bioterrorist events, improved and more secure communication systems, enhanced laboratory capacity, and a group of inoculated health professionals capable of responding to a smallpox outbreak: "In 2005, CDC will be awarding $862,777,000 to support state and local public health response efforts. Since these funds are intended to enhance detection and surveillance capabilities, improve laboratory diagnostic capacities, improve the delivery and quality of workforce training, improve outbreak control and containment strategies, and enable improved communication, it goes without saying that the basic public health infrastructure benefits from these investments" (J. Henderson, former CDC chief of program operations for bioterrorism preparedness and response, telephone interview, June 29, 2004).

While certain bioterrorism-specific reforms will undoubtedly remain, the early post-9/11 optimism regarding the new federal attention and funding has waned as state legislators, governors, and public health officials all come up against state and federal budget crises and shifting federal attention in the war against terrorism. This has been particularly true as budgetary crises in most states force legislators to make hard choices about their priorities for education, social welfare, direct health services, and population health more generally. Even level funding is inadequate to build up the public health infrastructure in a manner to address adequately the increased burden shouldered by public health departments to counter terrorism and bioterrorism. Many public health officials were bitterly disappointed that federal attention to upgrading the public health infrastructure waned as September 11 receded into the historical memory. Certainly, the nation's public and population health infrastructure has suffered as the Bush administration continually presses the nation to believe that the real war on terrorism—and therefore our budget priorities—is in Iraq.

Many in general government feared that a narrow focus on health as an adjunct to national defense could undermine their broader mission to provide a variety of services not necessarily tied to bioterrorism and emergency preparedness. The economic recessions that in some states had begun before September 11 strained state budgets and forced reduced spending in numerous sectors of the states' bureaucracies, including health. The budgetary problems were amplified by the federal mandate in late 2002 for a major smallpox inoculation campaign. Further, traditional public health surveillance techniques and disease reporting, if perceived as an infringement on personal liberties, can undermine public trust in the system as a whole.

The federal government, through the CDC, has accomplished a great deal to improve emergency response and bioterrorism preparedness. In addition to its aid to individual states and cities it has expanded the national Laboratory Response Network, increased the Strategic National Stockpile of pharmaceuticals and medical supplies and insured that they can be delivered to any place in the United States within twelve hours, and developed new technologies to improve the effectiveness of surveillance systems and other data-sharing systems. But, as Joseph Henderson put it in our 2004 interview: "The key concern today is to assure federal, state, and government leaders and elected officials don't sacrifice the ground gained since September 11 due to new priorities and shifting political interests. Significant resources are in place to support broad-based public health, including public health readiness. One cannot exist without the other. A solid public health system strives to reduce/eliminate illness, injury, and death every day, but especially when a catastrophic event occurs such as bioterrorism or SARS."

The maintenance of the public health infrastructure is probably the single most important means of preparing the nation for the myriad unpredictable crises arising from SARS, avian flu, and influenza epidemics, as well as from terrorist attacks. Without a strong permanent infrastructure, the best emergency planning will be inadequate. The financial crises of the various states, combined with the shifting focus of the federal government from bioterrorism and terrorism in general to smallpox and the war in Iraq more specifically have lessened the early potential to enhance the system of services that are essential for the improvement of the nation's efforts to address bioterrorism preparedness and the overall health needs of the American people.

References

Abate, T. 2001. Scared into Action. *San Francisco Chronicle*, October 8.
ANSER Institute for Homeland Security. 2003. Dark Winter. www.homelandsecurity.org/darkwinter/index.cfm (accessed July 29, 2003).

Burress, C. 2001. State Can't Handle Bioterrorist Attack. *San Francisco Chronicle*, November 7.

Centers for Disease Control and Prevention. 2001. Public Health's Infrastructure: A Status Report Prepared for the Appropriations Committee. Atlanta: Centers for Disease Control and Prevention.

———. 2002a. CDC and HRSA Bioterrorism and Response Grants, Illinois Homeland Security. www.100.state.il.us/security/ittf/terrorism report14.htm (accessed November 23, 2003).

———. 2002b. Media Relations, Office of Communication. Fact Sheet: Public Health Infrastructure. May 14. www.cdc.gov/od/oc/media/pressrel/fs020514.htm (accessed December 7, 2005).

Christian, S. E. 2001. Anthrax Scare: Health System's Weakness Exposed. *Chicago Tribune*, November 18.

Colmers, J. M., S. D. Pattison, and S. Peterson. 2005. State Health Expenditures before and after September 11. Manuscript. Author files.

Condon, G. 2002. Hospitals Team Up against Terrorism. *Hartford Courant*, November 15.

Connolly, C. 2001. Public Health System Is on War Footing. *Washington Post*, October 27.

Copeland, L. 2001. Local Public Health Officials Seek Help. *USA Today*, October 23.

Evans, G., B. Clements, and B. Shadel. 2001. We Can't Fight Bioterrorism on the Cheap. *St. Louis Post Dispatch*, November 28.

Fox, Daniel M. 2001. Foreword to *Public Health Administration: Principles for Population-Based Management*, ed. Lloyd F. Novick and Glen P. Mays. Gaithersburg, Md.: Aspen.

Freedberg, S. J. J., and M. W. Serafini. 1999. Be Afraid, Be Moderately Afraid. *National Journal* 31:812–813.

Gostin, L. O. 2000. *Public Health Law: Power, Duty, Restraint.* Berkeley: University of California Press; New York: Milbank Memorial Fund.

Graham, J. 2001. Money Woes Plague Nation's Health Labs. *Chicago Tribune*, November 23.

Guiden, M. 2002. Public Health Officials Prep for Bioterror with New Hires. *Stateline.org.* September 6. www.stateline.org (accessed December 7, 2005).

Hajat, A., C. K. Brown, and M. R. Fraser. 2001. Local Public Health Infrastructure: A Chartbook. October. www.naccho.org/files/documents/chartbook_frontmatter1–2.pdf (accessed Nov. 5, 2003).

Inglesby, T. V., R. Grossman, and T. O'Toole. 2001. A Plague on Your City: Observations from TOPOFF. *Clinical Infectious Diseases* 32:436.

Kampeas, R. 2002. States Adjust to Governing with Threat of Bioterror. *North County Times*, June 19. www.NCTimes.net (accessed December 7, 2005).

Kristof, N. 2001. This Is Not a Test. *New York Times*, December 28.

Nesmith, J. 2002. Health System's Bioterror Readiness Up. *Atlanta Journal and Constitution*, November 13.

Russell, S. 2001. Public Health Care under a Microscope: Bioterror Attacks Bring New Focus to Neglected Facilities. *San Francisco Chronicle*, December 2.

Satel, S. 2001. Public Health? Forget it; Cosmic Issues Beckon. *Wall Street Journal*, December 13.

Schwartz, J. 2001. Efforts to Calm Nation's Fears Spin Out of Control. *New York Times*, October 28.

Seibert, T. 2002. Bioterror to Be Top Priority for Grant; State Makes Plans for $16.3 Million. *Denver Post*, April 2.

Staiti, A., A. Katz, and J. F. Hoadley. 2003. Has Bioterrorism Preparedness Improved Public Health? *Center for Studying Health System Change.* Issue Brief no. 65: July. www.hschange.org/CONTENT/588/ (accessed December 7, 2005).

Stolberg, S. G. 2002a. The President's Budget Proposal: Buckets for Bioterrorism, but Less for Catalogue of Ills. *New York Times*, February 5.

———. 2002b. U.S. Will Give States $1 Billion to Improve Bioterrorism Defense. *New York Times*, January 25.

Terhune, C. 2001. Public Health Officials Say More Funding, Information Needed to Fight Bioterrorism. *Wall Street Journal*, October 23.

Thompson, S. H. 2001. Knowledge May Serve as Public Health Antidote to Bioterrorism Worries. *Tampa Tribune*, October 21.

Trust for America's Health. 2004. Ready or Not? Protecting the Public's Health in the Age of Bioterrorism—2004 State Public Health Budget Data. December 14. http://healthyamericans.org/reports/bioterror04 (accessed December 12, 2005).

U.S. Department of Health and Human Services. 2002. HHS Announces $1.1 Billion in Funding to States for Bioterrorism Preparedness. Press release. January 31. www.hhs.gov/news/press/2002pres/20020131b.html (accessed December 7, 2005).

Wolfe, C. 2002. Kentucky Plans Possible Bioterrorism Response. *Cincinnati Enquirer*, June 10.

Nicole Lurie, Jeffrey Wasserman, and
Christopher D. Nelson

Chapter 10

Public Health Preparedness

Evolution or Revolution?

Events at the dawn of the twenty-first century pushed public health emergency preparedness to the top of the U.S. national agenda. Concern intensified with the response to the 2005 Gulf Coast hurricanes and amid the growing possibility of an H5N1 influenza virus pandemic (bird flu). The federal government has responded with an investment of some $5 billion since 2001 to upgrade the public health system's ability to prevent and respond to large-scale public health emergencies, whether caused by terrorism or by natural agents.

However, the government's call to arms falls upon a system still in the process of recovering from years of being underresourced and often ignored by federal policy makers. The Institute of Medicine (IOM) termed the system "still in disarray" in 2003, despite the fact that the IOM had first articulated its concerns in 1988 (Institute of Medicine 1988, 2003). Moreover, the public typically has had a poor understanding of what public health systems are and of what governmental public health agencies do.

Heightened Expectations

The new emphasis on and funding for public health preparedness has heightened expectations about how the system should perform and has raised questions about the extent to which U.S. public health systems have evolved and improved in recent years. Congress and the taxpayers it represents want to know how the funds have been spent and whether the system is better prepared than before to protect the public in a public health emergency. Although the preparedness mission represents only a small part of what public health does, the changes that have occurred in public health during the past few years provide a vantage point from which to examine the status of the system as a whole and to identify ways of encouraging the evolution of—and even hastening a revolution in—public health.

Signs of Change

Between 2003 and 2006, RAND researchers have had the opportunity to examine the public health infrastructure through a series of interrelated projects: an assessment of California's public health preparedness; tests of a measure of health department performance; the development and conducting of tabletop exercises in thirty-two communities in twelve states; an examination of the public health–hospital interface; a study of the impact of variation in state and local relationships on preparedness; and a review of quality improvement efforts in public health. All told, the RAND team visited forty-four communities in seventeen states.[1] Taken together, these assessments suggest that public health is in the midst of a major transition, spurred in part by the addition of public health preparedness to the responsibilities of state and local public health agencies. Key signs of change include new partnerships, changes in the workforce, new technologies, and evolving organizational structures. Although each of these elements has had some positive impact on public health, none has been implemented without problems, and integration of preparedness with other public health functions remains a major challenge for many public health agencies. Furthermore, the preparedness mission has raised special challenges for public health in the areas of leadership, governance, quality, and accountability.

In a 2002 commentary, Nicole Lurie pointed out that much of our public health infrastructure has changed little over the past century and asked: "Do we want to rebuild a nineteenth-century system, even with twenty-first-century technology?" Although building a brand-new public health system from scratch is both impractical and politically untenable, we believe that public health preparedness can have a profound impact on how the U.S. public health system evolves. In this chapter we discuss key ways in which public health preparedness is affecting public health agencies and suggest that despite the challenges inherent in embracing this new responsibility, public health will become a stronger and more visible governmental partner as a result, better able to protect and improve population health.

Recent Changes in Public Health
New Partnerships

Partnerships between community entities, such as private health care facilities or schools and local government officials, are not at all new to public health. However, the process of preparing a community to meet the challenges of a potential public health emergency has required public health departments to build relationships with new kinds of partners, including emergency management agencies, law enforcement, and other first responders (Lasker 1997). The development of emergency response plans or participation in drills, for example, has required public health agencies to work closely with first responders and has stimulated agencies to develop stronger relationships with the hospital and health care community. Throughout our site visits and exercises, we observed repeatedly that preparedness planning has been instrumental in forging these new relationships and that communication and working relationships between many of these entities are better than in the pre-9/11 era.

But developing these relationships has not been without its challenges, largely because of differences in culture, work style, and mission. Emergency responders and police have emergency responses as a primary mission. They are used to making rapid decisions, acting quickly, and working in a hierarchical command structure—a culture that has been derisively described by some in public health as "ready-fire-aim." In contrast, public health departments are typically responsible for a range of activities, including many that involve slowly evolving and non-life-threatening problems; they have therefore been able to conduct much of their work in a more contemplative mode and at a relatively slower pace. In many public health agencies, a high priority is placed on reaching consensus before taking action. Agencies typically value collaboration skills, and many have reported discomfort when functioning in a hierarchical command structure. Indeed, some public health officials self-selected into collaborative organizations philosophically object to what they see as the "militarization of public health" and the use of incident command structures.

The relationships between public health agencies and hospitals have also been affected by different missions and experiences. From the personal health care delivery system perspective, hospitals have long had requirements for disaster preparedness, and hospital staffs often function hierarchically, especially in emergencies. In fact, many in the hospital community view public health agencies as latecomers to emergency planning and preparedness and are uncertain about agencies' role or what they offer (Wasserman et al. 2006). Nonetheless, taken together, collaboration with these partners is heightening the expectations for the role of public health in communities.

Changes in the Workforce

New Staff

Preparedness has resulted in several changes to the public health workforce, including adding new personnel and new responsibilities. First, all states and most metropolitan areas have hired bioterrorism or emergency preparedness coordinators. These staff often have backgrounds and experience in emergency response, law enforcement, or the military, and it has taken time for them to understand the culture of the public health enterprise and vice versa. At the same time, people in these roles are often responsible for bringing new ways of doing things to health departments, including exercises, drills, and after-action reviews. Many are comfortable in a command structure and willing to serve as incident commanders in an emergency. Although such traits can serve them well in their roles as preparedness coordinators, the background and perspective these personnel bring can sometimes create friction with public health leaders, who are often more reticent about stepping into these roles.

New Roles and Responsibilities

Nonpreparedness staff in many public health departments have been asked to take on new roles and responsibilities in the event of a public health emergency, and many are being cross-trained to do so. For many public health agencies, this represents the first time that the entire staff has been trained to work toward a focused, common public health goal outside their day-to-day roles. This training has provided public health personnel with an awareness of emergency preparedness that fully permeates health department workforces more than has the awareness of traditional public health missions, such as immunization, control of sexually transmitted diseases (STDs), or chronic disease prevention. However, the development and implementation of such training programs is still redundant and nonstandardized, and it is often unclear how well staff could actually perform their new roles in a crisis.

Staff Shortages

Most health departments we visited experienced challenges related to both staff availability and budget. Many states have hiring freezes in place. There is not a robust pipeline of trained personnel to work in public health agencies, and salaries for public health nurses, epidemiologists, laboratory professionals, and physicians are often not competitive with those of their private-sector counterparts. Several states we visited have dealt with these problems by contracting services out to nonprofit and private-sector entities. However, it is not clear that this strategy builds long-term internal capacity in health departments. In numerous instances, states and localities that have transferred staff in other nonpreparedness-related positions (for example, immunization coordinator) to senior preparedness roles have found that there was not a workforce available to replace them. All of this has led to a prevailing perception that public health emergency preparedness and other public health functions have a zero-sum relationship, in which increasing investment in one sector entails reducing investments in the other. In fact, our case studies and key-informant interviews revealed that senior state and local health department officials spend a substantial fraction of their time, often upward of 20 percent, on preparedness-related matters (Lurie, Valdez et al. 2004). Public health departments reported that cuts to local public health budgets have led to reduction in, and in some instances elimination of, important public health services and programs, including teen pregnancy prevention, tuberculosis (TB) screening, and STD contact tracing.

Aging Workforce

An aging workforce has compounded workforce shortages in public health. Moreover, because of overall shortages of qualified employees to fill key public health positions, health jurisdictions are competing with one another for scarce human resources. Often this focus on competition has kept departments from considering other alternatives for meeting workforce needs, such as using the available pool of employees more efficiently.

New Technologies

Technology has become increasingly important in the workplace, and preparedness efforts—as well as the infusion of federal funds—have allowed public health agencies to achieve technological gains in two important areas. First, many communities have made recent investments in technology that enables all parties, including public health, to communicate on the same radio frequencies even when power is not available. This technology allows public health officials to communicate with their counterparts in emergency medical services (EMS) and allows fire and police departments to communicate with one another. Second, funding has facilitated advances in the information technology (IT) infrastructure for public health. Improvements have ranged from the development of a national Health Alert Network and Laboratory Response Network, which strengthens electronic laboratory reporting of reportable diseases, to statewide systems to conduct surveillance and outbreak investigation, most of which feed into the Centers for Disease Control and Prevention (CDC). The latter type of system enabled Pennsylvania to respond effectively to a hepatitis A outbreak in 2003 (Stoto et al. 2005). In part, it is this infrastructure that has the potential to bring many revolutionary strategies to public health. For example, while not related directly to preparedness funding, New York City recently mandated reporting of hemoglobin A1C test results as part of its strategy to address the diabetes epidemic (Steinbrook 2006). Improved IT can help many jurisdictions with similar innovative approaches to controlling both acute and chronic diseases.

Integration of Preparedness with Other Public Health Functions

New partnerships, changes in the workforce, and new technologies have all made positive contributions to public health; however, integration of preparedness with other public health functions has remained a challenge. Because preparedness has been a new function with its own budget, its functions have often been kept separate from other public health functions. For example, vaccines and other components in the Strategic National Stockpile are tracked and distributed separately from other vaccines and medications handled by public health departments. In the face of concerns about pandemic influenza, for which the country is now preparing, we observed that some public health departments consider planning for a flu pandemic to be an entirely separate activity from general public health emergency preparedness. Also, such planning has involved only those responsible for annual influenza activities, with the unfortunate result that staff involved in the former activity did not take advantage of several years of work done by preparedness staff. We observed many similar instances in which public health departments missed opportunities to exploit the interface between bioterrorism surveillance and activities in other areas, ranging from patient safety and hospital nosocomial infections to chronic disease surveillance. However, increasing integration of these types of activities may well be building toward a tipping point in how public health activities are performed and could be another part of the revolution in public health practice.

Impact on Performance

In the course of our work, we found that when public health agencies had made strides to integrate preparedness with other public health functions, performance, at least judged by exercises, was improved. For example, one large health jurisdiction had only a skeletal preparedness staff and distributed the bulk of the preparedness resources it received through the CDC grants to existing units. Unit heads were told that preparedness objectives should shape everything they did and that, reciprocally, other functions should influence preparedness efforts. We found through both key-informant interviews and direct observation that these efforts to integrate preparedness with other functions were reflected in performance. In contrast, we found that less-well-integrated health departments tended to perform poorly on tabletop exercises or reported other challenges in responding to real events. For example, staff in one state reported major problems implementing a mass vaccination clinic during the 2004–2005 flu vaccine shortage, only to discover after the fact that its preparedness staff had already worked through the logistics of such an effort.

Impact on Epidemiology and Communications

Our research also found that integration of preparedness and other efforts seemed to have a positive effect on epidemiology and communications. In epidemiology, investments in laboratory capacity and reporting, IT, and the hiring of many more epidemiologists appear to have increased the epidemiological and investigative capacity of many health departments. Since public health emergencies on the scale of a bioterrorist attack or pandemic flu are thankfully rare, these staffs are available to fulfill general epidemiology tasks while maintaining the skills and capacity for a large-scale response. We are optimistic that over time, this will be reflected in greater outbreak detection, better investigation, and more rapid control of an outbreak. A similar phenomenon appears to have occurred regarding the use of incident command structures. Although some health departments have been resistant to using such a structure, several have embraced the concept and applied its principles to a range of activities, including outbreak investigation and budget planning. Particularly in the area of outbreak investigation, public health staff report improvements in both timeliness and completeness of outbreak management.

Effect on Risk Communication

The need for effective risk communication as a component of preparedness and response has led health departments to hire more public information officers. We saw several health departments in which such people used their communication skills not just to convey specific risk information, but also to improve communication among the health department, other partners, and the public and to raise awareness of other public health issues.

Major Challenges

Leadership

One clear and consistent finding that has emerged from our work concerns the role of strong leadership in public health preparedness. In our tabletop exercises, we repeatedly observed that strong leadership trumped all other factors in determining how jurisdictions fared when presented with a wide range of scenarios related to infectious disease outbreaks. The performance of health departments whose leaders were willing to take responsibility for, and make decisions in, a hypothetical situation was far better than that of those in which the leaders said they would be willing to be "co-in-charge" with others. Leaders were also important in facilitating organizational change, motivating staff, developing relationships with key community groups and other constituencies, training staff to assume various backup roles in the event of an outbreak, conducting strategic planning, and understanding when and where to hand off functions to officials from other agencies.

Although our work to date has not examined closely the best means of developing and promoting strong public health leadership, we noted that some successful health jurisdictions provided aggressive leadership training programs for employees. In one health department, for example, we were told about a program promoting public health leadership and cultural change, in which employees are taught how to assess performance and manage time, staff, and so on.

Quality and Accountability

The investment in public health preparedness has led to calls for accountability at a number of levels. First, Congress wants an accounting of how the funds were spent, and the CDC is responsible for monitoring preparedness—at least at the state level. Some state legislatures are making similar demands regarding local preparedness, and in some areas, the public, aided by the media and the recognition of large regional variations in preparedness, is asking important questions, such as, How prepared are we? and How do we know if we are prepared? Unfortunately, those questions are difficult to answer, in large part because of a lack of measures to define and assess preparedness and of a strong evidence base to support them.

Measuring Performance

In many ways the current state of quality of U.S. public health systems is reminiscent of the state of quality in the personal health care delivery system a quarter-century ago. In fact, we have argued that there is a "quality chasm" in public health that is analogous to that in the personal delivery system (Lurie 2006). Evidence for this quality chasm includes the marked variability in mission, scope, and performance of public health agencies; the duplication of efforts in many areas of preparedness, such as training; and the uneven protection of the public in the event of a public health emergency. Although public health has made major strides in the area of performance measurement in general, it has lacked the kinds of risk-adjustment methods that have been developed to compare outcomes across systems. In the area of preparedness, the lack of well-accepted, standardized measures and metrics makes it difficult to satisfy the demands for accountability, or even to gauge the level of preparedness.

Although there is not agreement about these measurement issues on a national level, many state and local health departments we have encountered are making solid progress in measuring key attributes of public health emergency preparedness. But measuring preparedness creates new and difficult challenges for public health personnel because it involves measuring the capacity to deal with situations that happen only rarely, if at all.

Assessing Structural Elements of Preparedness

Responses to this challenge generally involve one of two approaches. The first entails assessing the structural elements of preparedness, such as the presence and quality of plans or infrastructure. Preparedness plans, however, are often generated by a relatively small group of people within a jurisdiction, whereas actual responses are coproduced by larger groups—including the general public. Similarly, these assessments provide little opportunity to test jurisdictions' ability to adapt plans and resources to unexpected and changing circumstances—a shortcoming illustrated vividly in the response to the recent Gulf Coast hurricanes. Finally, the self-report formats used by many assessments of plans and infrastructures are subject to biases in self-perceived skill and ability. One paradox is that jurisdictions with a well-developed understanding of preparedness are often more self-critical than others that are less prepared.

A second method involves exercises and drills of processes, or of surrogate outcomes based on realistic scenarios. These provide at least approximate measures of outcomes and, we believe, are a better way to assess preparedness (as well as to prepare). Their use has spread considerably in recent years. Nevertheless, we have a number of concerns about these assessments as currently used. Most jurisdictions routinely produce after-action reports on their exercises, but their evaluations of performance are often implicit, lacking reference to clear standards and transparent measures. This can impede attempts to establish shared terms of reference that can guide improvement efforts. Furthermore, these reports often sit on the shelf, and results are not widely communicated. Although we have heard about many exercises that reveal preparedness gaps that had already been revealed during previous exercises, we have found few jurisdictions that could cite specific instances in which such identification was followed by corrective actions. Even among jurisdictions widely regarded as exemplary, use of systematic quality improvement strategies in public health preparedness appears to be rare.

Effective Quality Improvement Activities

We have, however, identified examples of quality improvement activities in other areas of public health, although they mainly concern clinical services provided by health departments (Seid et al. 2006). We have also identified several states that are taking actions to facilitate improved preparedness at the local level. For instance, some states have set standards that, among other things, seek to make the CDC guidance more accessible and relevant to local health departments. Others are seeking to facilitate measurement of preparedness by creating common indicator systems and investing in online reporting systems; in at least one case, this system is built on the same platform as the state's Health Alert Network. Other states require regular preparedness exercises as a condition of releasing federal funds. At least one state encourages follow-through on corrective actions by tracking gaps identified in after-action reports and building requirements for corrective actions into each jurisdiction's contract with the state.

Developing Systems of Accountability

An important precondition for the development of an effective accountability system is greater agreement among stakeholders at the federal, state, and local levels regarding who should do what. Unfortunately, the initial funds from the CDC were distributed so rapidly that there was little time to determine which level of government should be responsible for what. In the ensuing three or so years, there has been little clarification about the allocation of responsibilities between federal, state, and local public health agencies. This confusion was a recurrent theme in our tabletop exercises; responsibilities and handoffs among local, state, and federal levels were nearly always unclear. Resolving this ambiguity is an important prerequisite for holding various governmental entities accountable for their performance and spending.

Developing a robust system of accountability is no simple feat. To be meaningful, public health emergency preparedness concepts and doctrine must be operationalized in clear and consistent measures that allow stakeholders to monitor progress and identify and address strengths and weaknesses. A key measurement dilemma in public health emergency preparedness is that exercises and drills are often the best way to measure the capacity to implement and adapt response plans, but they can also be quite expensive. We believe that it is possible to develop a set of relatively small-scale drills and exercises focused around the most important preparedness components and to build an accompanying small number of standardized metrics. At the same time, it should be possible to take advantage of more routine activities, such as those surrounding annual flu vaccination or back-to-school immunization campaigns, to test other aspects of preparedness. In a similar vein, systems that rely on emergency room or physician notification and reporting could be tested by monitoring and following up reports of children with uncontrolled asthma instead of confining reporting to notifiable infectious diseases. Creative development of such drills has the potential to strengthen other aspects of public health (such as tobacco control and HIV/AIDS) as well as to increase preparedness.

Measurement by itself, however, will not improve public health emergency preparedness; it must be supplemented by efforts that identify and interpret gaps, to develop and implement corrective actions. The imperative to improve preparedness, if tied to appropriate incentives, can help transfer quality improvement knowledge and skills to other domains of public health.

Evolution or Revolution?

Although emergency preparedness has not been easily incorporated into public health, it is clearly stimulating the evolution of public health practice. Yet important barriers remain, including inadequate accountability systems, little consensus regarding who should be responsible for what, the lack of evidence-based performance measures, and the need to integrate public health preparedness with traditional public health activities and functions. We note, however, that the emphasis on preparedness, while helpful, will not solve all of the nation's public health problems.

Sustained funding for public health preparedness will be important. In addition to the fact that public health has been underfunded for a long time, as the workforce ages into retirement, it will be crucial to assure that an attractive career path exists for the best and brightest in public health (Gebbie and Turnock 2006).This cannot be accomplished without assurance that funding for the public health infrastructure is a long-term investment and not a year-to-year decision for Congress to make.

Second, a uniform definition of public health and of expectations for public health agencies are needed. As noted earlier, there exists today no clear national understanding of what public health is and does. Preparedness has helped create an understanding among Americans that all should be protected from the consequences of a public health emergency, whether due to bioterrorism or a new emerging infection such as pandemic influenza. The National Association of County and City Health Officials (2005) has taken steps to develop an operational definition of a local public health agency. If widely adopted, this definition should help reduce uncertainty about what the public can expect from such an agency and should encourage the analogous clarification of expectations from state health departments. The CDC could also clarify the aspects of preparedness for which it is accountable and, as is the case for expectations for state health departments, develop a set of performance measures for itself. Taken together, actions at these three levels can go a long way toward creating a more uniform standard of health protection for the country.

By importing new frameworks, practices, partnerships, and concepts into public health, the emergency preparedness mission can help public health leaders transform the U.S. public health system so that it can respond effectively and economically to the broadening spectrum of challenges it faces. However, the pace of evolution, at least in nature, is slow. Revolutionary thinking—and action—is necessary to move to a public health system prepared to meet and respond to the challenges of our twenty-first-century world.

Notes

1. The studies include Lurie, Wasserman et al. 2004; Dausey, Lurie, and Diamond 2005; Dausey, Lurie, Diamond et al. 2005; Davis et al. 2006; Wasserman et al. 2006; Seid et al. 2006. Because we promised confidentiality to participants in all the sites, we are unable to provide examples that name specific states or jurisdictions.

References

Dausey, David J., Nicole Lurie, and Alexis Diamond. 2005. Public Health Response to Urgent Case Reports. *Health Affairs* 24 (August 30): w412–w419. http://content. healthaffairs.org/cgi/content/abstract/hlthaff.w5.412.

Dausey, David J., Nicole Lurie, Alexis Diamond, Barbara Meade, Roger Molander, Karen Ricci, Michael Stoto, and Jeffrey Wasserman. 2005. *Bioterrorism Preparedness Training and Assessment Exercises for Local Public Health Agencies.* www.rand.org/pubs/ technical_reports/2005/RAND_TR261.pdf (accessed May 3, 2006).

Davis, Lois M., Jeanne S. Ringel, Sarah K. Cotton, Belle Griffin, Elizabeth Malcolm, Louis T. Mariano, Jennifer E. Pace, et al. 2006. *Public Health Preparedness: Integrating Public Health and Hospital Preparedness Programs.* www.rand.org/pubs/ technical_ reports/2006/RAND_TR317.pdf.

Gebbie, Kristine M., and Bernard J. Turnock. 2006. The Public Health Workforce, 2006: New Challenges. *Health Affairs* 25:923–933.

Institute of Medicine. 1988. *The Future of Public Health.* Washington, D.C.: National Academies Press.

———. 2003. *The Future of the Public's Health in the Twenty-first Century.* Washington, D.C.: National Academies Press.

Lasker, Roz D. 1997. *Medicine and Public Health: The Power of Collaboration.* New York: New York Academy of Medicine. (Reissued by Health Administration Press, 1999.)

Lurie, Nicole. 2002. The Public Health Infrastructure: Rebuild or Redesign? *Health Affairs* 21:28–30.

———. 2006. Is There a Quality Chasm in Public Health? Gordon H. DeFriese Lecture. University of North Carolina at Chapel Hill.

Lurie, Nicole, R. Burciaga Valdez, Jeffrey Wasserman, Michael A. Stoto, Sarah Myers, Roger C. Molander, B. David Mussington, Vanessa Solomon, and Steven M. Asch. 2004. *Public Health Preparedness in California: Lessons Learned from Seven Health Jurisdictions.* August. www.rand.org/pubs/technical_reports/2004/RAND_TR181.pdf (accessed May 3, 2006).

Lurie, Nicole, Jeffrey Wasserman, Michael Stoto, Sarah Myers, Poki Namkung, Jonathan Fielding, and Robert Burciaga Valdez. 2004. Local Variation in Public Health Preparedness: Lessons from California. *Health Affairs* 23 (June 2): w341–w353. http://content.healthaffairs.org/cgi/content/full/hlthaff.w4.341/DC1.

National Association of City and County Health Officials. 2005. *Operational Definition of a Functional Local Health Department.* www.naccho.org/topics/infrastructure/documents/OperationalDefinitionBrochure.pdf (accessed 1 June 2006).

Seid, Michael, Debra Lotstein, Valerie L. Williams, Christopher Nelson, Nicole Lurie, Karen Ricci, Allison Diamant, Jeffrey Wasserman, and Stefanie Stern. 2006. *Quality Improvement: Implications for Public Health Preparedness.* www.rand.org/pubs/technical_reports/2006/RAND_TR316.pdf (accessed May 16 2006).

Steinbrook, Robert. 2006. Facing the Diabetes Epidemic: Mandatory Reporting of Glycosylated Hemoglobin Values in New York City. *New England Journal of Medicine* 354:545–548.

Stoto, Michael A., David J. Dausey, Lois M. Davis, Kristin Leuschner, Nicole Lurie, Sarah Myers, Stuart Olmsted, et al. 2005. *Learning from Experience: The Public Health Response to West Nile Virus, SARS, Monkeypox, and Hepatitis A Outbreaks in the United States.* www.rand/org/pubs/technical_reports/2005/RAND_TR285.pdf (accessed May 3, 2006).

Wasserman, Jeffrey, Peter Jacobson, Nicole Lurie, Christopher Nelson, Karen A. Ricci, Molly Shea, James Zazzali, and Martha I. Nelson. 2006. *Organizing State and Local Health Departments for Public Health Preparedness.* www.rand.org/pubs/technical_reports/2006/RAND_TR318.pdf.

Blown Away

Health Care, Health Coverage, and Public Health after 9/11 and Katrina

Rarely does health care become more public than in the aftermath of disasters. Following a natural or human-made calamity, the medical needs of the affected population take immediate priority. Emergency workers, volunteers, government officials, and the military must gather the dead and aid the injured. The emphasis is on immediate needs, on giving as many people as possible as much help as possible as soon as possible. When we think of health care following a disaster, we think of first responders, of Red Cross tents, of hurry and desperate urgency.

All this was true of 9/11 and Hurricane Katrina, but these postmillennium disasters were also different from any that came before. The two events forced Americans to confront quieter, long-lived health care problems that quickly became emergencies in the face of disaster. These problems were the rise of chronic illness and the increasing number of people without health insurance in the United States.

Just a few weeks after the fall of the Twin Towers, New York politicians implemented dramatic changes in the state's Medicaid system to allow more people to get health coverage quickly. New York's leaders argued, and Washington agreed, that recovery from disaster required that survivors, and even residents not directly affected by the disaster, have access to health care.

For the more far-flung survivors of Hurricane Katrina in 2005, the need was even more urgent. The entire nation witnessed how the hurricane laid bare an epidemic of chronic disease and lack of insurance in New Orleans's low-income neighborhoods. We saw how the elderly and the sick were those most likely to lose their lives in the winds, the floods, and the long, hard wait for help. Then came the accounts of evacuees suffering from heart disease, cancer, or diabetes who could no longer get their medications or see a doctor. The nation's emergency response system had been slow to react to the immediate medical needs of survivors, but it was completely unprepared for the ongoing needs of the chronically ill and uninsured. But the political response was very different from that following 9/11. Congress refused to pass a bill to create a temporary extension of health coverage for Katrina survivors modeled on New York's.

This chapter examines the role of health coverage in the aftermath of 9/11 and Hurricane Katrina. It argues that these two disasters must force us to recognize, for the first time, that access to health coverage should be an important component of disaster preparedness and response, and that the lack of universal health care in the United States exacerbates the suffering of populations affected by disaster and makes recovery more difficult.

The Health Care Crises of 9/11

After the plane crashes in New York, Washington, and Pennsylvania, thousands of Americans lined up to give blood. However, it quickly became evident that the September 11, 2001, terrorist attacks would leave few survivors, and much of the collected blood had to be thrown away. Triage centers set up near the World Trade Center site sat nearly empty as rescue workers turned to the grim business of recovering bodies rather than the injured (Barry 2001). There was little that medical personnel, or anyone, could do to aid survival in the immediate aftermath of the calamities.

But in the days and weeks following the attacks, health problems began to emerge that would require more than the traditional disaster response. One immediate concern of survivors and neighbors of the disaster was the long-term effects of dust inhalation at and near the site. This concern bore an immediate relation to one of the most prevalent chronic health conditions in New York City: asthma, which is especially common among urban, low-income children. A New York occupational health physician warned that the dust "could impact everyone, but especially the very young, the very old and those with existing pulmonary disease." Large concentrations of both the young and the elderly lived in the neighborhoods surrounding the World Trade Center (Schneider 2002).

A director of the Children's Aid Society, which runs several clinics for the poor in New York, told a reporter that "parents of asthmatic children were calling the agency as early as the Wednesday morning after the attacks," including from neighborhoods distant from Ground Zero (Mallozzi 2001). The federal government offered financial assistance for cleanup, but some public health advocates argued that the cleaning of apartments needed to be supervised by environmental experts, not individual residents (Wasserman 2002). One disaster relief organization offered to clean the dust from the apartments of families with asthmatic children at no charge (Cadwalader, Wickersham, and Taft 2001).

Another long-term health concern emerging from the disaster was the loss of health insurance by people who had worked in the Twin Towers and their families. In the United States, people under age sixty-five are almost completely reliant on their employers for health benefits; in no other country is health coverage so closely connected to jobs. And the September 11 attacks were "tied to the workplace in a way few previous disasters have been" (Mercer 2001). The vast majority of the dead and injured were at the World Trade Center because they had to be there for work. The attacks also wiped out numerous other workplaces in Lower Manhattan. A crisis of lost jobs quickly became a crisis of lost health coverage, for the families of the dead as well as for survivors and their families.

Although the Federal Emergency Management Agency makes provisions for emergency medical care after disasters, continuation of health coverage is not part of the agency's disaster planning. For workers who lose a job with health benefits, the U.S. government offers only one guaranteed right, known as COBRA coverage. Under COBRA, a laid-off employee may continue paying into the employer's group health plan but must pay the full cost of the coverage, not just the employee's share. This requirement makes COBRA coverage unaffordable for many people. In addition, COBRA covers only workplaces with twenty or more employees.

In the stunning voluntary response to 9/11, many of the organizations and businesses offering aid recognized victims' need for continuation of health coverage as a priority. For example, the investment banking firm Cantor Fitzgerald, which lost nearly 70 percent of its New York workforce in the disaster, "pledged to continue health coverage for victims' spouses and children for at least 12 months at the company's cost." Labor unions, particularly service worker and public employee unions, also offered extended health benefits to survivors of the disaster and to the families of victims (Armour 2001).

Blue-collar and nonunionized employees had an even more difficult struggle. Many had no health coverage even before 9/11. Many were immigrants afraid to seek benefits. Smaller companies could not afford to come up with the types of benefits and services to victims that some of the WTC's wealthy employers offered. For example, the families of two security guards killed in the disaster complained that the private security companies had never even contacted them with condolences for the loss of their loved ones, much less

offered them help with finances or health care (Armour 2001). In addition to
the efforts of the service unions, some private organizations were created to
assist low-income survivors and victims' families, most notably Windows of
Hope, which raises money to aid the families of restaurant workers in the
World Trade Center. Windows of Hope has given financial help to more than
one hundred families and "committed to fund five years of health insurance
coverage for all of the families" (Windows of Hope Web site).

Loss of health insurance also became a problem for the thousands of workers who lost their jobs in New York's temporary economic downturn following
9/11. Economists estimated that the city "lost 79,700 jobs, predominantly in
low-wage industries, in the 4th quarter of 2001—as a direct consequence of the
September 11th events" (Tallon 2001). Hospitality employees, who are heavily
immigrant and minority, were especially affected. "Hotels lost their business,
taxis lost their business, resorts lost their business, restaurants lost their business," commented one union organizer in November of 2001. "So, the people
who were working in those . . . subsets of the economy were the first to lose
their jobs [and] . . . a large number of these people not only lost their jobs, but
have lost health insurance. Because these were people whose entire health
insurance [was] tied to their jobs" (Chishti 2001).

No record exists of exactly how many people lost their health insurance
following 9/11, but city and state officials clearly felt that a health care and fiscal crisis loomed. New York City was already home to high numbers of people
without health coverage; the added pressure of the newly uninsured threatened
to overwhelm the city's indigent care system and its medical budgets.
Government needed to expand health coverage, and quickly, argued the director of New York's Health and Hospitals Corporation, to ensure the "financial
stability of the city's health care system." The best and quickest way to do this
was through Medicaid. Not only would a Medicaid expansion cover many of
the uninsured, but any additional local Medicaid commitments would also
bring increased state and federal funding into New York (Tallon 2001).

There were other reasons why a rapid Medicaid expansion made sense for
New York. Ironically, the collapse of the Twin Towers created an immediate
opportunity for a major restructuring of the program: The computers housing
New York's Medicaid records were located in 7 World Trade Center and now
lay pulverized beneath the rubble. And New York State, long known for having
the most generous Medicaid eligibility and benefits in the country, had already
begun new expansions of its Medicaid program before September 11. The state
assembly in 2000 had passed Family Health Plus, which would expand
Medicaid eligibility to 600,000 working poor adults, but the program had been

delayed by objections from Washington that it would cost too much. New York governor George E. Pataki had also recently won federal approval for an expansion of the state's Child Health Plus program for children (Hernandez 2001; *New York Times* 2001; Cohen 2001).

Although New York had much experience with Medicaid expansion, the program it created following 9/11 was absolutely unprecedented. Disaster Relief Medicaid dropped the notoriously grueling application process in favor of a simple, one-page form, and "those eligible [got] a Medicaid card the same day" (Ruiz 2002). Normally, a program making it easier to get a government benefit would have faced an "avalanche of opposition" but, as *New York Times* reporter Katherine E. Finkelstein noted: "The uninsured and their advocates have found far more universal support after September 11, as New Yorkers have faced all kinds of medical needs, including mental health services and continuing medical treatment that had been interrupted by the attacks." The national sympathy for New York's plight, particularly the sympathy emanating from Washington, enabled Pataki and New York mayor Rudolph W. Giuliani to push through Disaster Relief Medicaid, a program that would have otherwise been unthinkable in the U.S. culture of hostility to welfare (Finkelstein 2001).

Disaster Relief Medicaid eventually enrolled 400,000 people in the state, 250,000 of them in New York City. Its expanded eligibility was based on the delayed Family Health Plus guidelines, which raised income maximums for parents from 87 percent of the federal poverty level to 133 percent (and from 50 percent to 100 percent for single and childless adults) and eliminated the asset test. A study of Disaster Relief Medicaid found that many New Yorkers who enrolled in the program had lost their jobs due to 9/11, and most had no previous health coverage. Some had applied for Medicaid previously and been turned down due to income limits. Although all the participants interviewed for the study had enrolled because they desired access to health care that had previously eluded them, many also saw the program as a public health measure. Disaster Relief Medicaid was created "because the pollution was so bad and people were sick" after the collapse of the World Trade Center, said one participant. "I have the understanding," said another, "that since there were so many deaths from the disasters and the environment is full of viruses and all those things, the government of the United States wants to prevent serious illnesses, possibly cancer and deaths, chronic diseases" (Perry 2002, iii–iv, 5, 9).[1]

Despite the specific linkage of Disaster Relief Medicaid with 9/11 and its aftermath, the program may have been most effective in relieving, if only partly, the longer-term crisis of chronic disease and uninsurance in the city. The program uncovered a "pent-up demand for health services" among New Yorkers.

Participants eagerly sought mammograms, dental care, and preventive check-ups; many were able to fill prescriptions regularly for the first time (Perry 2002, 16–17). Primary care physicians in New York reported that "patients with disaster-relief Medicaid have come in with complaints about everything from chronic abdominal pain to high blood pressure." A forty-two-year-old Bronx home health aide had always relied on emergency rooms to treat her asthma and had never been able to afford medication. Since joining Disaster Relief Medicaid, "she can get her own prescriptions, bought reading glasses and went to a dentist. 'I needed things but with no coverage, there was nothing I could do,'" she told a reporter (Purnick 2002). A Hispanic woman, also asthmatic, told the *Washington Post* that "she had gone without treatment for long periods, buying medicine when she could afford it, at times borrowing inhalers from friends," but under the new program, "'Oh yes, I can go to the doctor!'" (Russakoff 2001).

Disaster Relief Medicaid lasted only four months. Participants could then apply for Family Health Plus, whose income limits were identical to the temporary program's, although the application process was more elaborate. However, apparently some participants were not aware that they might still be eligible for Medicaid after their temporary benefits expired. As a result, some of those insured under Disaster Relief Medicaid may have lost coverage (Perry 2002, 20–22). Beyond Ground Zero, an organization for workers affected by September 11, argues that Family Health Plus has "severely limited coverage" and offers a poor substitute for the short-lived Disaster Relief Medicaid (Beyond Ground Zero 2007).

Still, Disaster Relief Medicaid was more effective than COBRA in ensuring that 9/11 survivors and victims' families received or maintained access to health coverage. By early 2005, a Massachusetts relief organization reported that many 9/11 families were "coming to the end of their current low-cost group insurance [under COBRA] and are now facing individual premium payments of up to $1200 per month. They are telling us that in addition to high premium payments, they are now forced to pay high out-of-pocket expenses for their mental health visits, as mental health benefits are often limited under the individual plans." In February 2005 Senator Ted Kennedy and Congressman Edward Markey of Massachusetts cosponsored a bill to enable the families to continue COBRA coverage indefinitely, but it received little notice in the media and died quietly in Congress. Markey's invocation of the nation's sympathy for 9/11's victims—"This bill allows us to express our thanks for the heroism that these families demonstrated in the face of tragedy"—could not overcome congressional and public indifference to, or ignorance about, people's long-term and continuing health coverage needs after disasters (Markey 2005).

The Health Care Crises of Katrina

The aftermath of 9/11 brought into the public eye some of the nation's endemic health problems that normally remain hidden. In 2005, Hurricane Katrina shockingly exposed these problems, for all the world to see, during the first hours and days of the disaster. One unforgettable image beamed from New Orleans showed "a woman in a wheelchair, her face and body covered by a plaid blanket, dead, and left next to a wall of the New Orleans convention center like a discarded supermarket cart" (Stanley 2005). The hurricane took its toll most swiftly on the elderly, the chronically ill, the housebound, the wheelchair bound, people confined to hospital and nursing home beds—those who found it difficult or impossible to escape. High rates of poverty in New Orleans and the Gulf Coast region meant that much of the population hit hardest by the hurricane suffered from chronic illness, but few had health insurance.

Before the hurricane, Louisiana had among the highest rates of uninsurance in the nation, with 26.4 percent of working adults lacking health coverage (only Texas was higher, with 30.7 percent) (State Health Access Data Assistance Center 2005). Health disparities in the state were especially severe; the Louisiana Department of Health reported that 11.9 percent of African Americans in the state had diabetes, compared with 7.2 percent of whites, and that 15.8 percent of those who lived in households with incomes of less than $15,000 per year had the disease. Even higher rates of diabetes showed up among hurricane evacuees. An endocrinologist visiting a shelter in Lafayette, Louisiana, found that "500 of the 2,000 to 3,000 people housed there" had the disease (Payne 2005). The *Washington Post* surveyed evacuees in Houston shortly after the hurricane and reported that half had no health insurance, and 40 percent had heart disease, diabetes, or high blood pressure or were disabled. "When illness or injury strike, they were twice as likely to say they had sought care from hospitals such as the New Orleans Charity Hospital than from either a family doctor or health clinic" (Morin and Rein 2005).

After Hurricane Katrina, it was chronic illness and poverty among evacuees, as much as the expected injuries that usually follow disasters, which challenged the medical resources of disaster agencies and volunteers. A physician at Houston's Katrina Clinic for evacuees explained to the *Houston Chronicle*: "We usually plan for a disaster involving explosions, trauma, wounds. We recognized this was not that kind of disaster. . . . We didn't need a (mobile) surgical hospital, we needed a big pharmacy. We needed a laboratory. We did not need an operating table, we needed an exam table." The *Chronicle* reported: "As the crisis phase passed, people too poor for easy access to medical care for less pressing problems in New Orleans sought it out in the Katrina

Clinic. People who barely escaped New Orleans with their lives could now get attention for ingrown toenails." Physicians fitted people with eyeglasses, gave immunizations, and filled countless prescriptions (Hopper 2005). *New York Times* columnist Nicholas Kristof (2005) spoke with a volunteer doctor who "discovered a previously undetected hole in a 4-year-old boy's heart. The mother said nobody had ever listened to the boy's chest before." As Disaster Relief Medicaid in New York had led to a surge in previously neglected primary care, so did hurricane evacuation clinics expose the vast medical needs of an uninsured population.

But temporary help could do little to stem the outpouring of demand for medical care in the wake of Katrina. To the ranks of the uninsured were added hundreds of thousands of survivors who lost their health insurance when their workplaces and jobs were wiped out by the hurricane. Katrina's victims were, according to the *Chicago Tribune*, "one of the largest groups to lose medical coverage because of a single event in the nation's history"—it is difficult to think of a larger one (Graham 2005b). BlueCross BlueShield of Louisiana estimated that "200,000 men, women and children in the state who had health insurance through the workplace will lose those benefits as financially stressed organizations terminate staff or go out of business altogether." The state quickly instituted a requirement that insurance companies keep customers' policies active until November, even if they did not receive premium payments. BlueCross voluntarily added another month to the extension, but by the end of 2005, companies were beginning to cancel policies (BlueCross BlueShield of Louisiana 2005).

In the weeks following the hurricane, its survivors scattered throughout Louisiana, Texas, and most states in the union. Most were newly unemployed, many newly uninsured, and those enrolled in Medicaid faced the possibility of losing their benefits by leaving their home states. Thousands dropped below the poverty line by Katrina turned to Medicaid for the first time. But in Louisiana, a majority found that they were not eligible for the program because of the state's strict income cutoffs: Applicants' incomes had to be below 20 percent of the official poverty level (20 percent of $16,000 for a family of three)— in some cases, as low as 13 percent. (This extraordinarily stringent standard helps explain the state's reliance on its charity hospital system to care for the poor.) As in most states, only certain categories of people were considered eligible for Medicaid, particularly single mothers with children; to qualify for Medicaid in Louisiana, the childless had to have an income of less than $174 a month (Seattle Times News Services 2006). (Before Katrina, Louisiana had achieved some success in reducing the number of uninsured children in the state through the Louisiana Children's Health Insurance program [Kaiser Commission on Medicaid and the Uninsured 2005a].)

As a result of Louisiana's requirements, more than half of the six thousand state residents who applied for Medicaid in the weeks after the storm were turned down. Many of these people formerly had private health insurance, and some had been undergoing lifesaving treatments. Several newspapers reported the story of Emanuel Wilson, a fifty-two-year old school bus driver from New Orleans, who survived the hurricane but had to stop chemotherapy injections for intestinal cancer when he was turned down for Louisiana Medicaid (Alonso-Zaldivar 2005). Another New Orleans resident, Albert Bass, forty-seven, formerly of the Lower Ninth Ward, was hospitalized for fever and liver problems right after the hurricane. His Medicaid application was denied, and, as the *Chicago Tribune*'s Judith Graham reported in October 2005: "Now, tens of thousands of dollars in medical bills await a man with no income. . . . His asthma has worsened, but he has no money to pay for medications."

On September 15, 2005, Senators Charles Grassley (R-Iowa) and Max Baucus (D-Montana) introduced a bill, S. 1716, to create a temporary Medicaid program for Katrina survivors. The Emergency Health Care Relief Act of 2005 would offer survivors in any state five months of Medicaid coverage, with simplified application procedures and greatly expanded eligibility—200 percent of poverty for children, pregnant women, and the disabled; 100 percent of poverty for all other adults. And, unlike the state-federal cost sharing of traditional Medicaid, the federal government would pay the full cost of the program (Kaiser Commission on Medicaid and the Uninsured 2005a).

The Grassley-Baucus bill received the enthusiastic support of health care providers and advocates for the poor. It was endorsed by the governors of the states most affected by the hurricane: Kathleen Blanco (D) of Louisiana, Haley Barbour (R) of Mississippi, and Bob Riley (R) of Alabama (Freking 2005). The plan was also expected to pass fairly easily because of its bipartisan sponsorship; Grassley was a major ally of the Bush administration. Congress could also look to the earlier success with New York's Disaster Relief Medicaid as a model. As the Senate met on Monday, September 26, Grassley and Baucus "expected the bill to pass by a voice vote," according to the *Los Angeles Times*, but it was blocked by Republicans John E. Sununu of New Hampshire and John Ensign of Nevada. Sununu claimed he opposed the Medicaid extension because it would increase the already burgeoning national deficit (Curtius 2005).

The next day, Secretary of Health and Human Services Michael Leavitt sent a letter to Senate leaders declaring the Bush administration's opposition to the Grassley-Baucus bill. He called the bill "inadvisable" and "a duplication of administration efforts." Leavitt argued that state-by-state waivers would allow hurricane survivors to receive Medicaid benefits without a massive new federal intervention. The Senate bill, on the other hand, "requires a new Medicaid entitlement for Katrina survivors, regardless of whether that will work best for those survivors or the states," Leavitt wrote (Curtius 2005).

The bill's supporters reacted with fury. Senator Blanche Lincoln (D-Ark.), whose state was dealing with thousands of evacuees from the Gulf States, attacked "the web of red tape that this administration is spinning over our ability to provide the basic needs of health care to people who have been devastated." "Could you please explain to us," Grassley and Baucus replied to Health and Human Services secretary Leavitt, "why the Katrina evacuees do not deserve the same assistance provided the people of New York" after 9/11? Grassley, who chaired the Senate Finance Committee, even threatened to block the administration's proposed cuts to the overall Medicaid program if the White House failed to withdraw its opposition to the Katrina health bill (Freking 2005).

But the administration refused to budge, and the bill failed to garner any further momentum. Grassley gave up the fight and even led Senate efforts to enact major cuts to Medicaid in the 2007 federal budget. Katrina survivors were left without a health coverage plan that would even come close to the benefits offered New Yorkers after 9/11.

The Medicaid waivers granted to states to aid Katrina survivors were a far cry from the benefit expansions of Disaster Relief Medicaid. The waivers, which were limited to five months, did little beyond allowing states to provide some coverage to recent arrivals who are not state residents. They continued to exclude all childless adults from Medicaid, except the elderly or disabled. Unlike Disaster Relief Medicaid, the waivers did not allow for replacement of the arduous application process. And although the federal government initially picked up the cost, the Medicaid waivers required evacuees' home states to then reimburse Washington—thus adding to, not relieving, the health care costs of the states most damaged by the hurricane (Kaiser Commission on Medicaid and the Uninsured 2005a; Baxter 2005).

September 11 and Katrina were major disasters that led to devastating losses of life and property. Although the first was a terrorist attack and the second a natural disaster, both events brought some of the nation's recurrent health problems squarely into the public eye. Despite the similarities, government's responses to the health care needs arising out of 9/11 and Katrina were strikingly different. After the terrorist attacks, Washington acted swiftly to ease access to health coverage for survivors and others who had lost jobs and health insurance.

Following Hurricane Katrina, however, federal policymakers rejected similar benefits for evacuees. Why were Katrina survivors in 2005 denied the support offered New Yorkers in 2001? For such recent events it is difficult to find a clear answer, but I would like to suggest some possibilities.

As a major terrorist attack on U.S. soil, 9/11 was an absolutely unprecedented event in American history. The immediate and massive outpouring of support, from blood donations to cash, came from Americans roused not just by concern for the victims, but by a revitalized patriotism. And, again for the first time in history, they gave too much. The Red Cross had not only to destroy huge supplies of blood, but also to divert millions of unneeded donations to other projects. Congress also sponsored a generous fund for victims and their families. The dead were portrayed repeatedly not just as disaster victims but also as heroes who died, however involuntarily, for their country. In the highly charged atmosphere of a national security emergency, all 9/11 victims, and even by extension all New Yorkers, came to seem absolutely deserving. In the service of these deserving heroes, Congress put aside partisan bickering to speed unprecedented amounts of aid.

Hurricane Katrina was also unprecedented in the scale of its destruction, and the American people also poured out their generosity to its victims. But this time the massive voluntary effort would not be matched by federal largesse. In contrast to the widely admired rescue, recovery, and cleanup effort following 9/11, the government response to Katrina was catastrophically slow and inept. While 9/11 victims became heroes, the primarily African American hurricane survivors in New Orleans appeared in the U.S. media as a helpless underclass, and some were even portrayed (in endlessly repeated video clips of looting) as dangerous, which may have slowed the government's move into the city.

The bipartisan congressional supporters of expanded health care following the hurricane tried to insist that evacuees were as deserving as the survivors and families of 9/11. But the White House and congressional leaders were unwilling to accept the comparison. Cost was certainly a major barrier; federally funded Medicaid for tens of thousands of evacuees would be considerably more expensive than the program in New York. But other structural and ideological issues were equally, if not more, important. Offering health coverage to hurricane evacuees would require, if only briefly, nationalizing Medicaid, a program whose eligibility and benefits traditionally differed state by state. Making it easier to apply for and receive benefits also would require Congress to supersede Medicaid's usual strictness and confront the program's limitations on a national scale.

But the greatest barrier was political. Hurricane Katrina came at a time when the White House and Congressional Republicans were already planning drastic cuts to Medicaid. New York, on the other hand, had been in the process of *expanding* its Medicaid program on 9/11. While 9/11 had inspired lawmakers to put aside partisan differences on behalf of disaster victims, Hurricane Katrina could not stem the determination of the Republican Congress to scale back the nation's public health care programs.

While temporary health coverage expansion succeeded after 9/11 and failed after Katrina, a larger question is whether these efforts might lead to permanent change in the health care system. Disasters have often been catalysts for reforms in U.S. history; industrial calamities such as the Cherry Mine fire early in the twentieth century led to the creation of workers' compensation laws, for example, and the Triangle Factory Fire in 1911 spurred a regime of workplace safety regulation. September 11 and Katrina did lead to some calls for structural reform in American health care. A Long Island activist group, for example, in a leaflet entitled "9/11 Proves It Again: More Than Ever, We Need a National Health Plan!" declared that effective emergency planning would be impossible without a public, universal health care system (Long Island Coalition for a National Health Plan 2001). *New York Times* columnist Nicholas Kristof (2005) called the Katrina disaster "a window into our broken health care system; . . . let's rebuild the levees, but let's also construct a health care system that works."[2]

The very success of Disaster Relief Medicaid in New York was an implicit, and sometimes explicit, critique of the limitations of the existing health care system. Why was it such a revelation for people in need to be able to get health coverage quickly and efficiently? The goals of the Grassley/Baucus bill— portability beyond state lines, continuity of care, full federal funding, a simplified application process, more generous eligibility—underscored the shortcomings of regular Medicaid, which offered none of those provisions. That states had to apply for waivers from the federal government simply to be allowed to address the most basic health care needs of evacuees points to the obstacles created by Medicaid's federalist structure.

Many policy makers, however, insisted that a temporary program need not, and indeed should not, spur more permanent reforms. A spokeswoman for the New York State Health Department said the state did *not* see in the successes of Disaster Relief Medicaid "lessons . . . for Medicaid generally. 'This was an extraordinary response to extraordinary circumstances,' she said, emphasizing that the computer disruption left the state with no other way to process regular applications as needs soared" after 9/11 (Russakoff 2001).

Senator Max Baucus, sponsor of health care relief for Katrina victims, noted that "one concern has been that the bill could lead to an expansion of Medicaid and that those survivors added to Medicaid would stay on the rolls. Let me reassure my colleagues that there would be no ongoing right to Medicaid under this bill. The bill creates a temporary, time-limited, emergency benefit of up to 5 months of coverage. That's it. Once the period of coverage ends, there would be no mandated right to coverage" (*U.S. Federal News* 2005). Here Baucus tried to assure the White House and other critics of his bill that disaster relief measures are not connected with long-term reform. In the atmosphere of budget cutting aimed at entitlement programs, particularly Medicaid, the permanent health care crises laid bare by 9/11 and Katrina once again faded from view, at least in Washington.

While our recent national calamities have not forced a rethinking of the health care system, perhaps they could still call attention to the neglected role of health care and health coverage in disaster preparation. Planning for future emergencies must take into account the growing ranks of the uninsured, the potential loss of health coverage for the insured, and the prevalence of chronic disease. If Katrina is any indication, the disruption of care for chronic illness can be as or more catastrophic than immediate injuries in disasters, especially in vulnerable populations such as the poor or aged. The most obvious measure would be carefully rehearsed planning for the evacuation of hospitals and nursing homes, as well as of the aged and disabled not in institutional care (lack of accommodation for the disabled in the World Trade Center added to the difficulties of escape). Following that, provision for continuity of health coverage and health care in the aftermath of a disaster could help, for example, a nationwide computerized pharmacy system to allow people to fill prescriptions even if they have lost or can't remember their medications. In addition to continuity, disaster survivors require portability of their health coverage. Both Medicaid recipients and more affluent people with insurance faced disruptions to their access to care because they could not take their coverage with them when they left their states or lost their jobs. Provisions for federally funded automatic health coverage extensions after disasters would help ease recovery for survivors and ensure payment for health care providers, as well as avoid extended political bickering.[3]

Of course, continuity and portability should be the hallmarks of health care for everyone, not just disaster survivors. Most Americans have neither. Lasting reform in the current political climate may be impossible unless the nation learns one of the lessons of 9/11 and Katrina: A fragmented and unequal health care system makes disasters worse.

Disasters and the Definition of Public Health

In 9/11 and Katrina, disasters of terrorism, environment, and climate also became health care crises. To a great extent, this happened because of the restricted definition of "public health" held by emergency planners and public and private officials. Public health preparation and response to disasters throughout the twentieth century focused, often with great success, on the prevention and control of epidemic outbreaks. Following earlier Gulf Coast hurricanes, governments and relief agencies responded rapidly to aid the injured and avert epidemic disease, and they generally congratulated themselves on their rapid response (Hurricane Betsy #1 1965 File. 1965; U.S. Department of Health, Education, and Welfare 1967; Wilds 1978, 105). Their prioritization of sewage, sanitation, and pest control helped avert thousands of deaths. But twentieth-century public health relief efforts rarely took into account the challenges of chronic illness and never considered issues of health coverage (New Orleans Health Department 1965, 1985).

This limited definition of public health has persisted, forcing disaster planning and relief into a narrow channel that neglects many of the populace's most urgent health needs. The major congressional report on the failure of Katrina relief efforts, for example, has a forty-four-page section on medical care, but it does not mention health coverage or continuity of care and refers to the chronically ill only as an evacuation problem rather than as a health care problem (U.S. Congress Select Bipartisan Committee 2006).

Disaster planners of the past counted their efforts a success if they were able to avert an epidemic of cholera or typhoid. Fears of such epidemics, prevalent in the early days after Katrina, proved unfounded. But planners did not predict what actually did happen: that chronic conditions like diabetes, cancer, and asthma would get worse because people couldn't maintain treatment. In addition, the appalling stress suffered by hurricane survivors seems to have further exacerbated these major health problems.[4] The director of New Orleans' health department reported in 2007 that death rates among the citizens of New Orleans continued to increase more than a full year after the hurricane, which he blames on a worsening of long-term medical conditions (Stephens 2007).

The overly narrow definition of public health and its relationship to disaster planning continues to have long-term effects. In both New York and New Orleans, public health agencies are struggling to deal with the medical aftermath of the disasters. New Orleans has not been able to address the issue of lack of health insurance, which is a *growing* crisis, as many evacuees return without coverage. Residents of the city are so desperate for medical care that when the New Orleans Health Department held a Health Recovery Week at Audubon Zoo in 2006, patients lined up the night before and waited for hours for the opportunity to see a volunteer doctor, fill a prescription, or get dental care. Unfortunately, "capacity for each day was reached within an hour of opening the registration," so thousands had to be turned away. Public health leaders in New Orleans attempted to fill the gap left by the lack of health coverage, the closing of Charity Hospital, and physicians' flight from the Gulf Coast, but their efforts only helped a tiny percentage of those who desperately needed it.[5] Dr. Evangeline Franklin (2007) of the Health Department testified before a congressional subcommittee that the physician volunteers who participated in Health Recovery Week said "that they had never seen so many people who were so very sick."

In New York, Disaster Relief Medicaid has expired, and a new health crisis has surfaced. Officials have finally conceded that thousands of new cases of lung disorders can be traced to the inhalation of dust from the World Trade Center collapse on 9/11. The city has taken the important step of establishing the W.T.C. Environmental Health Center at Bellevue Hospital to treat patients without charge. Nine hundred New Yorkers were being seen there in early 2007, and there was a waiting list of several hundred people, "including many low-income residents of Chinatown and the Lower East Side, and immigrant workers without health insurance." The waiting list is expected to grow substantially since city and federal officials announced the link between dust inhalation and severe breathing problems (DePalma 2007). Like the New Orleans Health Department's Recovery Week effort, a disaster's aftermath in New York has forced public health agencies to cross traditional barriers and take an active role in the provision of health care. But as the extreme waiting times and rejections show, these cities and their public health agencies simply do not have the resources to fully address the devastating medical conditions of disaster survivors.

The long-term health problems created and exacerbated by 9/11 and Katrina tell us that not only the definition of public health but also the meaning of the term "emergency" need to undergo drastic change. "Emergency" implies, of course, an immediate and short-term problem. But immediate and short-term planning and solutions are insufficient to either prepare for or recover from a disaster. The U.S. health care system as well as the disaster preparedness system are eager to respond to emergency situations and are usually (Katrina excepted) very good at it. There may be a parallel here in the federal law that requires emergency rooms to accept everyone—emergency care is the only type of medical care provided as a right (Hoffman 2006). But in this age of chronic medical conditions it is irrational and inefficient to provide emergency care only. The same holds true for disaster planning and recovery. It is no longer possible or desirable to fully separate "emergency" needs from longer-term ones. Both must be taken into account.

The defeat of Medicaid expansion for hurricane evacuees and the current struggles of New York and New Orleans to address the continuing medical crises of their citizens demonstrate that, despite their devastating effects, the disasters of 9/11 and Katrina have failed to break down the barriers between public health, health coverage, and health care. Such a breaking of barriers is absolutely essential if we are to better prepare for future disasters, as well as to provide the population with a decent level of health during less chaotic times.

Acknowledgments

I would like to thank the following: James Colgrove, Jerry Markowitz, and David Rosner for conceiving this project and letting me change my topic; David McBride for his helpful comments; archivists and librarians at the New Orleans City Archives, Rudolph Matas Medical Library, and the Louisiana State Archives; volunteers and patients at the Common Ground Algiers Health Clinic and tent city, New Orleans; Amy Forbes and Caroline Wiese for hospitality in Baton Rouge; and Lynn Rogut and the Investigator Awards Program of the Robert Wood Johnson Foundation for funding support.

Notes

1. The study, unfortunately, does not include specific numbers or percentages of respondents and only uses terms such as "many," "most," and "some."
2. On the role of disasters in the American welfare state, see Michele L. Landis, "Fate, Responsibility, and 'Natural' Disaster Relief: Narrating the American Welfare State," *Law and Society Review* 33, 2 (1999): 257–318.
3. Somewhat more modestly, the RAND Corporation has proposed providing portable health care vouchers to disaster survivors, while the Heritage Foundation suggests health care tax credits for evacuees. See www.rand.org/commentary/ 101005UPI.html and www.heritage.org/Research/HealthCare/bg1900.cfm.
4. Interview with staff member (name withheld), Common Ground Health Clinic, by the author, Algiers, New Orleans, March 16, 2006.
5. Interview of Jason (last name withheld), Common Ground volunteer coordinator, by the author, Upper Ninth Ward tent city, New Orleans, March 15, 2006.

References

Alonso-Zaldivar, Ricardo. 2005. A Long Road to Recovery; Shut Out on Healthcare after Storm. *Los Angeles Times*, October 9.

Armour, Stephanie. 2001. Bad Times Make Choice to Help Victims Tough. *USA Today*, October 7.

Barry, Dan. 2001. Hospitals: Pictures of Medical Readiness, Waiting and Hoping for Survivors to Fill Their Wards. *New York Times*, September 12.

Baxter, Tom. 2005. Evacuees Intensify Medicaid Burdens. *Cox News Service*, October 17.

Beyond Ground Zero. 2007. Health and Economic Effects of the September 11th Disaster on Low-Income New Yorkers. www.nmass.org/nmass/bgz/bgz.html, accessed 6/22/07.

BlueCross BlueShield of Louisiana. 2005. Memorandum to Providers. November 9. www.lsms.org.

Cadwalader, Wickersham, and Taft. 2001. *Handbook of Public and Private Assistance Resources for the Victims and Families of the World Trade Center Attacks.* November 30. New York. www.cadwalader.com/assets/pro_bono_pdf/WTC_Handbook_ Name.pdf.

Chishti, Muzaffar. 2001. UNITE Immigration Project, remarks at "Workers' Rights and Immigrant Communities," Asia Society, New York City, November 1. www.asiasource. net/asip/workers.cfm.

Cohen, Rima. 2001. From Strategy to Reality: The Enactment of New York's Family Health Plus Program. *Journal of Health Politics, Policy, and Law* 26:1375–1393.

Curtius, Mary. 2005. Senators Fume at White House Disdain for Katrina Healthcare Plan. *Los Angeles Times*, September 29.

DePalma, Anthony. 2007. After 9/11, Ailing Residents Find a Place to Turn. *New York Times*, February 21.

Finkelstein, Katherine E. 2001. Disaster Gives the Uninsured Wider Access to Medicaid. *New York Times*, November 23.

Franklin, Evangeline. 2007. Testimony before U.S. House of Representatives Subcommittee on Oversight and Investigations of the Committee on Energy and Commerce. March 13. See www.cityofno.com/portal.aspx?portal=1&load=~/PortalModules/ViewPressRelease.ascx&itemid=3799 (accessed June 22, 2007).

Freking, Kevin. 2005. Senators, Administration Battle over Care for Katrina Victims. *Associated Press State and Local Wire*, September 28.

Graham, Judith. 2005a. Hurricane-Battered Louisiana Mulls Deep Medicaid Cuts. *Chicago Tribune*, October 21.

———. 2005b. Storm Sweeps Away Health Insurance. *Chicago Tribune*, December 29.

Hernandez, Raymond. 2001. U.S. and Albany Agree to Provide Health Benefits to Uninsured Poor. *New York Times*, May 30.

Hoffman, Beatrix. 2006. Emergency Rooms: The Reluctant Safety Net. In *History and Health Policy: Bringing the Past Back In*, ed. Rosemary Stevens, Charles E. Rosenberg, and Lawton R. Burns. New Brunswick: Rutgers University Press.

Hopper, Leigh. 2005. Houston's "Katrina Clinic"; A Safety Net That Held Strong, Breaking the Fall of 15,000. *Houston Chronicle*, September 19.

Hurricane Betsy #1 1965 File. 1965. Mayor Victor Hugo Schiro Collection, 1957–1970. New Orleans City Archives.

Kaiser Commission on Medicaid and the Uninsured. 2005a. Health Coverage for Individuals Affected by Hurricane Katrina: A Comparison of Different Approaches to Extend Medicaid Coverage. October 10. www.kff.org.

———. 2005b. New Materials Related to Health Coverage and Hurricane Katrina. September 9. www.kff.org/medicaid/upload/transcript090905.pdf.

Kristof, Nicholas D. 2005. A Health Care Disaster. *New York Times*, September 25.

Long Island Coalition for a National Health Plan. 2001. Newsletter. November. www.911digitalarchive.org.

Mallozzi, Vincent M. 2001. For Asthmatic Children, an Extra Health Burden. *New York Times*, September 20.

Markey, Edward J. 2005. Statement of Introduction: Continuing Care for Recovering Families Act. February 1. www.house.gov/markey/Issues/iss_health_st050201.pdf.

Mercer, William. 2001. Health and Group Benefits in the Aftermath of September 11. *Mercer Report* 115, October 25. wrg.wmmercer.com/content_print.asp?article_id= 20016295&ext=.PDF.

Morin, Richard, and Lisa Rein. 2005. Some of the Uprooted Won't Go Home Again. *Washington Post*, September 16.

New Orleans Health Department. 1965. Hurricane Betsy Report. September 24. New Orleans Health Department Records, New Orleans City Archives.

———. 1985. 1985 Basic Emergency Operations Plan for the City of New Orleans, Health Department: General Responsibilities, Disaster File, 1983–87. New Orleans Health Department Records, New Orleans City Archives.

New York Times. 2001. Mr. Pataki Broadens Health Insurance. June 4.

Payne, January W. 2005. At Risk before the Storm Struck: Prior Health Disparities due to Race, Poverty Multiply Death, Disease. *Washington Post*, September 13.

Perry, Michael. 2002. *New York's Disaster Relief Medicaid: Insights and Implications for Covering Low-Income People.* Washington, D.C.: Kaiser Commission on Medicaid and the Uninsured and the United Hospital Fund.

Purnick, Joyce. 2002. The Doctor Will See You, for Now. *New York Times*, March 7.

Ruiz, Albor. 2002. Disaster Medicaid Plan Set to Expire. *New York Daily News*, January 24.

Russakoff, Dale. 2001. Out of Tragedy, N.Y. Finds Way to Treat Medicaid Need. *Washington Post*, November 26.

Schneider, Andrew. 2002. Public Was Never Told that Dust from Ruins Is Caustic. *St. Louis Post-Dispatch*, February 10.

Seattle Times News Service. 2005. Many Evacuees Rejected for Medicaid. *Seattle Times*, October 6.

Stanley, Alessandra. 2005. Cameras Captured a Disaster but Now Focus on Suffering. *New York Times,* September 2.

State Health Access Data Assistance Center. 2005. *Characteristics of the Uninsured: A View from the States.* www.rwjf.org/files/research/Full_SHADAC.pdf.

Stephens, Kevin. 2007. Testimony before U.S. House of Representatives Subcommittee on Oversight and Investigations of the Committee on Energy and Commerce. March 13. www.cityofno.com/portal.aspx?portal=1&load=~/PortalModules/ViewPressRelease. ascx&itemid=3796 (accessed June 22, 2007).

Tallon, James R. 2001. Disaster Relief Medicaid: Testimony of James R. Tallon, Jr., President, United Hospital Fund, before the New York State Assembly Standing Committee on Health. December 3. www.uhfnyc.org/homepage3219/homepage_ show.htm?doc_id=192218.

U.S. Congress. Select Bipartisan Committee to Investigate the Preparation for and Response to Hurricane Katrina. 2006. *A Failure of Initiative: Final Report of the Select Bipartisan Committee to Investigate the Preparation for and Response to Hurricane Katrina.* Congressional Reports: H. Rpt. 109–377. February 15. Washington, D.C.: U.S. Government Printing Office. www.gpoaccess.gov/serialset/creports/katrina.html.

U.S. Department of Health, Education, and Welfare. 1967. *Nurses Serve in Hurricane Betsy.* Health Mobilization Series 1–7. Washington, D.C.

U.S. Federal News. 2005. Sen. Baucus Fights for Katrina Health Package. October 19.

Wasserman, Joanne. 2002. Ailing at Ground Zero: Neighbors Suffer from Medical, Emotional Problems. *New York Daily News*, January 12.

Wilds, John. 1978. *Crises, Clashes, and Cultures: A Century of Medicine in New Orleans.* New Orleans: Orleans Parish Medical Society.

Windows of Hope. www.windowsofhope.org (accessed February 15, 2006).

Conclusion

Public Health Takes on Gun Violence:
A Dialogue on Contested Boundaries

The essays in this book have addressed a host of issues that have challenged the public health community to assess and reassess its mission and purpose. Historically, public health has been caught between countervailing tendencies of the American political tradition. On the one hand, it is dependent on a collectivist approach to addressing social, economic, and biological issues that affect the nation's well-being. On the other hand, it is forced to operate within a political culture that often denigrates collective action and idealizes individualism and personal responsibility. Hence, public health practitioners find themselves forced to negotiate a fine line between activism and accommodation as they confront resistance to governmental, particularly federal, interventions, which are often seen as interference with individual liberties or free market principles.

Part 1 of the book explored how market forces circumscribe what can be defined as legitimate public health interventions. While the imperatives of capitalism have often been seen as oppositional to good public health, these chapters showed a more complex picture. Part 2 presented five case studies of public health practitioners negotiating contested institutional, political, and conceptual boundaries of the biological and the social. These chapters examined the relationship of the field of public health to environmental health, homelessness, accident prevention, the research enterprise, and clinical medicine. Part 3 looked at more recent challenges to the profession of public health as practitioners have been drawn into an ever-expanding number of unnatural and (seemingly) natural disasters. Hurricane Katrina and bioterrorism have forced the field to squarely face the limitations of its historical foundations in infectious disease and laboratory science and to ground itself in the broader social and political realities of modern American life.

This final chapter brings the book's central themes into sharp relief. Here, two of the nation's leading experts on gun violence discuss their own very practical experience with the possibilities and limitations of integrating the public health and criminal justice perspectives on the issue. Jeremy Travis, former head of the National Institute of Justice, the research arm of the Department of Justice, and Mark Rosenberg, epidemiologist at the Centers for Disease Control and head of their initiative on gun violence, engage in a dialogue about their efforts in the 1990s to apply a public health model to understanding and addressing gun violence in America. Their experiences illustrate the deeply political and ideological context of policy formation evident as they confronted the realities of a strong gun lobby, powerful Republican opposition to gun control, and a long-standing distaste within the CDC for expanding the boundaries of public health beyond the laboratory and communicable diseases. Significantly, the discussion of gun violence as a public health issue arose during a period in the 1980s when chronic illness gained new prominence within the public health community and gave added weight to the importance of noncommunicable sources of morbidity and mortality. Ironically, as Rosenberg and Travis describe, the Justice Department under Janet Reno was more receptive to a public health model of gun violence than was the CDC itself. This chapter illustrates the unpredictable ways that the boundaries of public health may broaden or narrow and the varied circumstances that can facilitate or impede efforts to put forth an expansive vision of what public and population health should be.

Mark Rosenberg: Let me start with how I got involved in the intersection between the public health perspective and the criminal justice perspective on gun violence. I had been at CDC working on infectious diseases, on smallpox, on cholera, on a lot of diarrheal diseases and outbreaks and epidemics and was trained in epidemiology. I then left CDC, got more training in infectious diseases and psychiatry, and was asked to come back to CDC in 1983 by Bill Foege, then the director of CDC, to start looking at the problem of violence as a public health problem.

The reason Bill asked us to start this approach was because in the early eighties they reassessed CDC's mission. Traditionally public health had focused on infectious diseases, and 95 percent of what public health did was infectious disease control. Bill said, "Let's look at the burden of death, disease, and disability in America and see where it falls," and, lo and behold, when they looked, the infectious disease burden was pretty small, and the burden from violence and unintentional injuries was huge, and he said, "If CDC is going to keep up with protecting the public's health then we've got to go where the problem is. And one of the problems is violence. It takes a huge toll on lives in this country, and when you add violence or 'intentional' injuries together with 'unintentional' injuries, injuries become a leading cause of death for people from one to forty-four."

Foege said, "We've got to focus on this," and he asked me if I would come back and start a unit that looked at violence as a public health problem. He said, "You know, you've got to take this job. You're trained in epidemiology, so you understand how to approach it. You're trained in public policy"—I'd been at the Kennedy School—"this certainly involves public policy. You understand psychiatry, and that's going to be a key part of this." And he said, "Probably most important of all is you understand infectious diseases, so the other people who are here might think you're nuts but they'll still talk to you! And besides, if you don't take this job with your set of training you'll never find something else that fits everything, so you've got to come back."

So I came back, not knowing how we would approach this or where we would go except that we wanted to analyze the patterns of violence—its epidemiology—to develop this new area of violence epidemiology. I came back and we started looking at homicide and suicide, and we started to develop what we called "the public health approach."

We said, first of all the public health approach is characterized by three things. [First,] it is based on science, so we're going to use data and evidence to guide our approach. Second, it's focused on prevention, and we are going to look for how to prevent these deaths from happening. That's different from a health or a health care approach, which tries to take care of the victims after they've been injured or shot. It's different because we were going to focus on prevention. Third, we'll be collaborative. And we said, there is no real profession of public health, but public health is a multidisciplinary enterprise. It involves epidemiologists, engineers, anthropologists, sociologists, psychologists, physicians, nurses, and others. Many, many people need to work together, and to look at homicide we certainly need criminologists and to look at the other area of intentional injury deaths, suicide, we certainly need suicidologists and psychiatrists and psychologists. So those were the three principles that characterized our approach.

We also realized from the start that violence prevention was not a priority for public health. My office was in the sub-subbasement of Building 3, a converted bathroom that used to be the men's room. They had taken out the fixtures but all the plumbing still ran through there, and every time anyone on any of the higher floors flushed the toilet we had to stop talking! This was where Violence was housed originally at CDC, and we had a group of about seven people including administrative staff support. So we started saying that violence is a public health problem, and the reason we started saying this was because most of the people at CDC said, "What are you doing here? Violence isn't a public health problem. Diarrheal diseases, respiratory diseases, even diabetes and heart disease are public health problems, but violence is not." And they pointed to all the public health textbooks—they'd never had anything on violence—and the long history of CDC and public health that excluded violence. So we said, "Violence *is* a public health problem because it takes a huge toll, and we've got to include it within the range of problems that we look at." We said that so we could get this onto the public health agenda and be accepted. So that's where we started from.

To explain what we meant when we said our approach was based on science, we developed four questions that we asked about any problem, and we said this was the public health approach. The first question we asked is, What's the problem? And we would ask the questions that any good reporter would ask. Who's involved? When does it happen? Where does it happen? How does it happen? We would try to describe the pattern of the problem. The second question we asked was, What are the causes? In asking about the causes we wanted to know why it happens, what are the risk factors, and what leads up to it. The third question is, What works to prevent it? We wanted to find out what was known about interventions that work and how we could evaluate them vigorously and scientifically. The fourth question is, How did you implement it? We wanted to know how, when you have something that works to prevent violence, how do you get it done. And that characterized our public health approach to violence.

As we started to mention violence as a public health problem, we got pushback from people in the police departments and in criminal justice, and they said, "You're claiming violence as *your* problem, and it's really *our* problem. It doesn't belong to you. We've been here for several hundred years, and you just started last week! How can you say violence is a public health problem?" And we had to explain that we're not claiming it exclusively as ours. We're claiming it so that public health would include it. But that was a point we had to make again and again and again. So it's interesting.

Jeremy Travis: In thinking about our conversation today, Mark, I was brought back in time to the year 1990 when I was appointed deputy commissioner for legal matters and general counsel at the New York City Police Department by the new police commissioner at the time, Lee Brown, who had come to New York to be police commissioner from a similar position in Houston, Texas. Lee was known in policing circles as an intellectual. He had a Ph.D. in criminology from Berkeley, one of the first African American criminologists in fact, and was recognized as a thinker about policing who was engaged in some cutting-edge policing issues on the national scene. At the time in New York we were experiencing a really horrific year-to-year increase in violence that had started in the mideighties. We had a new mayor, David Dinkins, a new police commissioner, Lee Brown, and the public demand at the time was that this administration, of which I was then a new member, had to do something about violence, and in particular gun violence, particularly gun violence by young people. So Lee Brown comes to New York City as a proponent of community policing, which was one reason he was hired, and immediately upon his arrival started talking about gun violence as a public health problem.

The memory that came back to me this morning was those early conversations within the police department where our new commissioner and the new team were trying to adopt this language and this construct coming from the commissioner of gun violence as a public health problem, and I have to tell you this did not go over well. This was certainly a foreign concept to law enforcement professionals. It was seen by some as an attempt to sort of change the subject away from what we, the police department, should be doing, and shifting responsibility to others, particularly those in the health professions— [what they] should be doing. In the minds of most people, the public health framework didn't help us figure out what we in the police department should do differently about the gun violence epidemic. Even calling it an epidemic, which I think we came to later, involves borrowing language from the public health field.

Despite this resistance to the public health framework, over time what happened was that we started to develop a number of strategies within the police department that reflected—even though we may not have used this language—a public health approach. We tried to figure out where the violence was happening, where the hot spots were throughout the city, and what strategies we could adopt. Everybody was given responsibility for a piece of the problem of gun violence within the command staff of the police department, and as general counsel my piece was to develop an initiative to ban assault rifles in New York City. This effort was ultimately successful and put me on the NRA list of least favorite people.

This high-level accountability for doing something about gun violence also caused me and my team to do some research on gun trafficking, which ultimately resulted in an article I published in the *Fordham Urban Law Journal* entitled "A Modest Proposal to End Gun Running in America." This, in turn, required us to focus on the problem of federally licensed gun dealers in other states, the loose regulation of federal firearms licenses, and the phenomenon of straw purchasers. My colleagues on the enforcement side of the police department soon teamed up with the Bureau of Alcohol, Tobacco, and Firearms to bring criminal cases against these dealers and gun traffickers, while the lawyers in the department worked with Congress to design laws to shut down the illegal businesses.

The overall effect of this framework of problem analysis and problem iden-tification and strategy development within the police department was quite noticeable, and it came from a commissioner who thought that way, but it also came from his looking at the epidemic of violence through this other lens as a public health problem in addition to a law enforcement lens. Lee Brown was certainly unusual in New York. This was certainly unfamiliar language in New York. I subsequently learned that in certain policing circles this was a more common language and over time became more common, but it was not a New York City framework at all.

Seeing this as an epidemiological problem, looking for root causes, identi-fying sources of illegal guns, and trying to track locations of gun violence—this was all new for policing. This whole approach to thinking about crime was new for policing, so this ultimately fit comfortably within the community policing, problem-solving, hot-spots analysis way that the policing profession was start-ing to redefine its mission. So even though the public health idea may not have been the language or the frame, the policing profession itself was undergoing profound changes in the early 1990s, so the public health approach fit comfort-ably with those broader changes that were underway. I don't know quite where the police first came in contact with these public health ideas. Maybe Mark knows the answer here, but my hypothesis would be that ideas from the public health side were penetrating into the policing world. So if we're telling the story of the first introduction to violence and the public health paradigm, that's my initiation story.

Mark Rosenberg: When Jeremy says they got a negative reaction from the police in New York, we got a negative reaction from the police all over, because they felt we were saying, "It belongs to us," when we were actually trying to say "We need to look at this as well as the other things public health traditionally looks at." And then there's a very interesting connection with Lee Brown.

When we got to Atlanta, we said, "Let's actually apply this," so we started working with the commissioner of public safety here, and his name was George Napper. George was also a Ph.D. from Berkeley in sociology and one of the intellectuals in policing and a very good friend of Lee Brown, so he introduced me to Lee Brown, and then Lee Brown and I were on panels together, went to meetings together a number of times, and actually talked about this issue over a number of years. I don't know exactly what led him to ultimately say just what he did or to adopt this particular approach but we had a lot of contact and a lot of interaction, introduced through George Napper. George is a wonderful person and he was very supportive of our efforts here. He helped us put together public health and law enforcement here in Atlanta. We initially started looking at domestic violence and helping the police here to do analysis of their cases, looking for what might prevent some of the cases and how they could use data to develop a preventive approach. George Napper was a very good connection, helping me to make my initial connection with Lee Brown when he was in Atlanta in 1983 or 1984.

Jeremy Travis: Well let me give a little of the intervening history and then talk about my coming to Washington. One of the projects that emerged from our analysis of gun violence in New York that in some ways was a good exemplar of how this approach—whether you want to call it a problem-solving approach or a public health approach—was successful and changed the way we thought about things was that we started some discussions within the police department to try to identify where guns were coming from. This, again, was not the traditional starting point for law enforcement types. They would wait until something happened and make an arrest and hopefully get a good prosecution ready and assume that that had advanced the cause of public safety. But Lee pushed us to ask questions about where guns were coming from, and as Mark said, we started trying to do good research, which is not always the place where a police organization would start.

We started collecting data on the state of origin of guns seized by the police department and discovered pretty quickly that the vast majority—and I think we were talking about something like 90 percent of the guns seized by the New York City Police Department—were last sold legally by a gun dealer outside of New York State. So we had this mystery that we had to solve—New York has some of the toughest gun control laws in the country but was awash with guns. So we had to try to understand where they were coming from. What this analysis led us to do was to—and we could use a public health metaphor, like draining swamps for mosquitoes or something like that—but we figured out that there was actually a very small number of gun dealers in Virginia, North Carolina, and some identified states that were producing a large percentage of the guns.

We then found common cause with a federal law enforcement agency— Alcohol, Tobacco, and Firearms—because they had regulatory authority over those gun shops. So we mobilized an enforcement operation against those gun shops to try to make purchases that were illegal to affect their regulatory status, but also this translated into legislation that we advanced, and I testified on behalf of it in the early days of the Clinton administration, to reduce the number of federal firearms licenses. One strategy was to raise the fees. At the time, for thirty dollars, you could get a federal firearms dealer's license that would allow you to sell guns from your kitchen table. We changed all that, with Treasury Secretary Bentsen's strong support, and we saw over time that a lot of those rogue dealers dried up. So it was a combination of enforcement action, a regulatory review. and a lot of public awareness, just making the case about where these guns were coming form. That's not the traditional law enforcement way of thinking about this stuff, and it really flowed from this analytical work that we set about doing in those early days in the 1990s.

Mark Rosenberg: If I can add just an additional point here that Jeremy might not say: I think the traditional view of law enforcement from the public health perspective was that law enforcement traditionally focused on deterrence and punishment. It was a post facto approach: After the crime had been committed, they would enter the scene. We started saying that public health could be a very good complement to that approach because our focus was on prevention, so here was a natural alliance. I think the work that Jeremy did and then later brought to government very much changed that paradigm. I think that law enforcement in the area of gun violence started looking very seriously at prevention, not just deterrence and incarceration, and I think that was new, and I think that was a very big expansion of the paradigm.

Question: How did the two of you come to know each other and begin to work on this problem?

Jeremy Travis: Let me just tell my half of the story about how Mark and I met. I was named the director of the National Institute of Justice in 1994 and was confirmed in the fall of '94 by the Senate, and already under way within the Clinton administration was a serious look at violence, gun violence in particular. There was a cross-agency committee that had been created, cochaired by the deputy attorney general, Phil Heyman, and Peter Edelman, assistant secretary at the Department of Health and Human Services. Even before going to Washington I attended a White House conference on violence where I remember vividly somebody from—it may have been from CDC—unfolding this graph to great dramatic effect, to give proper credit for the marketing genius here, but unfolding slowly this graph that showed the high rates of morbidity among African American men attributed to gun violence. It just went on and on and on and on and on, so everyone kept waiting for the graph to end but it didn't quite end. So there was work under way in the Clinton administration around violence all at the same time that the '94 Crime Act was being debated and community policing was being put on the table. But for me the key support that

I got in making the connection with Mark was from Attorney General Janet Reno, and you had already connected with Janet.

Mark Rosenberg: Right.

Jeremy Travis: Mark was a minister without portfolio or without designation in the Justice Department, and I remember how remarkable it was for me to go into a meeting with the attorney general on gun violence and there would be sitting Dr. Mark Rosenberg from CDC, and I thought, Well, this is a little different! But then Mark and I very quickly found common cause, and you'll obviously have to tell this side of the story, Mark, but we met during a time when CDC was coming under some criticism for the work you were doing on gun violence, and NIJ, which I was heading up, had a history of doing work on violence. There was strong interest in seeing NIJ build on that history. Because we could claim our law enforcement credentials on this research agenda, in some ways we were able to pick up some of the slack that CDC couldn't. So we started funding research projects together, bringing our research grantees or PIs together on various things. I sent folks down to Atlanta. Mark would be in Washington a lot, and at the level of both knowledge production—the scholarship—but also through our practice, communities that we were in touch with, these two agencies started operationalizing this idea of our disciplines working together, much more than had been the case before.

Here's just a simple example of this: I created something at NIJ called the Research in Progress lectures, a monthly seminar series where we'd invite in an academic who was doing work on an NIJ-funded grant where the findings hadn't yet been published, hadn't gone through peer review. We wanted to have researchers come to the Institute when they were in the middle of their work, when they'd just had that eureka moment where the computer had printed out the data, they were excited and wanted to come and share it. Our first speaker was Al Blumstein—his presentation was on understanding the age dimensions of the rising levels of violence—and our second was Arthur Kellermann. So here we had Art Kellermann, a CDC-funded researcher doing work in Atlanta, coming to NIJ, speaking to an audience of justice folks, and his presentation was on . . .

Mark Rosenberg: I think the risk of firearm ownership.

Jeremy Travis: Exactly. Exactly. And what he was talking about—Were you at the presentation?—was the work he was doing in Atlanta on an intervention level, where the emergency room doctors were working with the police on ways to prevent the next shooting when somebody came in injured in what was clearly some gang-related incident. That approach—even that way of thinking—just sent a buzz through the law enforcement community. So our work—the NIJ lecture series, the tapes of the lectures, the write-ups of the talks—all got these research findings out to that world of practice very efficiently. So there was soon a lot of talk in policing and criminal justice circles about, "Okay, what can we do in the emergency rooms with the docs around the country?" So that idea was coming from lots of places, but certainly the Kellerman work accelerated it, and that idea became part of the new way of thinking about gun violence.

Mark Rosenberg: That's a good connection with Arthur there and with Janet Reno. I had been struck by two things when I came to CDC to look at violence. One was if you looked at the burden of injuries, there were two big causes of injury deaths and disability in the U.S.: One was car crashes, the other was guns, and these were roughly about the same level of burden. Later on, building up to the peaking of youth homicide rates in '93, there were many states where there were actually more gun deaths than car deaths, but they were roughly burdens of about the same size. Lots had been done to prevent road traffic deaths. In the 1960s the United States had started the National Highway [Traffic] Safety Administration. They had taken $300 million and said, "We're going to look at research. We're going to look at ways to prevent these road deaths because we don't want our kids dying in traffic crashes." And NHTSA became very important and was very, very effective in markedly reducing the road traffic death rate. That initial amount was matched every year by much, much more that was invested in preventing road deaths, but in the area of gun injuries we spent almost nothing. Nothing! There was no prevention research. The police intervened after shootings but there was no research on how they could be prevented. There wasn't even a lot of good research on who bore the burden or what were the causes or what strategies might be employed.

So in 1987 we started a research program. The other thing that was striking, as Jeremy mentioned, was the racial disparities, that young black men died at a rate of gun death eight times the rate of young white men. It was an incredible disparity in death. Most of the burden was born by the black community, and most of them were poor blacks, and most of the violence, as we started to analyze it, was black on black shootings. So the disparities, the huge burden, and the total lack of research in this field led us at CDC to say, "This is an area where we could really change things and make a big contribution and save lives by applying the same kind of science that had been applied to road traffic crashes."

So in 1987 we got some funding for a research program on injury prevention, and we decided that one of the things we wanted to look at scientifically was gun deaths, and one of the first applications we got was from Arthur Kellermann. He had done one previous study, and this time he proposed to look at the risk of having a firearm in the home, because gun proponents at that time said, "This is the way to protect you and your family against intruders and against injury," but a lot of people had the feeling that if you had a gun around, that in itself was dangerous. Arthur proposed to actually do a case control study and look and see whether a gun in the home protected you or whether it increased your risk of death.

What he found was that if you have a gun in the house, not only does it not protect you but it increases the risk of homicide to someone in that house by threefold. It triples your risk. It's more likely to be used to shoot a spouse or a child than an intruder. Or it will be used in a suicide, to shoot oneself—and that risk went up fivefold if you had a gun in the house. And the risk of its being used in domestic violence went up significantly as well. So Arthur's study was very important and was the beginning of a long research program where we tried to do scientific research and establish common ground. We thought that if we could depolarize this debate between the NRA and the gun controllers, if we could build a common ground based on science, we could start to bring people together and make real progress in prevention.

And it started to work. We started to build a real legitimate, scientific program, and we did make presentations to Janet Reno. I forget when that was but I had created a set of slides that showed how the homicide rate for young black men was so disproportionate that it went on and on and on with these slides. I remember it was a presentation to all of the U.S. attorneys that had come together in D.C. for their annual meeting. It felt odd because I was this doctor from Atlanta on a panel with all lawyers and criminologists, and it felt to me that I was giving some facts about a subject where I knew much less than they did. At the end of my talk, I was sitting up there still a little nervous, and a Secret Service person came up to me and said somewhat gruffly, "Are you Dr. Rosenberg?" I thought, Oh, my God, what did I do now? I thought they're going to give me the gong, get me off of here. And I said yes, and he said, "Here, this is for you." It was a little folded note from one of those spiral note pads—about 2 × 3 inches where you turn it over and write on the next page—and it said, "Dr. Rosenberg, that was fantastic. Thank you. Janet Reno." I could breathe again.

She was so interested in data and statistics and understanding. Do you remember that, Jeremy? It was so unusual for someone at her level to really want to understand the data and what it showed. What do we know about this? Most people came in with their preformed opinions and just wanted to make sure no one was going to contradict them, and she came in with questions and wanted answers. It was so refreshing and wonderful, and I think her interest in the issue really helped bring the two fields together. She was really instrumental in a very important way.

I think in 1994 things changed because Congress changed, and this is when our Republican congressman from here, Newt Gingrich, helped to engineer a big Republican victory and the NRA got much more control of the agenda. As Jeremy mentioned, the NRA tried to stop what we were doing because they thought that if we put the data together, that would be very threatening, and they didn't want that to happen. And so they tried to shut us down, and this went on for several years. They started up several groups specifically to get rid of us. One of them was called Doctors for Integrity in Science and Policy, led by someone who was a physician. He led this attack on us, trying to say that the science we did was all biased, picking out quotes out of context in talks that we gave, making up quotes that we never said, and publishing these regularly in the NRA journals and the other gun journals. They gave talks about this, and wrote to congressmen and senators, and many people started attacking us. The attacks got pretty bitter, and they went on in Congress.

We had started as this little branch in the sub-subbasement, and we had subsequently combined what we were doing with the people working on unintentional injury. By 1994 we had a National Center for Injury Prevention and Control. At one of our appropriations hearings the NRA had mobilized people in Congress who wanted to not only stop us from looking at gun violence but they wanted to do away with the whole center, and there were six senators who wrote a letter to the secretary of Health and Human Services (HHS) saying that the National Center for Injury Prevention and Control should be abolished and that I should be fired because the work we were doing was junk science. One of the headlines called us "the cesspool of junk science." That was how they characterized what we were doing, so the fact that Jeremy and NIJ were able to pick up on this issue where we were forced to stop any work that could be interpreted as "gun control" was important. Our research on gun violence included development of a surveillance system for collecting data on gun injuries and deaths. It was one of the most successful surveillance systems we had set up, and the funding for that was completely taken away.

Starting in 1994 we got attacked very seriously. David Satcher, as the director of CDC, strongly defended us. He was a real champion and went up and stood in front of the NRA surrogates in Congress and stood behind what we were doing. We had a scientific review of all the research we had done on gun violence, and the review said the research was absolutely credible, well done, and stood on its merits, but the NRA kept coming back stronger and stronger.

Then, a few years later, David Satcher moved up to become surgeon general and assistant secretary for health, and the CDC got a new director who was not ready to stand up and defend what we had been doing in the area of gun violence because the political atmosphere had changed totally. During that intervening period, from about 1995 on, we weren't allowed to do anything that could be interpreted as advocating gun control; now CDC is basically not even allowed to use the word "gun" in what it does. So the fact that NIJ came along here and stood up for gun violence prevention was really important.

Julius Richmond, the only person to have served simultaneously as both surgeon general and assistant secretary for health, talks about three components that are really important in advancing any cause and really solving any societal problem: You need scientific data, a social strategy, and political will. On the first—scientific data—we worked very closely with NIJ to help put the data together, and we explored new areas. We went into the area of domestic violence. Remember, Jeremy, that Linda Saltzman worked with people on your staff and we started to develop shared definitions of domestic violence, and we did a joint survey. This was a real "first" between NIJ and CDC on the incidence, prevalence, and risk factors for domestic violence in the U.S.

Jeremy Travis: It was a landmark.

Mark Rosenberg: It was really important, and it meant so much to our people to be able to work together. It helped us in the first of Julie's components of starting to establish the data. His second component is to put together a social strategy, and I think we started to devise joint strategies: prevention became intimately woven into the NIJ and Janet Reno's fabric and way of thinking about these things. And Janet Reno and Donna Shalala chaired a committee, a secretarial level committee, on domestic violence. As part of that they were looking at gun violence, and they supported legislation banning guns for policemen convicted of domestic violence offenses. So the coming together of the two departments helped in the data; it helped in the social strategy; and maybe even most important for us it helped in Julie's [Julius Richmond's] third component, which is developing political will.

I think this was also helped significantly by the work that Peter Edelman did with Phil Heyman, starting soon after Clinton took office and looking at violence in the U.S. and violence prevention. One of their subgroups was gun violence prevention. They backed that, and they said it was important and that it needed to be done, and they provided the political will. They said, "If it takes this many lives, this is a major problem. It needs to be addressed. It's solvable.

The disparities make it even more urgent, and we need to address it." So that political will was strengthened by both departments working together, and I think in 1994 we saw what happened when the NRA dominated the political scene, through the congressional elections, and dismantled, at least on our side, a lot of that machinery that had been set up. The political will to go on within Health, in HHS, really diminished. But I think bringing our departments together really helped in all three of those areas in very important ways.

Jeremy Travis: For us, Mark, 1994 was an important year for two reasons—it was not only the year that Congress changed hands, but it's the year that the '94 Crime Act was signed into law, which was a big initiative of the Clinton administration, and the ultimate version had some Republican pieces as well. From NIJ's point of view, the most important part of the '94 Crime Act was the community policing initiative, which ultimately pumped billions of dollars into the jurisdictions around the country, mostly direct grants to police departments to hire more police officers on the condition that those police officers would be used for community policing, and the whole department would shift towards a community policing philosophy.

So what that did at the local level was to create a relationship between the federal government—in this case, the Justice Department—where we could talk directly to the police agencies through the Community Oriented Policing Services, or COPS, office and NIJ about ways to reduce violence and how the community policing problem-solving methodology could be applied in these jurisdictions. We had in essence created this channel of communication between federal agencies that were thinking in the right direction and local law enforcement. So we held big national training conferences and convenings all around the country. The COPS office set up regional community policing training institutes.

From the NIJ point of view—this completes the other side of Mark's story— we worked out an arrangement with the COPS office, again with Janet Reno's full support and blessing, that we would take about one and a half percent of the money off the top of the federal funding program to fund research related to that federal funding program. So we all of a sudden, after being an agency that had a very small budget by any measure—I guess maybe $26 million a year at that time—we started having an infusion of money in the order of magnitude of about $7 million to $10 million a year for research on policing and related topics. And what was the number one topic? Violence.

So there we were in a time when Washington's political environment had changed following the Republican congressional victories in 1994, having created direct relationships with police agencies with the backing of a bipartisan group that had come together to support the '94 Crime Act, and with the specific backing of the attorney general to do research related to the Crime Act and the policing portion of the Crime Act, and with the most money for research that we'd ever had. In 1994, we should remember, crime hadn't yet started to come down more than one year in a row, and topic number one was still violence, and within that the most important area of concern was gun violence. So, when Mark was facing his difficulties with the new Congress, we were able, because we had this mandate from Congress, from the attorney general, and from the field, to start to fund a serious research agenda on violence.

Mark Rosenberg: And I think one really important thing you did, Jeremy, you really shifted the basis of research. I think the research that had been done before you got there at NIJ was very much seen as politically driven as a way to support policies of the administration and dominant members of Congress. It had been seen as a way to support important political actors but not as a way to conduct a legitimate scientific enterprise, and I think you really changed that, focusing the research on science and data. I think the other thing that you made clear to me in your discussion right here that's really important is that community policing represented a paradigm shift from law enforcement's approach to gun violence being deterrence and incarceration to prevention. Community policing was really shifting the focus to prevention in a very big and very important way, and the money that went into policing was much bigger than the money that went into research, but it was really a way to implement preventive approaches.

Question: When your funding was getting cut, did you find a lot of political support, or did you find the CDC staff and leadership kind of backing away from you and just reverting to the view that gun violence was really not something that CDC was deeply invested in?

Mark Rosenberg: Different people reacted differently. I think David Satcher, being an African American and very much in touch with the toll that violence took on the African American community, was a staunch defender of the need to apply science to gun violence prevention. He was really with us and behind us in trying to keep our opposition from demolishing, abolishing, and reducing the funding for our center.

But I think there were times when it even got too hot for David. There was a task force set up to look at disparities in health, and David chaired this, I think with Donna Shalala. They were looking for health indicators where there were big disparities between minorities and the majority. They found, for example, that in heart disease blacks suffered three times the frequency of heart disease at the same age or that hypertension was two and a half times worse in minority communities; diabetes, three times worse. I asked if they were going to include homicide because that was eight times worse—it was, in fact, the biggest disparity—and they said, "No, this is too hot to handle." So gun violence didn't even make it on to this list of the most important disparities in health.

I think people were wary of opening up CDC to too many attacks and too much criticism because they felt that if what we were doing on gun violence became an Achilles heel, people would threaten CDC in ways that could go beyond the injury center and beyond what we were doing. The NRA was gaining strength and momentum and they were really—I think the word is "emboldened"? Is that the right word for these days? They were emboldened to start threatening and attacking other parts that CDC saw as really central to its mission. I think when this question came up—I mentioned that we had been doing this firearm injury surveillance system and had started it on a pilot basis in a number of states—we had about maybe $200,000 or $300,000 in our budget for this system that was in the developmental stage. It was really going well but the NRA succeeded in getting Congress to just take $300,000 out of our budget.

I felt this work was too important for us to stop and went to the Robert Wood Johnson Foundation. Steve Schroeder was the president of the Robert Wood Johnson Foundation at that time, and they said, "We'll make up this money for you because this is really a critical issue, and you need to continue this line of scientific research." We put together with the RWJ staff a proposal and they were going to fund us for about $2.4 million over several years. We had worked this out in detail with their staff and president, and usually when you have their approval it's pretty much pro forma: Once you have the staff approval, the president takes it to the board, he knows his board, and it's usually pretty much a done deal. Steve called me and said, "It didn't pass," and it turned out that there was someone on the board who was an NRA member. And he vetoed this, a proposal that we had been working on for months, and Steve said, "I have never had this happen to me before." He had the rug pulled out from under him.

We were clearly disappointed but decided to try to find some other funding, I went to George Soros's foundation, and the person running the program said, "The one thing George said when he set up his foundation is he's never going to get into gun control. That's too political. He doesn't want to touch that." So I said, "Well, what we're going to do is science and shift the battle from gun control versus guns for all to just developing the science base." We went and we made our presentation to George Soros himself, and he said, "I'll give you $3 million for this." He also thought it was very important, and he saw the marked disparity in the burden of death and he was very interested in social justice. And so we went back to CDC and said, "George Soros wants to give us $3 million. We can continue this data-based surveillance program." We had a mechanism for taking the money, and CDC officials said, "No. George Soros is too controversial a figure, and this is really too controversial an issue. You cannot accept that $3 million." So we arranged for the money to go to Harvard School of Public Health, and a public health researcher there, David Hemingway, continued that work. But you asked what the general sense was at CDC: I think there was a lot of fear that they didn't want to do things that would offend powerful people in Congress.

Jeremy Travis: We at NIJ were certainly aware of what was going on and particularly aware of what was happening at CDC. At NIJ there is one program officer there, Lois Mock, who had shepherded the gun violence research portfolio for many, many years, and she had a relationship with the NRA which was actually quite good, always invited somebody from the NRA to be on her panel at the American Society of Criminology research conferences, so I think that stood us in good stead. At this point, over the seven, eight, or ten years of the little bit of gun research that the Institute had done, Lois had always maintained that sort of open-door policy.

But I think the larger point is that the research that we were funding was part of this overall federal initiative to transform police agencies to be more effective, and so that was the headline. We weren't out there saying, "Look at all the gun research we're doing." We were saying, "We're helping police agencies to be more effective in reducing violence." It was a distinguishing characteristic that set our research activities apart from those that might have been at a health agency. Our research agenda was carried out in a law enforcement and criminal justice context. I was able to say that Congress had passed the 1994 Crime Act, the 1994 Crime Act called for research, and we're the research agency and we're doing that research. So we already had that congressional authorization. Now if we'd been attacked like Mark was, this argument might not have protected us much, but there it was, and it was pretty clear.

Furthermore, the work that was being done was very local, around and in conjunction with police efforts to transform community policing and to address local crime issues. A particular strategy that I adopted that may have helped was to call upon the applicants for research funding to propose a partnership between a local agency—typically a police agency—and a local university. We called these the Local Initiated Research Partnerships. These partnerships were also a way of building a local buy in from two institutions that meant a lot to the local stakeholders, including elected officials, your university, and your police department. So the research that was being conducted was often very pragmatic and directly related to what was going on in that particular city, with direct involvement by both the university and the police. I was aware that that strategy would stand us in good stead, which it did, and it also made the research yield, in terms of practical outcomes, much higher than other strategies might have done.

In addition, Janet Reno was one of the most independent, strong-willed, not-to-be-swayed people in public life. She took attacks for eight years and left with her head high. She was a strong supporter of NIJ and science and, personally, of me. Mark, when you and I talk about Janet the way we do, we always say that she was so data oriented, so refreshingly open. I often remind people that she was a chemistry major in college before going to law school. She has a scientific mind from way back.

Mark Rosenberg: The collaborations between NIJ and CDC continued, but we moved from things that were directly gun violence to looking more at domestic violence.

Jeremy Travis: That's right. We had a really remarkable collaboration between our agencies at the level of the cabinet secretaries, and between our research institutes that Mark and I headed up, on the issue of violence against women. Again, we had strong congressional authorization here which set up that secretarial task force, a separate funding initiative for the violence against women research coming out of the National Academy of Sciences, which had issued a strong report that called for a sustained research agenda for the country on violence against women. I think it's fair to say, Mark, that we built on our preexisting relationship on gun violence to morph our collaboration into a very robust agenda on violence against women that had a number of explicitly collaborative research projects where we cofunded research, something that we hadn't really done much of in the gun violence area.

Mark Rosenberg: Yes. We cofunded, we cosponsored talks on it, and then we distributed together, published the results and distributed it as a joint publication, which was the first time that had ever been done. I also just want to say that these interdepartmental collaborations, I think, are very rare, and they're very hard to make work, and I think Janet Reno was extraordinary in welcoming input from HHS and from doctors and health people into the issue, and I think Jeremy as well was always open to us and valued us and respected us.

Those things don't always happen across departments in government. In fact, they're rare even between different agencies within a single department. Sometimes the turf issues and the competitiveness and the need to control is so dominant that the collaborative efforts may get lip service but little else, and I think, Jeremy, you were always so supportive of what we were trying to do. You always took calls, you always set up meetings, you kept this going, and I think the change in paradigm is an important part, but I think the personal leadership that people exert on an effort like this is also very important, and I think you had people that really felt passionate about doing the right thing, and I wouldn't want to skip that. I think both Janet Reno, and she had an assistant attorney general, Eldie Acheson—Right?—and some others.

Jeremy Travis: Laurie Robinson, the assistant attorney general for Justice Programs, was the other key person.

Mark Rosenberg: Yes, there were several people that Janet Reno had around her that I think really supported this effort, but I think the individuals who participated are also key to making something like that happen.

Question: What's the end of the story, for both you personally but also in terms of what has happened to the various collaborations? What do you think the long-term impact on the culture of both the criminal justice community as well as the health community has been?

Jeremy Travis: Well, I'll speak about the criminal justice community, and I'll talk specifically about policing. I think the policing profession is a transformed profession these days. It's much more analytical, much more results oriented, much more open to collaboration and partnership than ever before. So the typical police chief now doesn't shy away from talking about the crime phenomenon in his or her jurisdiction, doesn't shy away from being held responsible for making contributions toward reducing crime. Most police departments now have very sophisticated crime analysis operations. A lot of them are using GIS and crime-mapping technologies as a way of identifying problems. A sophisticated police department now takes as a given that it collaborates with others and recognizes that identifying a problem and designing strategies to address the problem requires partnerships with other sectors of society, and public health is often present at that partnership table. So I think the policing profession has changed substantially.

Part of, but not the total—certainly by far not the total—contributor to that result have been these influences from the public health world, but this was as the public health interest in violence was emerging, the timing was just right, because a new way of thinking was also emerging within the police world. You can trace the sort of intellectual lineage back to the Kansas City Preventive Patrol experiment in the midseventies, which basically said that the standard way of doing police business was not working. The reactive posture of the police, and the notion that crime prevention was seen as a consequence of just riding around in your patrol car. That's how prevention was defined, until the Kansas City study came out. So there's a thirty-year history of change in policing that we are talking about here.

The part of the story that we're telling right now is that when the level of violence got to be the most acute in this country, following the mideighties when we saw violence rates—gun violence, particularly in young people, doubled in seven years—and there was a real sense of crisis, that at that time of crisis we had the confluence of a number of important developments. We had leadership at the national level, congressional support—notwithstanding the attacks from the NRA—and a policing profession that was poised to think differently, and then the availability of an approach that I credit the public health folks with, and Mark in particular, that focused on violence in an entirely different way.

The focus was not on how we could change our sentencing structure to ramp up punishment one more notch so that maybe we'll get either some deterrence or incapacitation value from more people in prison; the public health approach was, Let's understand the problem first. It sounds so obvious. It sounds so rudimentary, like of course this is the way a profession should think about its core business, but in my way of looking at this history that analytical approach was novel and it came at a time when everything was lined up, at a time when frankly I think the nation needed this other way of thinking about things.

So we stand in a very different place today, compared to those scary years in the late eighties and early nineties. Today we have the lowest rates of violence in a generation, notwithstanding the recent upticks in a number of cities. We are trying to understand, again in an analytical way, what might have contributed to this good result. Certainly many things contributed to this good result, but I think the new approach within policing and within policing's partners, including public health partners, that was empirically informed, data driven, and problem solving in its methodology should receive much of the credit. Today, the country's just a very different place from where it was in the early nineties, and violence is not what it used to be.

Mark Rosenberg: I think that's a great summary. I think a couple of things happened here, too, to change the national picture. One was that violence, especially gun violence, changed in the public perception from being a problem that was blacks shooting blacks and therefore it could be ignored. When you had the sudden eruption of school violence and you started having shootings at schools— Columbine had not yet happened when President Clinton called a meeting, I remember this, a meeting. (Were you there, Jeremy?) President Clinton was there, Janet Reno was there, and it was to talk about school violence, and I remember we had done an analysis of these multiple school shootings, multiple death outbreaks, and there was a real pattern—they were increasing in an alarming way—and I had this big poster that I held up that showed how they were increasing and something was going to happen, and this was a month before Columbine. And then Columbine hit and blew the top off the problem, and youth violence and kids with guns started to be seen as something that was not just a black-on-black problem, and I think that was a very important change in public perception that lent support to the urgency of addressing this. School violence became another legitimate way of addressing the problem, and that also helped to bring the public health approach and criminal justice approaches together.

I also want to say, when we talked about criminal justice having focused more on intervention after the act, that's also true of medicine. If you look at the budget of how we spent our health dollars in this country, it's starting to change slowly, but up until maybe three years ago, of the trillion dollars that we spend on health in this country, 99 percent of it is spent on treatment and 1 percent is spent on prevention. So it's not just criminal justice that had that approach to the problem but so did medicine, and public health was the smaller partner of medicine in this very small budget. The budget started to increase with the notion of preparedness and counter-terrorism, but the focus on prevention is not the dominant strategy in either of the fields, but it has clearly started to change.

In looking back I think that another important part of this, from working together initially in the area of gun violence, we mentioned domestic violence, where I think it's been a very important partnership and a very important collaboration, and another very important part is child abuse and especially child sexual abuse. I think up until maybe ten years ago the standard approach to child sexual abuse was you wait until it happens and then you lock up the perpetrator and you put the kid in therapy, and there was no preventive approach. Now I think police and public health are both working on this approach that says we've got to identify perpetrators before it happens and get them help, get them services, and we can't rely on children to identify the perpetrators. It's usually a male in their family who's usually five feet higher than they are and they can't stand up and the adults have to take some responsibility for stopping it when they think it may happen or when it's happening. But a focus on prevention in child sexual abuse and child abuse and domestic violence, in a lot of these areas they've kind of gone hand-in-hand I think, criminal justice and public health, and I think that's been a very important and big contribution that was kind of forged in the area of working together on gun violence. But that spread to a number of other very important boundary crossings together.

Question: Is the CDC effort on gun violence still in the sub-subbasement bathroom?

Mark Rosenberg: No. It's been flushed! You won't hear. It's a four-letter word, and I don't think it's really mentioned, the work that CDC does. They still have each year in their appropriations language something that says, "None of the funds that CDC gets shall be used to advocate or promote gun control in any way," and that's still there. What CDC did with this gun injury surveillance system was to transform it into a violent injury surveillance system. The NRA said, "Why do you only want to look at guns? Why not look at knives and fists and metal mallets, whatever you can find? Why don't you look at all of these? Why focus your efforts on guns?" So CDC said, "Okay. We'll look at all violent deaths." So they're now developing a violent death reporting system. It's kind of like looking at a highway death reporting system, and people said, "Don't just look at cars. You need to include tricycles." "Okay, we'll include tricycles." But it's now going forward to looking at the violent death reporting system. It's gone slow, but it's moving. They're doing that, but I don't think they're funding any research on firearm injuries per se, and I think that's really dropped off the agenda—there's nothing happening, and they're not even allowed to attend meetings on the subject or on that issue.

Jeremy Travis: Mark, I wanted to make one other observation before we close. I wonder if you agree with this: I think another consequence of this shift in paradigm—and without trying to be too specific about exactly what caused this shift, I think we can all agree on it—is that the shift has enabled the country to move away from a demonization of young people, which was very much the public mood as the rates of violence were skyrocketing in the late eighties and early nineties. If we recall back to some of the statements about "superpredators" and "the coming blood bath" predicted by some academics who looked at some of the demographic trends, there was a sense, again fueled by the popular media, that there was something terrible happening within our population of young people and that these were not our children. There was, as you said eloquently a number of times in this conversation, a significant racial overtone to those observations.

So the different framing of the issue that was made possible by both the public health contribution and the community policing contribution said, "We have a problem that we have to do something about, and there are many contributors to that problem. Let's figure out what those contributors might be and address them as best we can and have a strategy for each." This approach had a salutary effect, I think, by shifting the focus away from the young people who were either shooting or being shot as the problem.

You may remember a report I did at the Urban Institute where we looked at the rise and fall in rates of violence in America. What was particularly interesting about that report was the finding that the decrease in violence that started in '93 was led by our young people, that the sharpest levels of decline were in the lower age groups. So we now are able to say, ten years later, that, yes, true, in the late eighties the upsurge in violence was led by young people—the sharpest increases in violence could be seen in the younger age groups—but the good news is that the decline in violence after the peak in '92–'93 was also led by young people.

So we are now able to, I think, talk about young people in a very different way, and it's because we, through a number of mechanisms, were able to shift the focus from an unrelenting focus on youth crime, which led to all of these awful things that we now are paying a price for, such as lowering the age of criminal responsibility, shifting more cases into the adult system, saying if you did the crime you have to do the time, all those things. We still have that legacy that came from the late eighties, and it was because the country allowed itself to focus on perpetrators rather than on causes.

Mark Rosenberg: I think that's a wonderful point. It also, I think, made it clear that there are many more causes to these problems than we would see if we adhered to our normally strict disciplinary vision, and that we really needed to broaden the way we thought about these problems. I think that's one of the advantages of these porous boundaries between public health and criminal justice, is that we can each start to look from the other's perspective and see new causes and see new ways to solve the problem. What I've seen individually, and it wasn't just a case—as you said so clearly, it wasn't just a case of rounding up the usual suspects. We each had our usual suspects, but in looking at the reasons for the increase in crime or the decrease in crime, now we're starting to see, hey, maybe there were new suspects we had never really reached before and it provides new answers.

I think one other part of just looking at this crossing the boundary here that I thought was very important is that for us in public health having partners in criminal justice who would acknowledge that what we were doing was valuable and important made a huge difference for us in being able to persevere, whether it was against the personal attacks of the NRA or the congressional attacks against our budget or just the traditional refusal of most public health people to admit that violence was a public health problem. Beginning to work with Jeremy and Janet Reno and people at the Department of Justice helped strengthen our resolve and really boosted us. I hope that there was a similar effect, because I think sometimes these were kind of very lonely and very difficult areas to push ahead, but just having the collaborators, having partners makes it much easier to do, this kind of mutual support that you can get from cross-disciplinary work.

I also think in health it's starting to become obvious that problems that we used to think were just health problems—we never thought that violence was just a health problem, but things like AIDS—now it's very clear that there are many other sectors that have to be involved, whether its labor or law enforcement for some measures here, but that most of the problems that traditionally we thought were just health problems now really require us to collaborate with other areas. The clearest example is in the area of bioterrorism. In preparing this, no one sector can do that alone, and it forces us to improve those linkages and connections if you want to be able to respond in any rational and productive way.

Jeremy Travis: Mark, it's so great to be back in touch with you, and it brings back wonderful memories. You were a great colleague personally and to my agency when we needed all the credibility that people with MDs after their names are able to bring to a struggling profession like law enforcement when it was trying to figure out how to do its job better. It was a great collaboration and it's just great to be talking with you again.

Mark Rosenberg: I would say ditto, totally.

Contributors

Ronald Bayer is professor and codirector in the Center for the History and Ethics of Public Health at the Mailman School of Public Health, Columbia University. Through his work on AIDS, tuberculosis, tobacco control, and public health surveillance, he has sought over the past two decades to articulate an ethics of public health that is distinct from bioethics.

Phil Brown is professor of sociology and environmental studies at Brown University, where he leads the Contested Illnesses Research Group, directs the Community Outreach Core of Brown's Superfund Basic Research Program, and directs the Societal Impacts Component of Brown's NSF project on Biocompatibility and Toxicity of Nanotechnology. He is the author of *No Safe Place: Toxic Waste, Leukemia, and Community Action*, coeditor of the collection *Illness and the Environment: A Reader in Contested Medicine*, and author of the recent *Toxic Exposures: Contested Illnesses and the Environmental Health Movement*. His current research includes labor-environment coalitions, connections between breast cancer activism and environmental justice, and biomonitoring.

Işıl Çelimli is a Ph.D. candidate in sociology at Columbia University. Her interests are urban and cultural sociology and qualitative methods. Currently, she is completing her dissertation.

James Colgrove is an assistant professor in the Center for the History and Ethics of Public Health at Columbia University's Mailman School of Public Health. He is the author of *State of Immunity: The Politics of Vaccination in Twentieth-Century America* (University of California Press, 2006) and coauthor, with Amy Fairchild and Ronald Bayer, of *Searching Eyes: Privacy, the State, and Disease Surveillance in America* (University of California Press, 2007).

Amy L. Fairchild is an associate professor in the Department of Sociomedical Sciences at Columbia University's Mailman School of Public Health. Her work at the intersection of history and policy addresses broad questions regarding the functions and limits of state action in the realm of public health and has recently appeared in *Health Affairs, New England Journal of Medicine*, and the *Journal of Social History*. She is the author of *Science at the Borders: Immigrant Medical Inspection and the Shaping of the Modern Industrial Labor Force* (Johns Hopkins University Press 2003) and coauthor, with Ronald Bayer and James Colgrove, of *Searching Eyes: Privacy, the State, and Disease Surveillance in America*.

Sherry Glied, a health economist, is professor and chair in the Department of Health Policy and Management of Columbia University's Mailman School of Public Health. She is the author of numerous articles and two books, *Chronic Condition* (Harvard University Press, 1998), an analysis of U.S. health care policy;

and, with Richard Frank, *Better but Not Well* (Johns Hopkins University Press, 2005), an examination of changes in the well-being of people with mental illness in the United States since 1950.

Marianne M. Hillemeier received her MPH in Maternal and Child Health from Harvard University and her doctorate in sociology and demography at the University of Michigan. Her research interests focus on socioeconomic and race/ethnic disparities in children's health and functioning.

Beatrix Hoffman, associate professor of history at Northern Illinois University, is writing a history of the right to health care in the United States.

Marian Moser Jones received an undergraduate degree from Harvard University and an MPH from Columbia University's Mailman School of Public Health. She worked for twelve years as a journalist covering health, science, and legal issues. Currently, she is a Ph.D. candidate in history and ethics/sociomedical sciences at Columbia, where she is writing her dissertation on the history of the American Red Cross and disaster relief.

Mary Clare Lennon is professor in the Ph.D. program in sociology, the Graduate Center, City University of New York. Her research interests focus on social disadvantage and health. Recent projects include an examination of the temporal dynamics of homelessness and a study of the consequences of economic disadvantage in childhood for child development and well-being.

Nicole Lurie is the Paul O'Neill Professor of Policy Analysis and codirector of the Center for Domestic and International Health Security at RAND in Arlington, Virginia.

Gerald Markowitz is a Distinguished Professor of History at John Jay College of Criminal Justice and the Graduate Center, City University of New York. He is the recipient of numerous grants from private and federal agencies, including the Milbank Memorial Fund, National Endowment for the Humanities, and the National Science Foundation. Together with David Rosner, he has authored and edited numerous books and articles on environmental and occupational safety and health, including *Deceit and Denial: The Deadly Politics of Industrial Pollution* (2002).

William McAllister is a senior research fellow at the Institute for Social and Economic Research and Policy, Columbia University and a codirector of the Research Methods Core of the Columbia Center for Homeless Prevention Studies, Columbia University. In addition to studying homeless prevention, he is carrying out research to understand the nature, causes, and impacts of the temporal structure of the lives of homeless people and of the recruitment process for U.S. political elites.

Christopher D. Nelson is senior political scientist and the Thomas Lord Distinguished Scholar at the RAND Corporation, where he focuses on performance measurement, standards, and quality improvement methods for public health emergency preparedness. He has also worked on issues related to occupational safety and health policy and education reform.

David Rosner is Ronald H. Lauterstein Professor of Sociomedical Sciences History at Columbia University and director of the Center for the History of Public Health at Columbia's Mailman School of Public Health. He and Gerald Markowitz are the authors of *Are We Ready? Public Health since 9/11* and *Deceit and Denial: The Deadly Politics of Industrial Pollution.* He received his MPH from the University of Massachusetts and his doctorate from Harvard in the history of science. He was formerly University Distinguished Professor of History at the City University of New York. In addition to numerous grants, he has been a Guggenheim Fellow, a recipient of a Robert Wood Johnson Investigator Award, a National Endowment for the Humanities Fellow, and a Josiah Macy Fellow.

Dennis P. Scanlon is an associate professor in Penn State's Department of Health Policy and Administration. He received his Ph.D. from the University of Michigan and holds a master's degree in economics from the University of Pittsburgh. Professor Scanlon has authored several articles on health plan quality, performance measurement and quality improvement, competition, purchasing, and consumer choice of health insurance plans. Recently he completed a federally funded research project examining the state of quality improvement activities at managed care plans, and the degree to which plans are using performance measures for quality improvement activities. He is currently the principal investigator for the evaluation of the Robert Wood Johnson Foundation's Aligning Forces for Quality initiative, and for the Center for Health Care Strategies' Regional Quality Improvement initiative.

Alvin R. Tarlov is professor of medicine, University of Chicago. Prior appointments include chair, Department of Medicine, University of Chicago; president, Henry J. Kaiser Family Foundation; professor of medicine at Tufts University and professor of public health at Harvard University; and from 2000 to 2005, director, Texas Program for Society and Health, James A. Baker III Institute for Public Policy, Rice University. His interests are in public policies to reduce social inequalities and thus to improve population health.

Nancy Tomes is professor of history at Stony Brook University. She is the author of several books, including *The Art of Asylum Keeping: Thomas Story Kirkbride and the Origins of American Psychiatry* (rev. ed., 1994) and *The Gospel of Germs: Men, Women, and the Microbe in American Life* (1998). At present she is completing a book titled *A Patient Paradox: The Making of the Modern Health Consumer, 1930–1980.*

Jeffrey Wasserman is a senior policy researcher at the RAND Corporation. His research interests lie primarily in the areas of public health preparedness, health care reform, and health promotion and disease prevention. Professor Wasserman is also an instructor in the University of Southern California's International Public Policy and Management Program, School of Policy Planning, and Development.

Index

ABATE (A Brotherhood Against Totalitarian Enactments), 116, 117
Abourezk, Sen. James, 117
Acheson, Eldie, 275
advertising, 72–73
Advisory Committee on Childhood Lead Poisoning Prevention, 103
Advisory Committee on Genetic Testing, 103
Agency for Toxic Substances and Disease Registry, 95
AIDS, 7, 8, 35, 170–171, 216, 219. *See also* HIV surveillance
AIDS Action, 216
Aid to Families with Dependent Children (AFDC), 129
air pollution, 69, 87, 88, 96, 102–103
Akhtar, Mohammed, 205
Alaska, 90, 168, 169
Alaska Community Action on Toxics, 90
Aleutian-Pribilof Islands Association, 90
Alliance for a Healthy Tomorrow, 92
Alternatives for Community and Environment (ACE), 87–88
American Cancer Society, 67, 90
American Enterprise Institute, 205
American Journal of Public Health (*AJPH*), 74, 76, 118
American Medical Association (AMA), 60, 65–66, 67, 73
American Motorcycle Association, 113–114, 115, 116
American Public Health Association (APHA), 6, 71–72, 73, 205
ANSER Institute for Homeland Security, 211
anthrax scare (2001), 206, 213; as spur to public health preparedness, 36, 206, 207–208, 209, 215, 218
antibiotics, 23
antiterrorism responsibilities. *See* bioterrorism preparedness
Arizona, 208–209
Arkansas, 121
Arrow, Kenneth, 16

asthma, 87–89, 240–241
Astra-Zeneca, 90–91
Atlanta, Ga., 262–263, 265–266
automobile safety, 110, 112, 266

Baker, Susan, 118
Barbour, Haley, 247
Baucus, Max, 247, 251
Bauer, W. W., 67
Beitsch, Leslie M., 216
Belmont principles, 161. See also *Belmont Report*
Belmont Report (1979), 165–166, 172n1
Benjamin, Georges C., 212–213, 216, 218–219
Bentsen, Lloyd M., 264
Beyond Ground Zero, 244
bioterrorism preparedness, 15, 204–206, 219–223; and anthrax scare, 36, 206, 207–208, 209, 215, 218; conflicting meanings of, 206–207, 220–221; and federal funding, 206, 207, 210, 212, 215–218, 221, 222; and public health infrastructure, 205–206, 212–223; before September 11 attacks, 210–212; and smallpox inoculation campaign, 206, 218–219, 233
Blanco, Gov. Kathleen, 247
BlueCross BlueShield of Louisiana, 246
Blumstein, Al, 265
body burden testing, 99–102
Boston, Mass., 87–88, 91
Boyce, W. Thomas, 193
Brady, Joseph, 166
Breast Cancer Action, 91
Breast Cancer Awareness Month, 90–91
breast milk monitoring, 100
Breslow, Lester, 74
Bridges to Excellence program, 46
Brissett, Dennis, 77
Britain, 111, 182, 185
Brown, Lee, 260–262
Brown University, 92
budgetary crises, 217–218, 222, 223

Buehler, Jim, 170

Bureau of Alcohol, Tobacco, and Firearms, 261

Bush, George W., 214. *See also* Bush administration

Bush administration, 102–105, 222; and environmental health, 102–105; and Hurricane Katrina response, 247–248, 249

Cabot, Hugh, 66

Cairns, Hugh, 111

California, 112–113, 121, 208, 211; environmental health activism in, 91, 92–93, 94

Canadian Institute for Advanced Research, 8

Cancer Industry Tours, 91

Cates, Ronald, 207, 209

Center for Health, Environment, and Justice, 93–94

Center for Strategic and International Studies, 211

Centers for Children's Environmental Health and Disease Prevention Research, 96

Centers for Disease Control and Prevention (CDC), 7, 50, 209, 216; and environmental health, 95, 96, 97–98, 99, 100; and local and state health departments, 209–210, 212, 213, 214, 222, 230; and public health preparedness, 206, 214, 221–222, 233, 235, 236–237; and research on violence, 258–260, 265, 266–269, 272, 273, 278; and surveillance issues, 162–171

Centers for Medicare and Medicaid Services, 44, 45, 51

Centers for Preventive Research, 36

Central Florida Health Care Coalition, 45

Chadwick, Edwin, 8

Chafee, Sen. John, 119, 121

Chalmers, Thomas, 165

Chandler, Harriette, 207–208

charity, 18. *See also* corporate philanthropy

Checkoway, Barry, 75

chemicals, toxic. *See* toxic chemicals

Chicago, Ill., 22–23, 214, 215–216

Child Health Association, 67

Children's Aid Society (New York City), 240

chronic illness, 5, 26–27, 216; and disasters, 239–241, 243–244, 245–246, 251, 252. *See also specific diseases*

citizen/consumer involvement, 74–76. *See also* citizen-science alliances

Citizen's Board of Inquiry into Health Services for Americans, 73

citizen-science alliances, 94–97. *See also* environmental health activism

Claybrook, Joan, 117–118

climate change, 103–104

Clinton, Bill, 277. *See also* Clinton administration

Clinton administration, 263–265, 269–270. *See also* Reno, Janet

COBRA continuation health coverage, 241, 244

Cold War, 68

Collaborative on Health and the Environment (CHE), 93

Colmers, John M., 217–218

Colorado, 110, 113, 173n22, 211

Columbia Center for Children's Environmental Health, 88–89, 96

Columbia University, 62. *See also* Columbia Center for Children's Environmental Health

Columbine High School massacre (1999), 277

Committee on the Costs of Medical Care (CCMC), 65–66

Commonweal (California organization), 93, 99

Commonwealth Fund, 41

Communities for a Better Environment, 92

community-based participatory research (CBPR), 89, 95–97

"community medicine" (term), 79n9

Community Oriented Policing Services (COPS), 270

community policing, 270, 271

conceptual models of health, 36–37. *See also* economic model of health

Concerned Citizens of Tillery, 92

Congress. *See* U.S. Congress

Congressional Budget Office, 47

Connecticut, 211, 212

Cornely, Paul, 6, 72–73

Coron, Angela, 208

corporate philanthropy, 49

Council for International Organizations of Medical Sciences (CIOMS), 161–162, 165

Council of State and Territorial
Epidemiologists (CSTE), 166, 168, 169–170
courts, 113–115. *See also* U.S. Supreme Court
Cranston, Sen. Alan, 117
Crime Act of 1994, 264, 270–271, 273
Cushing, Harvey, 65

Dahlgren, Goran, 37
Dark Winter exercise, 211
Daubert v. Merrell Dow (1993), 104
Davey, Bruce, 116–117
Declaration of Helsinki (1964), 161, 165,
172n8
Defense Department (U.S. Department of
Defense), 95
Denno, Willard, 61
DHHS. *See* U.S. Department of Health and
Human Services
diabetes, 90, 230, 245, 272
Dinkins, David, 261
Disability Adjusted Life Years (DALYs), 179
Disaster Relief Medicaid, 243–244, 247, 248,
250, 253
disasters, 250. *See also* Hurricane Katrina;
public health preparedness; September 11
attacks
disease advocates, 170–171
disease management programs, 46–47
disparities. *See* health disparities
District of Columbia, 110
domestic violence, 131, 263, 269, 274
Donabedian, Avedis, 176

Easyriders (magazine), 115–116
economic model of health, 15; and
externalities, 17–19, 27; and health
production, 16–19; and public goods
(or bads), 17–29
Edelman, Peter, 264, 269
Eden, Catherine, 208–209
Edgley, Charles, 77
Ehrenreich, Barbara, 73
Ehrenreich, John, 73
Ellis, Bruce J., 193
"emergency" (term), 253–254
Emergency Health Care Relief Act of 2005
(Grassley/Baucus bill), 247–248, 250
emergency preparedness. *See* public health
preparedness

emergency responders, 205–206, 228
Employee Retirement Income Security Act
(ERISA), 41
employers: and disease management
programs, 46–47; and health insurance,
41–46, 48, 51–52nl; and health
promotion, 46–47; motives of, 39–41,
48–51; relation of, to public health,
32–41, 47–52
Engelthaler, David, 208
Ensign, John, 247
environmental health, 85; and Bush
administration, 102–105; and public
health, 85–87, 97, 105–106. *See also*
environmental health activism
environmental health activism, 85–87,
93–97; and air pollution, 87, 88, 96,
102–103; and breast cancer, 90–93; and
environmental justice, 85–93; and
participatory research, 89, 94–97, 99–102
Environmental Health Perspectives, 104
environmental justice movement, 85–86,
87–93
Environmental Protection Agency (EPA), 95,
96, 98, 101, 103
Environmental Working Group (EWG),
99–100, 101
epidemics, 5, 204, 252
epidemiology, 20–21, 100, 161, 232
Epstein, Richard, 3
Europe, 30n9, 94, 111, 119. *See also* Britain
Evans, Robert G., 36
externalities, 17–19, 27

Falkenrath, Richard, 215
Family Health Plus, 242–243, 244
Farm Security Administration, 66
fast-food industry, 4–5
Federal Data Quality Act (2002), 103
Federal Emergency Management Agency
(FEMA), 241
federal funding: for environmental health
research, 95, 96, 98, 99; for preparedness,
99, 206, 207, 210, 212, 215–218, 221, 222,
226; and public health infrastructure, 99,
206, 214–217, 218, 236; and
research/practice distinction, 166–167
Fee, Elizabeth, 60, 61, 62
Finkelstein, Katherine E., 243

Fishbein, Morris, 65

Florida, 45, 115, 121, 122

Foege, Bill, 258–259

Food and Drug Administration (FDA), 66

Food, Drug, and Cosmetic Act (1938), 66

food security, 89–90

Ford, Gerald, 117

Ford, Robert, 120–121

Fox, Daniel, 9

Frank, John, 8

Franklin, Evangeline, 253

"free rider" problem, 17–18, 28

General Accounting Office, 121

General Electric Corporation, 46

General Motors Corporation, 42, 45

genetic influences, 181, 185–187, 193–194

geographical information systems (GIS), 106

Gibbs, Lois, 94

Gilchrist, Mary, 213–214

Gingrich, Rep. Newt, 268. *See also*
    "Gingrich revolution"

"Gingrich revolution," 121

Giuliani, Rudolph W., 243

Graham, Judith, 247

Grassley, Charles, 247

Grassley/Baucus bill, 247–248, 250

Great Lakes Chemical Corporation, 101

Great Society programs, 74

Greenpeace, 101–102

Griscom, John, 8

Grossman, Michael, 16. *See also* Grossman
    model

Grossman model, 16–19, 29n3

gun violence, 258, 276–277; CDC and,
    258–260, 265, 266–269, 272, 273, 278;
    Clinton administration and, 263–265,
    267–268, 269, 270, 274, 275, 277; and
    National Institute of Justice, 264,
    265–266, 268, 269, 270, 271, 273; and
    police departments, 260–264, 265–266,
    273–274, 275; and public health model,
    258–260, 261, 279–280

Gyle, Norma, 211, 212

Harnish, Anne, 207

Harvard School of Public Health, 273

Health Alert Network, 212, 230

health behaviors, 182, 185. *See also*
    nutrition; smoking

health, definitions of, 3, 86

health departments. *See* state and local
    health departments

health disparities, 35–36, 97, 176, 245;
    influences on, 180–194; in other
    countries, 176, 185; racial, 266, 271–272

Health Employer Data Information Set
    (HEDIS), 44

health insurance, 40, 41–43, 48, 67, 68, 241;
    employers' role in, 41–46, 48, 51–52n1;
    loss of, in disasters, 239, 241–244,
    245–251, 252–254; value-based
    purchasing of, 43–46

health production, 16–19, 194–196; and
    health disparities, 180–194

Health Resources and Services
    Administration (HRSA), 206, 214, 221

Healthy Home Healthy Child campaign,
    88–89

Healthy People 2000, 95

Healthy People 2010, 36, 47–48, 50, 95

Healthy Tomorrow (Massachusetts), 94

heart disease, 128, 272

helmet laws. *See* motorcycle helmet laws

Helms, Sen. Jesse, 117

Hemingway, David, 273

Henderson, Joseph, 223

hepatitis A, 169, 230

Herzog, William, 76

Hewitt Associates, 42, 46

Heyman, Phil, 264, 269

Hilleboe, Herman, 69–70

HIV/AIDS. *See* AIDS

HIV surveillance, 162, 163–164

homelessness, 127–128; and disease,
    147–148; and public health, 141–142,
    147–149. *See also* homeless prevention

homeless prevention: individual strategies
    for, 128–135, 137–147, 148–149;
    structural-level strategies for, 135–147,
    148–149

Hospital Quality Alliance, 44

hospitals, 44–45, 228

Howard, Rep. James, 117

HUD (U.S. Department of Housing and
    Urban Development), 95

Huff, James, 104–105
Hughes, James M., 203, 215
human development, 190–191
human subjects research, 161–171
Hurricane Katrina, 78, 239–241, 245–251,
    252–253
hypertension, 272

Illich, Ivan, 182
Illinois, 110, 113, 213
immunization, 25–26; compulsory, 118, 120
Imperial Chemical Industries, 90
incident command structures, 232
individualism, 58, 122
industrial hygiene, 69
inequality. See health disparities
infant mortality, 35
infectious diseases, 21, 23, 216. See also
    epidemics; specific diseases
influenza, 226, 231
informed consent, 161, 162–164, 171
information technology (IT), 230–231
infrastructure. See public health
    infrastructure
Institute of Medicine (IOM), 44; 1988 report
    by, 1, 3, 35, 69, 77, 205, 226; 2003 report
    by, 3, 32–34, 35, 36, 37–38, 39, 226
institutional review boards (IRBs), 163, 164,
    167–168
insurance, 27. See also health insurance
Insurance Institute for Highway Safety, 119,
    122
Iowa, 110, 209, 213–214
Italy, 119

Jackson, Richard, 103
Jacobson v. Massachusetts (1905), 118
Jeffords, Sen. James, 120
Johns Hopkins Center for Civilian
    Biodefense Studies, 211
John Snow, Inc. (Boston), 95
Journal of the American Medical
    Association (JAMA), 65
Justice Department (U.S. Department of
    Justice), 258. See also Reno, Janet

Kampeas, Ron, 213
Katz, Jay, 165

Kellermann, Arthur, 265, 267
Kennedy, Donald, 103
Kennedy, Sen. Ted, 244
Kentucky, 121–122, 209
Kessler, Ron, 38
Kindig, David, 9
Knowles, John H., 112
Koplan, Jeffrey, 10
Kramer, Mary, 209
Kristof, Nicholas, 246, 250

laboratories, 211, 213–214
Laboratory Response Network, 223, 230
Lalonde, Marc, 8, 112
Lancet, 3
Larimore, Granville, 69–70
Lawrence, Regina, 58
lawsuits, 4–5
Leach, Rice, 209, 210
lead poisoning, 4, 104
Leapfrog Group, 44–45
Leavitt, Michael, 247–248
Lee, Philip, 211
Lenihan, Patrick, 215–216
Levine, Robert, 161, 166, 172n9
life course, 187–190
life expectancy, 35, 182
Lincoln, Blanche, 248
local health departments. See state and local
    health departments
Loka Institute (Amherst, Mass.), 95
Long Island Coalition for a National Health
    Plan, 250
Los Angeles, Calif., 24, 214
Louisiana, 121–122, 245–247. See also New
    Orleans
Love Canal, N.Y., 94, 95
Lumpkin, John, 213

mammography, 90
Marin Breast Cancer Watch, 91
Markey, Edward, 244
Martin, Marsha, 216
Maryland, 49
Massachusetts, 49, 207–208, 244;
    environmental health activism in, 87–88,
    91–92, 94; and motorcycle helmet law,
    112, 113, 114–115, 120

Massachusetts Breast Cancer Coalition, 91–93
McCormack, Joseph N., 60
McEwen, S. Bruce, 191–192
McKeown, Thomas, 182
McKinney, Rep. Stewart, 117
Medicaid, 217; and disasters, 239, 242–244, 246–248, 249–251, 253
medical care, 43–44, 182–183; attempts to measure, 44–46
medical profession, 60–61, 86; and public health, 5–6, 60–61, 70, 73, 75, 176–180, 195–196. *See also* American Medical Association
mental illness, 127, 131, 143, 145
mercury, 101–102
Michigan, 112, 113–114
Middaugh, John, 168
Milio, Nancy, 77–78
Milne, Tom, 213
Minnesota, 173n12
Missouri, 207
Mock, Lois, 273
Model Public Health Privacy Act, 170
Model State Emergency Health Powers Act, 206
Modified Motorcycle Association, 116
monitoring, 97–102
Moore, Harry Hascall, 63–65
Morris, Jerry, 8
motorcycle helmet laws, 110–112, 117; and Congress, 112, 116–117, 119–121; courts and, 113–115; effectiveness of, 117–119, 121–122; for minors, 110, 122–123; opposition to, 112–117, 118, 120–121; in other countries, 111, 119
motorcycles, 111–112, 115. *See also* motorcycle helmet laws
Moulton, Anthony, 209–210
Mount Sinai School of Medicine, 99
Moynihan, Sen. Daniel Patrick, 120, 121
Mustard, J. Fraser, 187

Nader, Ralph, 112
Napper, George, 262–263
National Academy of Sciences, 274
National Association of County and City Health Officials (NACCHO), 212, 236

National Association of State Budget Officers, 217
National Business Coalition on Health, 45
National Cancer Institute, 90, 91
National Center for Environmental Health (NCEH), 103
National Center for Infectious Diseases (CDC), 203
National Center for Injury Prevention and Control, 268
National Children's Study (NCS), 98
National Commission for the Protection of Research Subjects of Biomedical and Behavioral Research, 165–166. See also *Belmont Report*
National Committee for Quality Assurance, 44
National Custom Cycle Association, 116
National Electronic Disease Surveillance Network, 36
National Foundation for Infantile Paralysis, 67
National Health Planning and Resources Development Act (1974), 74
National Highway Fatality and Injury Reduction Act of 1989, 119–121
National Highway Safety Act (1966), 112, 117
National Highway Traffic Safety Administration (NHTSA), 110, 266; and motorcycle helmet laws, 116, 117–118, 122
National Human Research Protections Advisory Committee, 103
National Institute of Environmental Health Sciences (NIEHS), 91, 92, 95, 96, 98, 104
National Institute of Justice (NIJ), 270–271; research by, on violence, 264, 265–266, 268, 269, 270, 271, 273
National Institute of Occupational Safety and Health (NIOSH), 96
National Institutes of Health, 103, 105, 164, 166. *See also* National Cancer Institute; National Institute of Environmental Health Sciences; Office for the Protection from Research Risks
National Public Health Performance Standards Program, 36
National Public Health Training Network, 36

National Research Act (1974), 164

National Research Council, 104

National Rifle Association (NRA), 261, 268–269, 270, 272, 273

National Science Foundation, 92

National Toxicology Program, 104–105

National Tuberculosis Association, 67

Nationwide Health Tracking Act, 99

Nebraska, 211

neoclassical economics. *See* economic model of health

New Deal, 66

New Hampshire, 110

New Orleans, La., 252–253; and Hurricane Katrina, 239–240, 245–246, 249, 252–253

New York City, 168–169, 170, 214, 230; environmental health activism in, 87–89, 92, 96; and gun violence, 260–262, 263–264; homelessness in, 129, 130, 140, 143; in September 11 aftermath, 240–242, 243–244, 253

New York State, 112, 113, 131; Medicaid program of, 239, 242–243, 244, 247, 248, 250, 253; and public health surveillance, 167, 169, 170

Nordhaus, William D., 16

North Carolina, 92

North Carolina Medical Journal, 118

nutrition, 89–90

obesity, 4–5, 27, 89–90, 128

Occupational Safety and Health Act of 1970, 39

Office for the Protection from Research Risks (OPRR), 162–164, 165, 166–167, 168

Ohio, 207

Oklahoma National Memorial Institute for the Prevention of Terrorism, 211

Organization for Economic Cooperation and Development (OECD), 35, 176

Overton, Frank, 61

participatory research, 89, 95–97

partnerships, 47–51, 227–228, 273–274, 279–280

Pataki, George E., 243

paternalism, 3, 111, 122–123

Pattison, Scott D., 217–218

pay-for-performance (P4P) mechanisms, 45–46

PBDEs (polybrominated diphenyl ethers), 101, 102

Pennsylvania, 121

perchlorate pollution, 105

Perkins, Richard, 118

Perrotta, Dennis, 208

"personal responsibility," 7

Peterson, Sheila, 217–218

Pew Charitable Trusts, 98

philanthropy, corporate, 49

Philipson, Tomas, 23

physicians. *See* medical profession

planning boards, 75–76

police departments, 228; and gun violence, 260–264, 265–266, 273–274, 275

polio, 209

"population health," 15, 36–37, 97, 195–196, 203; and expanded mission of public health, 2, 3, 7–9, 179

precautionary principle, 92, 94

Precautionary Principle Project, 92

preparedness. *See* public health preparedness

President's Council on Bioethics, 103

prevention. *See* homeless prevention

Privacy Act (1974), 164

Procter & Gamble company, 46

Progressive Era, 61, 69

public goods (or bads), 17–29

public health: boundaries of, 1–5, 10–11, 28–29, 204–207; definitions of, 2–3, 15, 19–20, 236, 252–254; and environmental health, 85–87, 97, 105–106; and the market, 58–59, 72–73, 77–78; and the medical profession, 5–6, 60–61, 70, 73, 75, 176–180, 195–196; workforce of, 2, 28, 228–230, 236. *See also* public health infrastructure; public health preparedness

public health infrastructure, 2, 36, 37, 209–210, 226–227; and federal funding, 99, 206, 214–217, 218, 236; and state budgetary crises, 217–218, 222, 223; weaknesses in, 212–214, 217–218, 219, 233–234. *See also* laboratories; state and local health departments

public health preparedness: and changes in workforce, 228–230, 236; difficulty of measuring, 235–236; and federal funding, 99, 226, 230, 233, 235, 236 (*see also under* bioterrorism preparedness); impact of, on state and local health departments, 226–237; integration of, with other public health functions, 231–232; and partnerships, 227–228. *See also* bioterrorism preparedness
Puerto Rico, 110, 112

Quality Adjusted Life Years (QUALYs), 179

racial disparities in health, 266, 271–272
radioactive materials, 183
RAND Corporation, 227
Reagan, Ronald, 7
Red Cross, 249
redistribution, 18–19, 24, 25, 29n5
Reforming States Group, 217
Reno, Janet, 265, 267–268, 269, 270, 274, 275, 277
research: distinction between, and public health practice, 161–171; and environmental health, 91, 92–93, 95–97, 102–105; on motorcycle helmets, 117–119, 121–122; participatory, 89, 92–93, 95–97; political limits on, 102–105, 268–269, 270, 271–273, 278; on violence, 265–269, 271, 272–275, 279
"research right-to-know," 100
respiratory disease, 96. *See also* asthma
restaurant inspection, 24–25
Richmond, Julius, 269
Richmond, Calif., 92–93
rights revolutions, 70
Riley, Gov. Bob, 247
"risk factors," individual, 8, 134
Robert Wood Johnson Foundation, 10, 272
Robinson, Laurie, 275
Rockefeller Foundation, 62
Roosevelt, Franklin D., 66
Rose, Sir Geoffrey, 148, 195
Roxbury Environmental Empowerment Project (REEP), 88

Safe Cosmetics Campaign, 94
Saltzman, Linda, 269
Satcher, David, 215, 268–269, 271–272

Scheele, Leonard A., 68–69
schools of public health, 62, 93
Schroeder, Steve, 272
Schuster, Rep. Bud, 117
"science shops," 95
Selecky, Mary, 215
September 11 attacks: health crisis in aftermath of, 240–242, 243–244, 253; impact of, on field of public health, 15, 36, 57, 78, 212, 219–223
sewage treatment, 21
sexually transmitted diseases, 26
Shalala, Donna, 269, 271–272
Shelby Amendment (1999), 103
Silent Spring Institute (SSI), 91–92, 95, 106
Simon v. Sargent (1972), 113, 114–115
"sin taxes," 4
Sistahs United, 92
smallpox, 5, 23; inoculation campaign against (2002–2003), 206, 218–219, 223
smoking, 6, 27, 30n9, 35
Snider, Dixie, 164
Snow, John, 85
social-health gradient, 180, 185–187. *See also* health disparities
social insurance programs, 27. *See also* health insurance
"social medicine" (term), 79n9
Society of Environmental Journalists, 101
Soros, George, 272–273
Speers, Marjorie, 164, 165, 166
Spengler, Jack, 101–102
Stang, Paul, 38
state and local health departments, 5, 15, 19, 66–67, 69; and budgetary crises, 217–218, 222, 223; and new responsibilities for preparedness, 204–223, 226–237; in Progressive Era, 5, 61; and research/practice distinction, 167–170. *See also* public health infrastructure
Steckler, Allen, 76
Steward, William H., 70
Stoddart, Greg L., 9, 36
Strategic National Stockpile, 223, 231
stress reactivity, 193–194
Sununu, John E., 247
Suomi, Stephen J., 193
Supreme Court. *See* U.S. Supreme Court

surgeons general, 6. *See also* Richmond, Julius; Satcher, David

surveillance, 161–171. *See also* monitoring

Susser, Mervyn, 8

swine flu, 7

syphilis experiment, 7, 70

tax policies, 4, 19, 27, 41, 49

Teret, Stephen, 118

terrorism. *See* bioterrorism preparedness

Texas, 121, 208, 245

Texas Medicine, 119

Thatcher, Margaret, 7

Thompson, Tommy, 104, 205, 206

Thurow, Lester, 17, 18

Titmuss, Richard, 8

tobacco industry, 4, 6

TOPOFF exercise, 210

toxic chemicals, 69, 104–105, 183; environmental health activism and, 90–93, 94, 97–102

Toxics Action Center (New England), 94

Toxics Link Coalition, 91

Toxic Substances Control Act, 99

Toxics Use Reduction Institute (TURI), 94

traffic safety. *See* automobile safety; motorcycle helmet laws

Translational Research Program, 95

Trust for America's Health (TFAH, previously Health-Track), 98

tuberculosis, 5, 209

Tuskegee syphilis experiment, 7, 70

typhoid, 167

Union of Concerned Scientists (UCS), 105

University of Massachusetts, Lowell, 94

UPS (United Parcel Service), 46

Urban Institute, 279

U.S. Congress, 270–271; and motorcycle helmet laws, 112, 116–117, 119–121

U.S. Department of Defense, 95

U.S. Department of Health and Human Services (DHHS), 98, 103, 161, 270. *See also specific DHHS agencies*

U.S. Department of Housing and Urban Development (HUD), 95

U.S. Department of Justice, 258. *See also* Reno, Janet

U.S. Government Accounting Office, 131

U.S. Public Health Service, 7, 10, 15, 70. *See also specific USPHS agencies*

U.S. Supreme Court, 104, 113, 114, 118

vaccines, 231. *See also* smallpox: inoculation campaign against

value-based purchasing (VBP), 43–46

van der Gaag, Jacques, 187

violence, research on, 265–269, 271, 272–275, 279. *See also* gun violence

Virchow, Rudolph, 8

Wagoner, Rick, 42

Wallack, Lawrence, 58

Wal-Mart, 42

Washington, D.C., 110

water systems, 22–23, 105

Weatherall, D. J., 181

Weisbrod, Burton, 16

West Harlem Environmental Action (WE ACT), 87–89, 92, 96

West Nile virus, 212–213

White, Kerr, 62

Whitehall studies, 8, 185

Whitehead, Margaret, 37

Whitman, Christine, 104

Windows of Hope, 242

Winslow, Charles-Edward Amory, 68

Woburn, Mass., 95

Wollschlager, Warren, 212

workers' compensation, 39

workforce. *See* public health: workforce of

World Health Organization (WHO), 3, 86, 111

World War II, 111

Yale University, 62

Y2K, 211